Study and Review Guide to accompany

ANATOMY & PHYSIOLOGY

Eighth Edition

Kevin T. Patton
Gary A. Thibodeau

Written by: Linda Swisher, RN, EdD

ELSEVIER
MOSBY

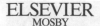

ELSEVIER
MOSBY

3251 Riverport Lane
St. Louis, Missouri 63043

Study and Review Guide to accompany
Anatomy & Physiology, 8th edition   ISBN: 978-0-323-08370-6

Notices

Knowledge and best practice in this field are constantly changing. As new research and experience broaden our understanding, changes in research methods, professional practices, or medical treatment may become necessary.

Practitioners and researchers must always rely on their own experience and knowledge in evaluating and using any information, methods, compounds, or experiments described herein. In using such information or methods they should be mindful of their own safety and the safety of others, including parties for whom they have a professional responsibility.

With respect to any drug or pharmaceutical products identified, readers are advised to check the most current information provided (i) on procedures featured or (ii) by the manufacturer of each product to be administered, to verify the recommended dose or formula, the method and duration of administration, and contraindications. It is the responsibility of practitioners, relying on their own experience and knowledge of their patients, to make diagnoses, to determine dosages and the best treatment for each individual patient, and to take all appropriate safety precautions.

To the fullest extent of the law, neither the Publisher nor the authors, contributors, or editors, assume any liability for any injury and/or damage to persons or property as a matter of products liability, negligence or otherwise, or from any use or operation of any methods, products, instructions, or ideas contained in the material herein.

Previous editions copyrighted 2010, 2007, 2003, 1999, 1996, 1993, 1987 by Mosby, Inc., an affiliate of Elsevier Inc.

ISBN: 978-0-323-08370-6

Content Strategist: Kellie White
Content Manager: Rebecca Swisher
Content Development Specialist: Joe Gramlich
Content Coordinator: Emily Thomson
Publishing Services Manager: Deborah Vogel
Project Manager: John Gabbert

Printed in the United States of America

Last digit is the print number: 9 8 7 6 5 4 3 2 1

Introduction

This *Study and Review Guide to accompany Anatomy and Physiology*, eighth edition, is designed to help you be successful in learning anatomy and physiology. Before attempting to complete any chapter in the *Study and Review Guide*, thoroughly read the corresponding chapter in the textbook, learn the key terms listed at the beginning and end of each textbook chapter, and study your lecture notes. You will then be prepared to complete the questions and exercises that are provided for each chapter.

Each chapter in the *Study and Review Guide* begins with a brief overview of the chapter concepts. A variety of questions is offered to help you cover the material effectively. These questions include multiple choice, true-false, matching, short answer, clinical challenges, labeling, and crossword puzzles. After completing the exercises in a chapter, you can check your answers in the back of the book. Each answer is referenced to the appropriate text page. Additionally, questions are grouped into specific topics that correspond to the text. Each major topic of the *Study and Review Guide* provides references to specific areas of the text, so if you are having difficulty with a particular grouping of questions you have a specific reference area to assist you with remedial work. This feature allows you to identify your area of weakness accurately.

Multiple Choice

For each multiple choice question, there is only one correct answer out of the choices given. Circle the correct choice.

True or False

Read each statement carefully and write true or false in the blank provided.

Matching

Match each numbered term or statement in the left-hand column with its corresponding lettered term or statement in the right-hand column. Write the correct letters in the blanks provided.

Fill in the Blanks

Fill-in-the-blank questions ask you to recall missing word(s) and insert it (them) into the answer blank(s). These questions may involve sentences or paragraphs.

Identify the Term that Does Not Belong

In questions that ask you to identify the incorrect term, three words are given that relate to each other in structure and function, and one more word is included that has no relationship to the other three terms. You are asked to circle the term that does not relate to the others. An example might be: iris, stapes, cornea, and retina. You would circle stapes because all other terms refer to the eye.

Application Questions

Application questions ask you to make a judgment based on the information in the chapter. These questions may ask you how you would respond to a situation or to suggest a possible diagnosis for a set of symptoms.

Labeling Exercises

Labeling exercises present diagrams with parts that are not identified. According to the directions given, fill in the appropriate labels on the numbered lines or match the numbers with the list of terms provided.

Crossword Puzzles

Vocabulary words from the Key Terms section in each chapter of the text have been developed into crossword puzzles. This exercise encourages recall and proper spelling.

One Last Quick Check

This section selects questions from throughout the chapter to provide you with a final review. This mini-test gives you an overview of your knowledge of the chapter after completing all of the other sections. It emphasizes the main concepts of the unit, but should not be attempted until the specific topics of the chapter have been mastered.

Acknowledgments

I wish to express my appreciation to the staff at Elsevier, and especially to Tom Wilhelm, Jeff Downing, Kellie White, Rebecca Swisher, Joe Gramlich, and Emily Thomson for their guidance and support. My continued admiration and thanks to Kevin Patton for another outstanding edition of the text and to Gary Thibodeau who sets the bar for us all to achieve. The time and dedication to science education that you both have given will undoubtedly help improve the quality of health care for our future and instill in each student a deep appreciation for the wonders of the human body.

My thanks to Brian and Sam—Your encouragement kept me on task, the discussions kept my creative juices flowing, and your love makes my life special.

Finally, this book is dedicated in memory of my beloved husband Bill—my beautiful connection to the past, and to my grandchildren Billy, Maddie, and Heather—the sunshine of my life and my link to the future.

Linda Swisher, RN, EdD

Contents

CHAPTER 1

Organization of the Body

The study of anatomy and physiology involves the structure and function of an organism and the relationship of its parts. It begins with a basic organization of the body into different structural levels. Beginning with the smallest level (the cell) and progressing to the largest, most complex level (the system), this chapter familiarizes you with the terminology and the levels of organization needed to facilitate the study of the body in parts or as a whole.

It is also important to be able to identify and describe specific body areas or regions as we progress in this field. The anatomical position is used as a reference when dissecting the body into planes, regions, or cavities. The terminology defined in this chapter allows you to describe the areas efficiently and accurately.

Finally, the process of homeostasis is reviewed. This state of relative constancy in the chemical composition of body fluids is necessary for good health. In fact, the very survival of the body depends on the successful maintenance of homeostasis.

I—ANATOMY AND PHYSIOLOGY AND CHARACTERISTICS OF LIFE

Multiple Choice—select the best answer.

1. *Anatomy* refers to:
   a. using devices to investigate parameters such as heart rate and blood pressure.
   b. investigating human structure via dissection and other methods.
   c. studying the unusual manner in which an organism responds to painful stimuli.
   d. examining the chemistry of life.

2. *Systemic anatomy* refers to anatomical investigation:
   a. at a microscopic level.
   b. that begins in the head and neck and concludes at the feet.
   c. that approaches the study of the body by systems: groups of organs having a common function.
   d. at the cellular level.

3. *Physiology* refers to the:
    a. nature of human function.
    b. structure of the human form.
    c. evolution of human thought.
    d. accuracy of measuring the human physique.

4. The removal of waste products in the body is achieved by a process known as:
    a. secretion.
    b. excretion.
    c. circulation.
    d. conductivity.

5. *Metabolism* is the:
    a. exchange of gases in the blood.
    b. formation of new cells in the body to permit growth.
    c. sum total of all physical and chemical reactions occurring in the body.
    d. production and delivery of specialized substances for diverse body functions.

▶ *If you had difficulty with this section, review pages 1-6.*

II—LEVELS OF ORGANIZATION

Multiple Choice—select the best answer.

6. Beginning with the smallest level, the levels of organization of the body are:
    a. cellular, chemical, tissue, organelle, organ, system, organism.
    b. cellular, chemical, organelle, organ, tissue, organism, system.
    c. chemical, cellular, organelle, organ, system, organism.
    d. chemical, organelle, cellular, tissue, organ, system, organism.

7. Molecules are:
    a. combinations of atoms forming larger chemical aggregates.
    b. electrons orbiting a nucleus.
    c. a complex of electrons arranged in orderly shells.
    d. composed of cellular organelles.

8. Mitochondria, Golgi apparatus, and endoplasmic reticulum are examples of:
    a. macromolecules.
    b. cytoplasm.
    c. organelles.
    d. nuclei.

9. Blood production is a function of which system?
    a. circulatory
    b. respiratory
    c. skeletal
    d. urinary

10. Support and movement are functions of which systems?
    a. respiratory, digestive, and urinary systems
    b. reproductive and urinary systems
    c. skeletal and muscular systems
    d. cardiovascular and lymphatic/immune systems

Matching—match the term with the proper selection.

a. many similar cells that act together to perform a common function
b. the most complex units that make up the body
c. a group of several different kinds of tissues arranged to perform a special function
d. collections of molecules that perform a function
e. the smallest "living" units of structure and function

11. _____ organelle

12. _____ cells

13. _____ tissue

14. _____ organ

15. _____ systems

Matching—match each system with its corresponding functions.

a. support and movement
b. communication, control, and integration
c. reproduction and development
d. transportation and defense
e. respiration, nutrition, and excretion

16. _____   integumentary system

17. _____   skeletal system

18. _____   muscular system

19. _____   nervous system

20. _____   endocrine system

21. _____   digestive system

22. _____   respiratory system

23. _____   cardiovascular system

24. _____   lymphatic system

25. _____   urinary system

26. _____   reproductive system

▶ *If you had difficulty with this section, review pages 7-10.*

III—ANATOMICAL POSITION, BODY CAVITIES, BODY REGIONS, ANATOMICAL TERMS, BODY PLANES AND SECTIONS

Multiple Choice—select the best answer.

27. In the anatomical position, the subject is:
    a. seated with the head facing forward.
    b. standing with the arms at the sides and palms facing forward.
    c. seated with arms parallel to the ground.
    d. standing with the arms at the sides and palms facing backward.

28. The dorsal body cavity contains the:
    a. brain and spinal cord.
    b. abdominal organs.
    c. pelvic organs.
    d. thoracic organs.

29. The ventral body cavity contains the:
    a. thoracic and abdominopelvic cavities.
    b. thoracic cavity only.
    c. abdominopelvic cavity only.
    d. brain and spinal cord.

30. The axial portion of the body consists of:
    a. arms, neck, and torso.
    b. neck, torso, and legs.
    c. torso, arms, and legs.
    d. head, neck, and torso.

31. The abdominopelvic cavity contains all of the following *except* the:
    a. kidneys.
    b. pancreas.
    c. lungs.
    d. urinary bladder.

32. The mediastinum contains all of the following *except* the:
    a. esophagus.
    b. aorta.
    c. lungs.
    d. trachea.

33. Visceral peritoneum would cover which of the following organs?
    a. heart
    b. liver
    c. lungs
    d. brain

34. A sagittal section would divide the body into:
    a. upper and lower parts.
    b. right and left sides.
    c. front and back portions.
    d. none of the above.

35. A coronal section would divide the body into:
    a. upper and lower parts.
    b. right and left sides.
    c. front and back portions.
    d. none of the above.

36. *Inguinal* is a term referring to which body region?
    a. anterior portion of elbow
    b. armpit
    c. posterior knee
    d. groin

Circle the correct answer.

37. The stomach is (superior or inferior) to the diaphragm.

38. The nose is located on the (anterior or posterior) surface of the body.

39. The lungs lie (medial or lateral) to the heart.

40. The elbow lies (proximal or distal) to the forearm.

41. The skin is (superficial or deep) to the muscles below it.

42. A midsagittal plane divides the body into (equal or unequal) parts.

43. A frontal plane divides the body into (anterior and posterior or superior and inferior) sections.

44. A transverse plane divides the body into (right and left or upper and lower) sections.

45. A coronal plane may also be referred to as a (sagittal or frontal) plane.

Matching—select the correct term from the choices given and insert the letter in the answer blank.

a. ventral cavity   b. dorsal cavity

46. _____ thoracic

47. _____ cranial

48. _____ abdominal

49. _____ pelvic

50. _____ mediastinum

51. _____ pleural

Labeling—using the terms provided, label the anatomical directions on the illustration below.

anterior (ventral)
lateral
posterior (dorsal)
proximal

sagittal plane
frontal plane
superior
inferior

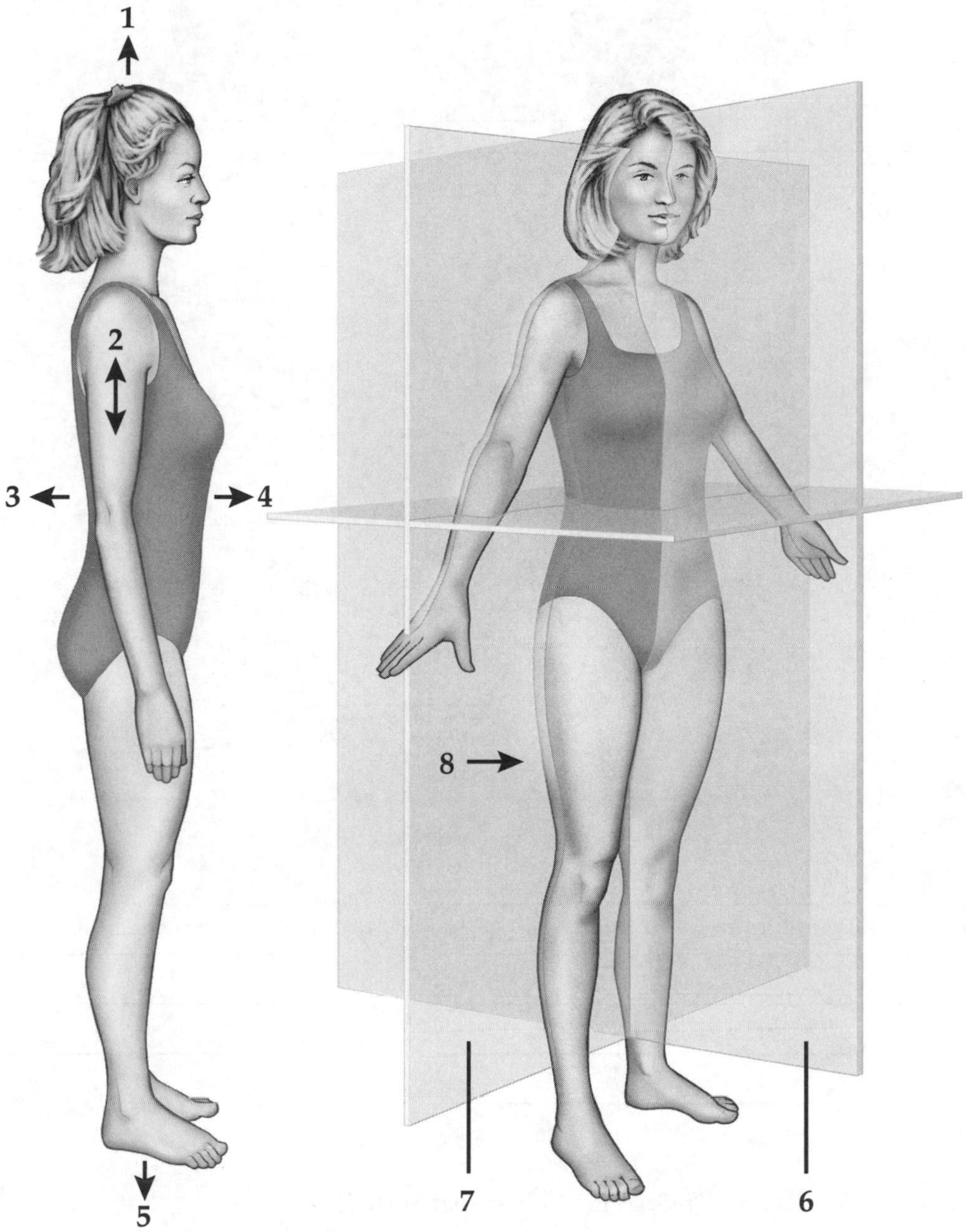

1 _____
2 _____
3 _____
4 _____

5 _____
6 _____
7 _____
8 _____

Labeling—label the various body cavities on the diagram below.

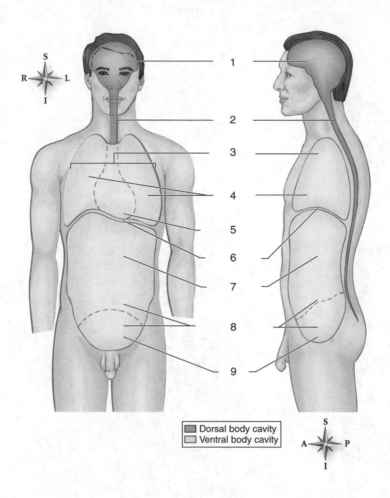

1	_____	6	_____
2	_____	7	_____
3	_____	8	_____
4	_____	9	_____
5	_____		

▶ *If you had difficulty with this section, review pages 10-18.*

IV—HOMEOSTASIS AND HOMEOSTATIC CONTROL MECHANISMS

Multiple Choice—select the best answer.

52. *Homeostasis* can be defined as the:
    a. relatively constant state maintained by the body.
    b. overall contribution of an organ system.
    c. external stimuli that evoke a disruption to an organism.
    d. lack of cytoplasm within a plasma membrane.

53. Which of the following is *not* a component of a feedback control loop?
    a. sensory mechanism
    b. integrating, or control center
    c. effector mechanism
    d. stressor stimulator

54. Negative feedback control systems:
    a. oppose a change.
    b. accelerate a change.
    c. ignore a change.
    d. none of the above.

55. Positive feedback control systems:
    a. oppose a change.
    b. accelerate a change.
    c. ignore a change.
    d. none of the above.

True or false

56. _____ Any given physiological parameter will never deviate beyond the set point.

57. _____ In the thermostatically regulated furnace example of negative feedback, the furnace functions as the sensor.

58. _____ Negative feedback systems are inhibitory.

59. _____ The process of childbirth, in which the baby's head causes increased stretching of the reproductive tract, which in turn feeds back to the brain, thus triggering the release of oxytocin, is an example of positive feedback.

▶ *If you had difficulty with this section, review pages 18-24.*

V—MECHANISMS OF DISEASE

Matching—match the term with the proper selection.

a. subjective abnormalities
b. study of disease
c. collection of different signs and symptoms that present a clear picture of a pathological condition
d. study of factors involved in causing a disease
e. objective abnormalities
f. undetermined causes
g. disease native to a local region
h. symptoms appear suddenly and for a short period
i. affects large geographic regions
j. actual pattern of a disease's development

60. _____ pathology

61. _____ signs

62. _____ symptoms

63. _____ etiology

64. _____ syndrome

65. _____ idiopathic

66. _____ acute

67. _____ pandemic

68. _____ endemic

69. _____ pathogenesis

Fill in the blanks.

70. _____ is the organized study of the underlying physiological processes associated with disease.

71. Many diseases are best understood as disturbances of _____.

72. Altered or _____ genes can cause abnormal proteins to be made.

73. An organism that lives in or on another organism to obtain its nutrients is called a _____.

74. Abnormal tissue growths may also be referred to as _____.

75. Autoimmunity literally means _____ _____.

▶ *If you had difficulty with this section, review pages 24-30.*

Crossword Puzzle

Across

1. Study of body function
5. "Staying the same"
9. _____ feedback is inhibitory
10. Total of chemical and physical reactions
11. Divides the body into sections
12. Group of similar cells

Down

2. Heart is an example
3. Organs arranged to perform a function
4. Basic unit of the body
6. Sum of its parts
7. Physique
8. Study of body systems

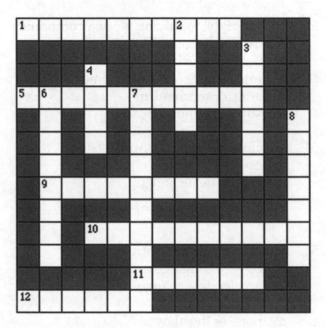

APPLYING WHAT YOU KNOW

76. Laurie has had an appendectomy. The nurse is preparing to change the dressing. She knows that the appendix is located in the right iliac inguinal region, the distal portion extending at an angle into the hypogastric region. Place an X on the diagram where the nurse will place the dressing.

77. Penny noticed a lump in her breast. Dr. Reeder noted on her chart that a small mass was located in the left breast medial to the nipple. Place an X where Penny's lump would be located.

78. Madison was injured in a bicycle accident. X-ray films revealed that she had a fracture of the right patella. A cast was applied beginning at the distal femoral region and extending to the pedal region. Place an X where Madison's cast begins and ends.

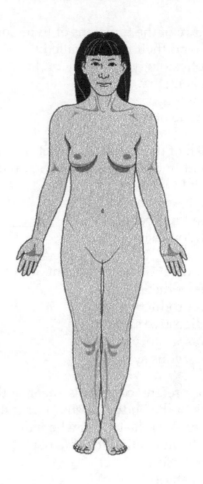

DID YOU KNOW

- Many animals produce tears but only humans weep as a result of emotional stress.
- Men notice subtle signs of sadness in a face only 40% of the time; women pick up on them 90% of the time.

ONE LAST QUICK CHECK

Multiple Choice—select the best answer.

79. The body's ability to continuously respond to changes in the environment and maintain consistency in the internal environment is called:
    a. homeostasis.
    b. superficial.
    c. structural levels.
    d. none of the above.

80. The regions frequently used by health professionals to locate pain or tumors divide the abdomen into four basic areas called:
    a. planes.
    b. cavities.
    c. pleural.
    d. quadrants.

81. A lengthwise plane running from front to back that divides the body into right and left sides is called:
    a. transverse.
    b. coronal.
    c. frontal.
    d. sagittal.

82. A study of the functions of living organisms and their parts is called:
    a. physiology.
    b. chemistry.
    c. biology.
    d. none of the above.

83. Which of the following structures does *not* lie within the abdominopelvic cavity?
    a. right iliac region
    b. left antecubital region
    c. left lumbar region
    d. hypogastric region

84. The dorsal body cavity contains components of the:
    a. reproductive system.
    b. digestive system.
    c. respiratory system.
    d. nervous system.

85. If your reference point is "nearest the trunk of the body" versus "farthest from the trunk of the body," where does the elbow lie in relation to the wrist?
    a. anterior
    b. posterior
    c. distal
    d. proximal

86. The buttocks are often used as injection sites. This region can also be called:
    a. sacral.
    b. buccal.
    c. cutaneous.
    d. gluteal.

87. Which of the following is *not* a component of the axial subdivision of the body?
    a. upper extremity
    b. neck
    c. trunk
    d. head

88. A synonym for medial is:
    a. toward the side.
    b. in front of.
    c. midline.
    d. anterior.

Fill in the blanks.

89. A principle of standardizing terminology is the avoidance of _____, or terms based upon a person's name.

90. The term _____ _____ means that the right and left sides of humans are mirror images of each other and only one plane can divide the body into left and right sides.

91. _____ refers to an inner region of an organ.

92. The narrow tip of an organ is the _____ portion.

93. Hereditary material called _____ carries the chemical blueprint of the body.

94. The endocrine system regulates internal environment by secreting _____ via the blood to target areas.

95. Processes for maintaining or restoring homeostasis are known as _____ _____ _____.

96. _____ _____ is the concept that information may flow ahead to another process to trigger a change in anticipation of an event that will follow.

97. _____ _____ mechanisms operate at the tissue and organ levels.

98. The study of aging is known as _____.

99. Tiny, primitive cells that lack nuclei and may cause infection are _____.

100. An inherited trait that puts one at greater than normal risk for development of a specific disease is a(n) _____ _____.

CHAPTER 2

The Chemical Basis of Life

A lthough anatomy can be studied without knowledge of chemistry, it is hard to imagine an understanding of physiology without a basic comprehension of chemical reactions in the body. Trillions of cells make up the various levels of organization in the body. Our health and survival depend upon proper chemical maintenance in the cytoplasm of our cells.

Chemists use the terms *elements* or *compounds* to describe all of the substances (matter) in and around us. Distinguishing these two terms is the fact that an element cannot be broken down. A compound, on the other hand, is made up of two or more elements and has the ability to be broken down into the elements that form it.

Organic and inorganic compounds are equally important to us. Without organic compounds such as carbohydrates, proteins, and fats, and inorganic compounds such as water, we could not sustain life.

Because we cannot see many of the chemical reactions that take place daily in our bodies, it is sometimes difficult to comprehend the principles involved in initiating them. Chemicals are responsible for directing virtually all of our bodily functions. It is therefore important to master the fundamental concepts of chemistry.

I—BASIC CHEMISTRY

Multiple Choice—select the best answer.

1. Which of the following is *not* one of the major elements present in the human body?
   a. oxygen
   b. carbon
   c. iron
   d. hydrogen

2. Which of the following is *not* a subatomic particle?
   a. proton
   b. electron
   c. isotope
   d. neutron

3. The total number of electrons in an atom equals the number of:
   a. neutrons in its nucleus.
   b. electrons in its nucleus.
   c. protons in its nucleus.
   d. ions in its nucleus.

4. An atom can be described as *chemically stable* if its outermost electron shell contains:
   a. three electrons.
   b. five electrons.
   c. six electrons.
   d. eight electrons.

5. Isotopes are atoms of elements that differ in their number of:
   a. protons.
   b. electrons.
   c. neutrons.
   d. nuclei.

6. Ionic bonds are chemical bonds formed by the:
   a. sharing of electrons between atoms.
   b. donation of protons from one atom to another.
   c. transfer of electrons from one atom to another.
   d. acceptance of protons from one atom by another.

7. Chemical bonds formed by the sharing of electrons are called:
   a. ionic.
   b. covalent.
   c. hydrogen.
   d. electronic.

8. A chemical reaction in which substances combine to form more complex substances is called:
   a. synthesis.
   b. decomposition.
   c. exchange.
   d. reversible.

True or false

9. _____ *Matter* is a term used by chemists to describe all the materials or substances around us.

10. _____ *Mass number* refers to the number of protons plus the number of neutrons in the atom's nucleus.

11. _____ Sodium chloride is an example of a covalent bond.

12. _____ Hydrogen bonds form from an equal charge distribution within a molecule.

13. _____ The digestion of food is an example of a decomposition reaction.

Identify the following elements:

14. O _____

15. Ca _____

16. K _____

17. Na _____

18. Mg _____

19. Fe _____

20. Se _____

▶ *If you had difficulty with this section, review pages 33-41.*

II—METABOLISM

Matching—select the best answer.

a. breaks down larger food molecules into smaller units
b. the form of energy that cells generally use
c. all the chemical reactions that occur in body cells
d. joins simple molecules together to form more complex ones
e. key chemical reaction during anabolism

21. _____ catabolism

22. _____ anabolism

23. _____ ATP

24. _____ metabolism

25. _____ dehydration synthesis

▶ *If you had difficulty with this section, review pages 41-42.*

III—INORGANIC MOLECULES

Multiple Choice—select the best answer.

26. Water plays a key role in such processes as:
    a. cell permeability.
    b. active transport of materials.
    c. secretion.
    d. all of the above.

27. Which of the following is *not* a property of water?
    a. strong polarity
    b. high specific heat
    c. high heat of vaporization
    d. strong acidity

28. Acids:
    a. are proton donors.
    b. dye litmus blue.
    c. release hydrogen ions when in solution.
    d. accept electrons when in an aqueous solution.

29. Substances that accept hydrogen ions are referred to as:
    a. acids.
    b. bases.
    c. buffers.
    d. salts.

30. The constancy of the pH homeostatic mechanism is caused by the presence of substances called:
    a. salts.
    b. bases.
    c. buffers.
    d. acids.

True or false

31. _____ The pH scale indicates the degree of acidity or alkalinity of a solution.

32. _____ Milk is acid on the pH scale.

33. _____ Litmus will turn red in the presence of an acid.

34. _____ The basic substance of each cell is water.

35. _____ Oxygen and carbon dioxide are examples of organic compounds.

▶ *If you had difficulty with this section, review pages 42-45.*

IV—ORGANIC MOLECULES

Multiple Choice—select the best answer.

36. Which of the following is *not* a type of carbohydrate?
    a. monosaccharides
    b. disaccharides
    c. megasaccharides
    d. polysaccharides

37. Which of the following is *incorrect* in reference to carbohydrates?
    a. They include substances referred to as *sugars*.
    b. They serve critical structural roles in RNA and DNA.
    c. They represent a primary source of chemical energy for body cells.
    d. They are replete with nitrogen atoms.

38. Proteins are composed of ____ commonly occurring amino acids.
    a. 8
    b. 12
    c. 21
    d. 24

39. Amino acids frequently become joined by:
    a. peptide bonds.
    b. phospholipid reactions.
    c. degradation synthesis.
    d. none of the above.

40. Which of the following is *not* an example of proteins?
    a. hormones
    b. antibodies
    c. urine
    d. enzymes

41. A structural lipid found in a cell membrane is a:
    a. triglyceride.
    b. phospholipid.
    c. steroid.
    d. prostaglandin.

42. Which of the following is the correct example of DNA base pairing?
    a. adenine-cytosine
    b. guanine-adenine
    c. adenine-thymine
    d. guanine-thymine

43. A DNA molecule contains each of the following *except:*
    a. sugar.
    b. nitrogenous base.
    c. phosphate.
    d. lipid.

44. DNA differs from RNA in that:
    a. RNA contains ribose instead of deoxyribose.
    b. RNA contains thymine instead of uracil.
    c. RNA contains a double polynucleotide strand.
    d. There is no structural difference between DNA and RNA.

True or false

45. _____ Steroids are poorly distributed throughout the body.

46. _____ High-density lipoprotein (HDL) is also called the "good" cholesterol.

47. _____ Protein compounds have no role in defending the body against harmful agents.

48. _____ The nonessential amino acids can be produced from the other amino acids or from simple organic molecules.

49. _____ Enzymes are proteins that function by the "lock and key" model.

50. _____ Prostaglandins are "tissue hormones."

▶ *If you had difficulty with this section, review pages 45-61.*

Crossword Puzzle

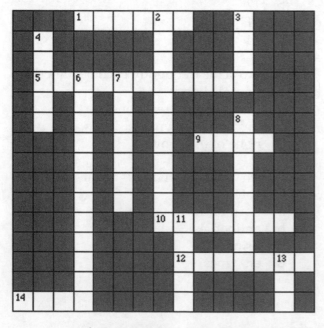

Across
1. Acts as a reservoir for H^+ ions
5. DNA or RNA (two words)
9. Small particle of an element
10. Simple form of matter
12. Amino acid
14. Tastes bitter

Down
2. Dissociates in solution to form ions
3. Releases hydrogen when in solution
4. _____ bond/electrocovalent bond
6. Sugar or starch
7. Chemical catalysts
8. _____ bond/shares electron pairs between atoms
11. Fat
13. Electrically charged atom

APPLYING WHAT YOU KNOW

51. Amanda and Steve own a home that was recently discovered to contain very high levels of radon. Where in the house would these levels be greatest? What could be done to eliminate the radon? What is the family at greatest risk for?

52. Shelley just finished preparing a meal of pan-fried hamburgers for her family. While the frying pan was still hot, she poured the liquid grease into a metal container to cool. Later she noticed that the liquid oil had solidified as it cooled. Explain the chemistry of why the now room-temperature fat was solid.

DID YOU KNOW

- After a vigorous workout, your triglycerides fall 10–20% and your HDL increases by the same percentage for 2–3 hours.

- The only letter not appearing on the Periodic Table is the letter "J."

- Hydrogen is the most abundant element in the universe (75%).

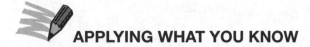

ONE LAST QUICK CHECK

Matching—identify each term with its corresponding description or definition.

a. atomic number
b. base pairs
c. electrolyte
d. high-energy bonds
e. isotopes
f. nucleotide
g. octet rule
h. polarity
i. polymers

53. _____ Atoms of the same element but with different mass number (because their nuclei contain different numbers of neutrons).

54. _____ Adenine-thymine and guanine-cytosine are examples of _____ present in DNA.

55. _____ Atoms with fewer than eight electrons in their valence shell will attempt to lose, gain, or share electrons with other atoms to achieve stability.

56. _____ The number of protons in an atom's nucleus.

57. _____ Any large molecule made up of many identical small molecules.

58. _____ Components of DNA and RNA that are composed of sugar, a nitrogenous base, and a phosphate group.

59. _____ Chemical property that allows water to act as an effective solvent.

60. _____ Large group of inorganic compounds including acids, bases, and salts.

Matching—select the best answer.

a. protein
b. carbohydrate
c. lipid

61. _____ ribose

62. _____ steroids

63. _____ amino acid

64. _____ glycerol

65. _____ monosaccharides

66. _____ phospholipids

67. _____ enzymes

Matching—select the best answer.

a. acid   b. base

68. _____ litmus turns blue

69. _____ "proton donor"

70. _____ bitter taste

71. _____ "proton acceptor"

72. _____ releases a hydrogen ion

CHAPTER 3

Anatomy of Cells

Cells are the smallest structural units of living things. Therefore, because we are living, we are made up of a mass of cells. Human cells, which vary in shape and size, can only be seen under a microscope. The three main parts of a cell are the cytoplasmic membrane, the cytoplasm, and the nucleus. As you review this chapter, you will be amazed at the resemblance of a cell to the body as a whole. You will identify a miniature circulatory system, reproductive system, digestive system, lymphatic system, skeletal system, and many other structures that will aid in your understanding of these and other body systems in future chapters.

I—FUNCTIONAL ANATOMY OF CELLS

Multiple Choice—select the best answer.

1. Which of the following is *not* a main cellular structure?
   a. plasma membrane
   b. interstitial fluid
   c. cytoplasm (including organelles)
   d. nucleus

2. All of the following are examples of the plasma membrane function *except:*
   a. boundary of cell.
   b. self-identification.
   c. receptor sites.
   d. "power plants" of cell.

3. Which of the following is a functional characteristic of ribosomes?
   a. provision of ATP
   b. protein synthesis
   c. DNA replication
   d. binding site for steroid hormones

4. Production of ATP occurs within which organelle?
   a. smooth endoplasmic reticulum
   b. Golgi apparatus
   c. lysosomes
   d. mitochondria

5. Preparation of protein molecules for cellular exportation is the function of which of the following organelles?
   a. Golgi apparatus
   b. microvilli
   c. peroxisomes
   d. mitochondria

6. In nondividing cells, DNA appears as threads that are referred to as:
   a. chromatin.
   b. nucleoplasm.
   c. nucleolus.
   d. none of the above.

7. The nucleolus is composed chiefly of:
   a. DNA.
   b. rRNA.
   c. tRNA.
   d. none of the above.

True or false

8. _____ The plasma membrane can be described as a triple layer of phospholipid molecules.

9. _____ The process by which cells translate the signal received by a membrane receptor into a specific chemical change in the cell is called *signal transportation*.

10. _____ Each and every cell always has one nucleus.

11. _____ Generally, the more active a cell is, the more mitochondria it will contain.

12. _____ Membranous bags that temporarily contain molecules for transport or later use are known as *peroxisomes*.

Matching—identify each cell structure with its corresponding function.

a. nucleolus
b. lysosome
c. cytoplasm
d. plasma membrane
e. endoplasmic reticulum
f. ribosome
g. mitochondria
h. nucleus

13. _____ forms ribosomes

14. _____ separates the cell from its environment

15. _____ acts as the cell's "digestive system"

16. _____ acts as a "protein factory"

17. _____ contains organelles

18. _____ contains DNA

19. _____ act as "power plants" of the cell

20. _____ classified as both smooth and rough

Labeling—from memory, label the parts of the typical cell on the diagram below.

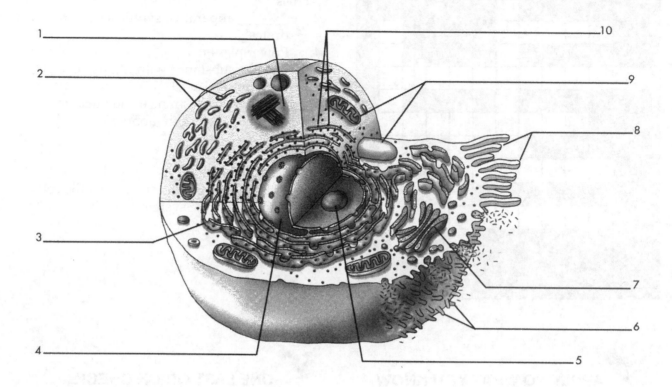

Animal cell.

▶ *If you had difficulty with this section, review pages 66-79.*

II—CYTOSKELETON

Fill in the blanks.

21. _____ is the cell's internal supporting framework.

22. _____ are the smallest cell fibers.

23. The thickest of the cell fibers are tiny, hollow tubes called _____.

24. The _____ is an area of the cytoplasm near the nucleus that coordinates the building and breaking of microtubules in the cell.

25. _____, _____, and _____ are cell extensions that appear on certain types of cells.

26. When membrane channels of adjacent plasma membranes connect to others, the formation is known as _____ _____.

27. _____ hold skin together.

▶ *If you had difficulty with this section, review pages 79-85.*

Crossword Puzzle

Across

2. _____ apparatus, synthesizes carbohydrates
4. Power plants
5. Gel-like substance within the cell
7. Contains DNA
8. Area of cytoplasm near the nucleus
9. Rough and smooth (abbrev.)

Down

1. Protein factory
3. _____ membrane, surrounds the cell
6. Cell's digestive system

APPLYING WHAT YOU KNOW

28. Brian is a sedentary, overweight cigarette smoker who has chest pain whenever he exerts himself. Upon examination, his cardiologist determines that Brian is suffering from heart disease. Which receptors in the cells that line the blood vessels of his heart are responsible? What type of cholesterol is responsible?

    What other diseases may he be at risk for?

29. After several weeks of exercising in the weight room, Valerie notices that she has not only become stronger, but quite muscular as well. Which organelle has increased its density in the cytoplasm of the cells of her muscles in response to a greater demand for ATP production?

DID YOU KNOW

- The largest single cell in the human body is the female sex cell, the ovum. The smallest single cell in the human body is the male sex cell, the sperm.

ONE LAST QUICK CHECK

Multiple Choice—select the best answer.

30. Which of the following cellular extensions are required when absorption is important?
    a. cilia
    b. microvilli
    c. flagella
    d. none of the above

31. Movement of the ovum within the female reproductive tract is largely as a result of:
    a. the flagella extending from the ovum.
    b. the cilia extending from the ovum.
    c. the cilia lining the uterine tubes.
    d. none of the above.

32. Skin cells are held tightly together by:
    a. gap junctions.
    b. desmosomes.
    c. tight junctions.
    d. adhesions.

33. Ribosomes are attached to:
    a. lysosomes.
    b. rough endoplasmic reticulum.
    c. peroxisomes.
    d. cilia.

34. The phospholipid area of the plasma membrane of a cell is:
    a. single-layered.
    b. bilayered.
    c. trilayered.
    d. multilayered.

Matching—identify each term with its corresponding definition.

a. release hormones
b. transport oxygen
c. destroy bacteria
d. contract for movement
e. detect changes in the environment

35. _____ nerve cells

36. _____ muscle cells

37. _____ red blood cells

38. _____ gland cells

39. _____ immune cells

Fill in the blanks.

40. A typical or _____ cell exhibits the most important characteristics of cell types.

41. _____ is the term meaning "water-loving."

42. _____ is the process that allows a message to be carried across a membrane.

43. _____ detoxify harmful substances that enter cells.

44. The _____ is one of the largest cell structures and occupies the central portion of the cell.

45. Embedded within the phospholipid bilayer of the cell membrane is a variety of _____ _____ _____ (IMPs).

CHAPTER 4

Physiology of Cells

Cells, just like humans, require water, food, gases, elimination of wastes, and numerous other substances and processes in order to survive. Cells must transport the substances within the cytoplasm and across cell membranes. The movement of these substances in and out of the cell is accomplished by two primary methods: passive transport and active transport. In passive transport, no cellular energy is required to effect movement through the cell membrane. However, in active transport, cellular energy is necessary to provide movement through the cell membrane.

Once nutrients enter the cells, a series of chemical reactions is necessary to prepare the materials to be utilized by the body. The chemical reaction that breaks down larger, more complex substances into simpler substances and releases energy from the food molecules is known as *catabolism*. Energy is essential because it provides the body with the power (ATP) to perform its tasks and to maintain body temperature.

Cellular respiration is the process by which cells break down glucose, or a nutrient that has been converted to glucose or one of its simpler products, into carbon dioxide and water. As the molecule breaks down, energy is released. Three main pathways are available to the cell to accomplish cellular respiration. These pathways are glycolysis, the citric acid cycle, and the electron transport system. The anatomy and physiology of the cells allow us to adapt successfully to our environment and maintain health. By working together harmoniously, the various structures and functions of cells assure survival.

I—MOVEMENT OF SUBSTANCES THROUGH CELL MEMBRANES

Multiple Choice—select the best answer.

1. Which of the following is *not* a passive transport process?
   a. dialysis
   b. osmosis
   c. filtration
   d. pinocytosis

2. Diffusion of water through a selectively permeable membrane in the presence of at least one impermeant solute is referred to as:
   a. diffusion.
   b. osmosis.
   c. phagocytosis.
   d. dialysis.

3. The trapping of bacteria by specialized white blood cells is an example of:
   a. pinocytosis.
   b. exocytosis.
   c. phagocytosis.
   d. none of the above.

4. A hypertonic solution is one that contains:
   a. a greater concentration of solute than the cell.
   b. the same concentration of solute as the cell.
   c. a lesser concentration of solute as the cell.
   d. none of the above.

5. The force of a fluid pushing against a surface could be described as:
   a. facilitated diffusion.
   b. hydrostatic pressure.
   c. hypostatic pressure.
   d. none of the above.

True or false

6. _____ Facilitated diffusion is a metabolically expensive process.

7. _____ The sodium-potassium pump is an example of an active transport process.

8. _____ Cellular secretion can be achieved by exocytosis.

9. _____ Solutes are particles dissolved in a solvent.

10. _____ Osmosis is a form of filtration that results in the separation of small and large solute particles.

Matching—identify each item with its corresponding description.

a. isotonic
b. hypertonic
c. hypotonic
d. diffusion
e. endocytosis

11. _____ solution that draws water from a cell

12. _____ two fluids that have the same potential osmotic pressure

13. _____ solution that causes cells to swell

14. _____ passive transport

15. _____ active transport

▶ *If you had difficulty with this section, review pages 90-102.*

Labeling—match each term with its corresponding number in the following diagram of cellular respiration.

_____ aerobic

_____ glucose

_____ mitochondrion

_____ anaerobic

_____ pyruvic acid

_____ citric acid cycle

_____ lactic acid

_____ O_2

_____ ATP

_____ transition

_____ H_2O

_____ acetyl CoA

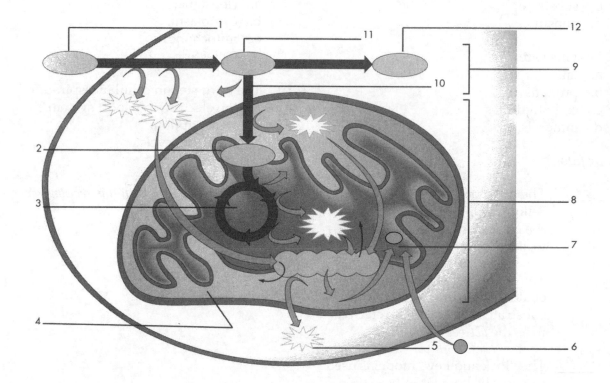

II—CELL METABOLISM

Multiple Choice—select the best answer.

16. Enzymes that cause essential chemical reactions to occur are called:
    a. metabolic agents.
    b. catalysts.
    c. substrates.
    d. initiators.

17. Molecules that are acted upon by enzymes are known as:
    a. diploid.
    b. hypertonic.
    c. introns.
    d. substrates.

18. In naming enzymes, the root name of the substance whose chemical reaction is catalyzed is followed by the suffix:
    a. -ase.
    b. -cin.
    c. -ose.
    d. -ous.

19. Most enzymes:
    a. are specific in their action.
    b. can alter their function by changing the shape of the molecule.
    c. are synthesized as inactive proenzymes.
    d. all of the above.

20. Which of the following activates enzymes by means of an allosteric effect?
    a. end-product inhibition
    b. kinases
    c. substrate
    d. pepsin

21. Enzymes are:
    a. fats.
    b. proteins.
    c. carbohydrates.
    d. minerals.

True or false

22. _____ The three processes that comprise cellular respiration are glycolysis, the citric acid cycle, and the electron transport system.

23. _____ The portion of an enzyme molecule that chemically "fits" the substrate molecule(s) is referred to as the *active site*.

24. _____ The "lock and key" model is used to describe how DNA base pairs align.

25. _____ Protein anabolism is a major cellular activity.

26. _____ The citric acid cycle is also known as the *Krebs cycle*.

27. _____ Glycolysis is aerobic.

Multiple Choice—select the best answer.

28. Which of the following statements is *not* true of glycolysis?
    a. It occurs in the cytoplasm of the cell.
    b. It is also known as the *Krebs cycle*.
    c. It is anaerobic.
    d. Glycolysis splits one molecule of glucose into two molecules of pyruvic acid.

29. The Krebs cycle takes place in the:
    a. ribosome.
    b. cytoplasm.
    c. mitochondria.
    d. Golgi apparatus.

30. The third step in cellular respiration is:
    a. the electron transport system.
    b. transcription.
    c. the Krebs cycle.
    d. glycolysis.

▶ *If you had difficulty with this section, review pages 102-109.*

Crossword Puzzle

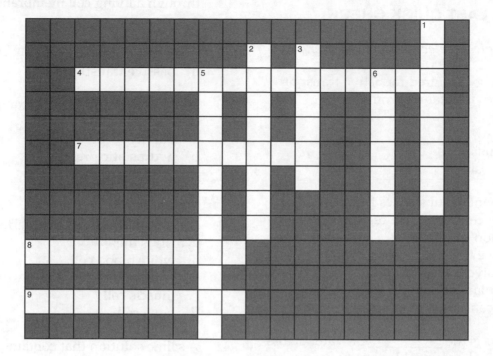

Across

4. Movement that requires cell energy (two words)
7. Sum of chemical reactions in a cell
8. Passive process
9. Requires no oxygen

Down

1. Metabolism that breaks down molecules
2. Concentration _____ measures differences in concentration from one area to another
3. Chemical catalyst
5. "Traps" extracellular material and brings it into cell
6. Diffusion of water

APPLYING WHAT YOU KNOW

31. Nurse Bricker was instructed to dissolve a pill in a small amount of liquid medication. As she dropped the capsule into the liquid, she was interrupted by the telephone. On her return to the medication cart, she found the medication completely dissolved and apparently scattered evenly throughout the liquid.

    This phenomenon did not surprise her because she was aware from her knowledge of cell transport that _____ had created this distribution.

32. Bobbi ran in the Boston marathon. During the race, she lost a lot of fluids through perspiration and became dehydrated. Would you expect her cells to shrink, swell, or remain the same?

DID YOU KNOW

- A human can detect one drop of perfume diffused throughout a three-room apartment
- The longest-living cells in the body are brain cells, which can live an entire lifetime.

ONE LAST QUICK CHECK

Multiple Choice—select the best answer.

33. The energy required for active transport processes is obtained from:
    a. ATP.
    b. DNA.
    c. diffusion.
    d. osmosis.

34. Movement of substances from a region of high concentration to a region of low concentration is:
    a. active transport.
    b. passive transport.
    c. cellular energy.
    d. concentration gradient.

35. Osmosis is the _____ of water across a selectively permeable membrane.
    a. filtration
    b. equilibrium
    c. active transport
    d. diffusion

36. A molecule or other agent that alters enzyme function by changing its shape is called:
    a. an allosteric effector.
    b. a kinase.
    c. an anabolic agent.
    d. a proenzyme.

37. Glycolysis is a catabolic pathway that begins with glucose and ends with:
    a. oxygen.
    b. filtration.
    c. pyruvic acid.
    d. sodium.

38. Which movement always occurs down a hydrostatic pressure gradient?
    a. osmosis
    b. filtration
    c. dialysis
    d. facilitated diffusion

39. The "uphill" movement of a substance through a living cell membrane is:
    a. osmosis.
    b. diffusion.
    c. active transport.
    d. passive transport.

40. Membrane pumps are an example of which type of movement?
    a. gravity
    b. hydrostatic pressure
    c. active transport
    d. passive transport

41. An example of a cell that performs phagocytosis is the:
    a. white blood cell.
    b. red blood cell.
    c. muscle cell.
    d. bone cell.

42. A saline solution that contains a higher concentration of salt than living red blood cells would be:
    a. hypotonic.
    b. hypertonic.
    c. isotonic.
    d. homeostatic.

43. A red blood cell becomes engorged with water and will eventually lyse, releasing hemoglobin into the solution. This solution is _____ to the red blood cell.
    a. hypotonic
    b. hypertonic
    c. isotonic
    d. homeostatic

MATCHING

Matching—match the statement with the proper selection. (Only one answer is correct.)

a. molecule able to diffuse across a particular membrane
b. protein "tunnels"
c. enzyme
d. facilitated diffusion
e. "cell drinking"
f. phagocytosis
g. type of membrane channel
h. enzymes that add or remove carbon dioxide
i. glycolysis

44. _____ membrane channels

45. _____ endocytosis

46. _____ pepsin

47. _____ carboxylases

48. _____ pinocytosis

49. _____ aquaporins

50. _____ carrier-mediated passive transport

51. _____ first stage of cellular respiration

52. _____ permeant

CHAPTER 5

Cell Growth and Reproduction

Cell reproduction completes the study of cells. A basic explanation of DNA, the "hereditary molecule," gives us a proper respect for the capability of the cell to transmit physical and mental traits from generation to generation. Cell reproduction is essential for an organism to maintain itself or grow. When a cell divides, it must be able to replicate the DNA in its genome so that the two daughter cells have the same genetic information as the parent cell. Reproduction of the cell—mitosis—is a complex process requiring several stages. These stages are outlined and diagrammed in the text to facilitate learning. Understanding cell growth, reproduction, and physiology will assist you in your comprehension of the physiology of the body as a whole.

I—PROTEIN SYNTHESIS AND CELL GROWTH

Multiple Choice—select the best answer.

1. Protein synthesis:
   a. is required for cell growth.
   b. begins with reading of the genetic "master code" in the cell's DNA.
   c. influences all cell structures and functions.
   d. all of the above.

2. In the DNA molecule, a sequence of three base pairs forms a(n):
   a. codon.
   b. anticodon.
   c. polymerase.
   d. none of the above.

3. Transcription can best be described as the:
   a. synthesis of tRNA.
   b. reading of mRNA codons by tRNA.
   c. synthesis of mRNA.
   d. synthesis of polypeptides at a ribosomal site.

4. Which of the following statements is true?
   a. Complex polypeptide chains form tRNA.
   b. The site of transcription is within the nucleus, whereas the site of translation is in the cytoplasm.
   c. Uracil is present in DNA in the place of thymine.
   d. None of the above is true.

5. A DNA molecule is characterized by all of the following *except:*
   a. double-helix shape.
   b. obligatory base pairing.
   c. ribose sugar.
   d. phosphate groups.

6. Which of the following is *not* a characteristic of RNA?
   a. It is single-stranded.
   b. It contains uracil, not thymine.
   c. The obligatory base pairs are adenine-uracil and guanine-cytosine.
   d. Its molecules are larger than those of DNA.

7. Nucleic acids are synthesized directly on the DNA molecule with the help of:
   a. enzymes.
   b. prophase.
   c. neoplasms.
   d. lipids.

Matching—identify the term related to protein synthesis with its corresponding definition.

a. mRNA
b. ribosome
c. tRNA
d. translation
e. transcription
f. complimentary base pair

8. _____ Process that occurs when the double strands of a DNA segment separate and RNA nucleotides pair with DNA nucleotides

9. _____ The type of RNA that carries information in groups of three nucleotides called *codons*, each of which codes for a specific amino acid

10. _____ The type of RNA that has an anticodon and binds to a base pair–specific amino acid

11. _____ The process involving the movement of mRNA with respect to the ribosome

12. _____ Uracil-adenine

13. _____ The site of translation

Labeling—label the following illustration of a DNA molecule.

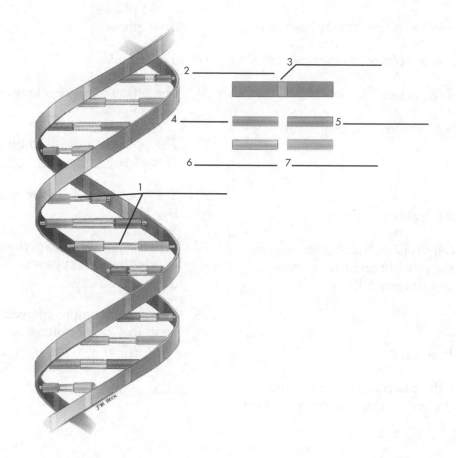

▶ *If you had difficulty with this section, review pages 113-123.*

II—CELL REPRODUCTION

Circle the word or phrase that does **not** *belong.*

14. mitosis	meiosis	M phase	enzyme
15. anaphase	end phase	apart	2 chromosomes
16. meiosis	sex cells	telophase	oogonia
17. zygote	mitosis	diploid	46 chromosomes
18. metaphase	prophase	telophase	interphase

Multiple Choice—select the best answer.

19. The correct order of mitosis is:
    a. prophase, metaphase, anaphase, telophase.
    b. anaphase, telophase, metaphase, prophase.
    c. prophase, anaphase, metaphase, telophase.
    d. none of the above.

20. The total of 46 chromosomes per cell is referred to as:
    a. haploid.
    b. diploid.
    c. myoid.
    d. none of the above.

21. A type of cell division that occurs only in primitive sex cells during the process of becoming mature sex cells is:
    a. mitosis.
    b. meiosis.
    c. gamete.
    d. differentiation.

22. Splitting of the plasma membrane and cytoplasm into two during cell reproduction is called:
    a. mitosis.
    b. meiosis.
    c. anaphase.
    d. cytokinesis.

23. Cell reproduction is sometimes referred to as the:
    a. A phase.
    b. R phase.
    c. M phase.
    d. X phase.

Fill in the blanks.

24. The phase of mitosis known as the "completion phase" is _____.

25. The phase of mitosis known as the "apart phase" is _____.

26. The "position-changing phase" of mitosis is _____.

27. When a cell is not experiencing mitosis and is "between phases," it is said to be in _____.

28. When a cell begins to divide, it is said to be in the "before phase" or _____.

Labeling—on the following diagram, label the phases of mitosis. Remember that interphase and DNA replication occur before mitosis begins!

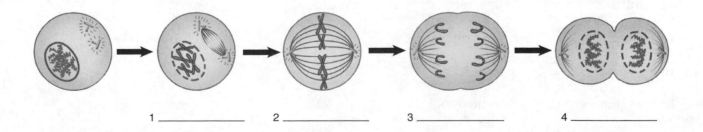

1 _____ 2 _____ 3 _____ 4 _____

▶ *If you had difficulty with this section, review pages 123-127.*

III—MECHANISMS OF DISEASE

True or false

29. _____ *Atrophy* refers to a decrease in cell size.

30. _____ Genetic disorders are mutations in a cell's genetic code.

31. _____ Cell death due to injury or a pathologic condition is known as *necrosis*.

32. _____ Viruses do not contain DNA or RNA.

33. _____ A blood disease caused by the production of abnormal hemoglobin is known as *sickle cell anemia*.

▶ *If you had difficulty with this section, review pages 126-128.*

APPLYING WHAT YOU KNOW

34. Mrs. McWilliam's home pregnancy test indicated that she was pregnant. She made an appointment with her doctor to confirm the results. While she was there, she inquired about ordering genetic testing while she was pregnant. What information might these tests reveal?

35. Dan broke his arm playing high school football and had to wear a cast for 6 weeks. When the doctor finally removed his cast, he was shocked to see that his arm had shrunk remarkably. His shock and disappointment were visible to the doctor. What should the doctor tell him about his arm?

DID YOU KNOW

- Our entire DNA sequence would fill two hundred 1,000-page New York City telephone directories.

- A complete 3 billion base genome would take 3 gigabytes of storage space.

Crossword Puzzle

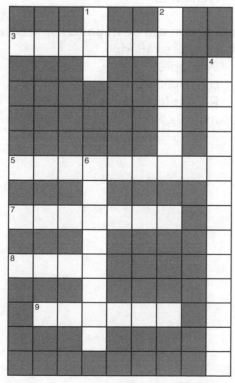

Across
3. Always pairs with thymine in a DNA molecule
5. Also known as the growth phases of a cell (2 words)
7. Cell reproduction
8. Segment of the DNA molecule
9. Mature sex cell

Down
1. Deoxyribonucleic acid
2. Sex cell reproduction
4. Synthesis of RNA molecule
6. Complete set of proteins synthesized by a cell

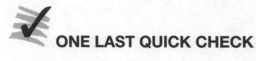

ONE LAST QUICK CHECK

Multiple Choice—select the best answer.

36. The genetic code for a particular protein is passed from DNA to mRNA by a process known as:
    a. transcription.
    b. translation.
    c. interphase.
    d. genome.

37. If a strand of DNA has a base sequence of AGGC, the complementary pair for that strand will be:
    a. TCCG.
    b. CCTG.
    c. TTCG.
    d. TUUG.

38. The spindle fibers attach to each chromatid during which stage of mitosis?
    a. prophase
    b. anaphase
    c. telophase
    d. metaphase

39. Which of the following is *not* true of RNA?
    a. It is a single strand.
    b. It contains uracil rather than thymine.
    c. The base pairs are adenine and uracil and guanine and cytosine.
    d. It contains deoxyribose sugar.

40. During which stage of mitosis does the cleavage furrow begin to develop?
    a. prophase
    b. metaphase
    c. anaphase
    d. telophase

41. All of the DNA in each cell of the body is called the:
    a. tissue typing.
    b. genome.
    c. gene.
    d. genetic code.

42. If the sequence of bases in a nucleic acid were AUCGA, which of the following statements would be true?
    a. The nucleic acid would contain deoxyribose.
    b. It is a strand of DNA.
    c. It is a strand of RNA.
    d. It will remain in the nucleus of the cell.

43. In which stage of mitosis do chromosomes move to opposite ends of the cells along the spindle fibers?
    a. anaphase
    b. metaphase
    c. prophase
    d. telophase

44. The synthesis of proteins by ribosomes using information coded in the mRNA molecule is called:
    a. translation.
    b. transcription.
    c. replication.
    d. crenation.

45. Translation can be inhibited or prevented by a process called:
    a. cytokinesis.
    b. cell division.
    c. RNA interference.
    d. meiosis.

*Circle the word or phrase that does **not** belong.*

46. DNA   adenine   uracil   thymine

47. RNA   ribose   thymine   uracil

48. translation   protein synthesis mRNA   interphase

49. cleavage furrow   anaphase   prophase   2 daughter cells

50. metaphase   prophase   telophase   gene

Fill in the blanks.

51. The DNA molecular structure allows only two combinations of bases to occur. This is known as _____ _____ _____.

52. The complete set of proteins synthesized by a cell is called the _____ of the cell.

53. The shape of a DNA molecule is referred to as a _____ _____.

54. _____ is the type of cell division that occurs only in primitive sex cells during the process of becoming mature sex cells.

55. Mature sex cells are called _____.

CHAPTER 6

Tissues

After successfully completing the study of the cell, you are ready to progress to the next level of anatomical structure: tissues. Four principal types of tissue—epithelial, connective, muscle, and nervous—perform multiple functions to assure that homeostasis is maintained. Among these functions are protection, absorption, excretion, support, insulation, conduction of impulses, movement of bones, and destruction of bacteria. This variety of functions gives us a real appreciation for the complexity of this level.

A macroscopic view confirms this statement as we marvel at the fact that soft, sticky, liquid blood and sturdy compact bone are both considered tissues. Our study continues with the discussion of body membranes and their function for the body. Membranes are thin layers of epithelial and/or connective tissue that cover and protect the body surfaces, line body cavities, and cover the internal surfaces of hollow organs. These major membranes—cutaneous, serous, mucous, and synovial—are also critical to homeostasis and body survival. An understanding of tissues and membranes is necessary to successfully bridge your knowledge between the cell and the study of body organs.

I—PRINCIPAL TYPES OF TISSUES

Multiple Choice—select the best answer.

1. A tissue is:
   a. a membrane that lines body cavities.
   b. a group of similar cells that perform a common function.
   c. a thin sheet of cells embedded in a matrix.
   d. the most complex organizational unit of the body.

2. The four principal types of tissues include all of the following *except:*
   a. nervous.
   b. muscle.
   c. cartilage.
   d. connective.

3. The most complex tissue in the body is:
   a. muscle.
   b. blood.
   c. connective.
   d. nervous.

4. In tissues, the material between cells that is made up of water and a variety of proteins is referred to as:
   a. intercellular material.
   b. extracellular matrix.
   c. lacunae.
   d. none of the above.

5. Which of the following is *not* a primary germ layer?
   a. endoderm
   b. periderm
   c. mesoderm
   d. ectoderm

6. Which tissue lines body cavities and protects body surfaces?
   a. epithelial
   b. connective
   c. muscular
   d. nervous

True or false

7. _____ The biology of tissues is referred to as *histology*.

8. _____ Proteins in the extracellular matrix include various types of structural protein fibers such as collagen and elastin.

9. _____ Sweat and sebaceous glands are formed by connective tissue.

10. _____ During embryonic development, new kinds of cells can be formed from a special kind of undifferentiated cell called a *stem cell*.

▶ *If you had difficulty with this section, review pages 131-135.*

II—EPITHELIAL TISSUE

Multiple Choice—select the best answer.

11. Which of the following is *not* a function of membranous epithelium?
    a. secretion
    b. protection
    c. absorption
    d. all are functions of the membranous epithelium

12. Which of the following is *not* a structural example of epithelium?
    a. stratified squamous
    b. simple transitional
    c. stratified columnar
    d. pseudostratified columnar

13. The simple columnar epithelium lining the intestines contains plasma membranes that extend into thousands of microscopic extensions called:
    a. villi.
    b. microvilli.
    c. cilia.
    d. flagella.

14. Epithelial cells can be classified according to shape. Which of the following is *not* a characteristic shape of epithelium?
    a. cuboidal
    b. rectangular
    c. squamous
    d. columnar

15. Keratinized stratified squamous epithelium is found in the:
    a. mouth.
    b. vagina.
    c. skin.
    d. all of the above.

16. Endocrine glands discharge their products into:
    a. body cavities.
    b. blood.
    c. organ surfaces.
    d. none of the above.

17. Which of the following is *not* a functional classification of exocrine glands?
    a. alveolar
    b. apocrine
    c. holocrine
    d. merocrine

18. The functional classification of salivary glands is:
    a. endocrine.
    b. apocrine.
    c. holocrine.
    d. merocrine.

19. This epithelial tissue readily allows diffusion, as in the linings of blood and lymphatic vessels.
    a. simple squamous
    b. stratified squamous
    c. simple columnar
    d. pseudostratified columnar

True or false

20. _____ Epithelial tissue is attached to an underlying layer of connective tissue called the *basement membrane*.

21. _____ Epithelium is rich with blood supply.

22. _____ Exocrine glands discharge their products directly into the blood.

Matching—identify the arrangement of epithelial cells with its corresponding description.

a. simple squamous
b. simple cuboidal
c. simple columnar
d. pseudostratified columnar
e. stratified squamous
f. stratified cuboidal
g. stratified columnar
h. transitional

23. _____ single layer of cube-shaped cells

24. _____ multiple layers of cells with flat cells at the outer surface

25. _____ single layer of cells in which some are tall and thin and able to reach the free surface and others are not

26. _____ layers of cells that appear cube-like when an organ is relaxed and flat or distended by fluid

27. _____ single layer of flat, scalelike cells

28. _____ single layer of tall, thin cells that compose the surface of mucous membranes

Labeling—label the following images and identify the principal tissue type of each. Be as specific as possible. Consult your textbook if you need assistance.

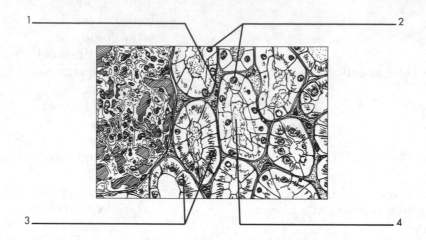

1 ⎯⎯⎯⎯⎯⎯⎯⎯⎯⎯⎯⎯⎯⎯⎯ 2

3 ⎯⎯⎯⎯⎯⎯⎯⎯⎯⎯⎯⎯⎯⎯⎯ 4

Tissue type: _____

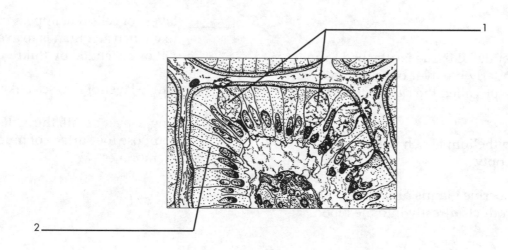

1

2 ⎯⎯⎯⎯⎯⎯⎯⎯⎯⎯⎯⎯⎯⎯⎯

Tissue type: _____

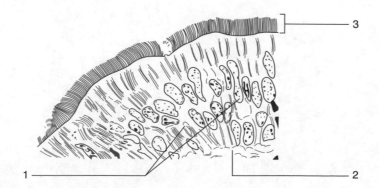

3

1 ⎯⎯⎯⎯⎯⎯⎯⎯⎯⎯⎯⎯⎯⎯⎯ 2

Tissue type: _____

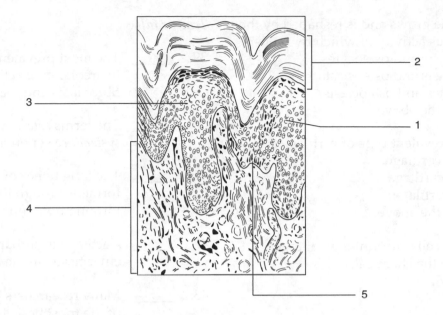

Tissue type: _____

▶ *If you had difficulty with this section, review pages 135-143.*

III—CONNECTIVE TISSUE

Multiple Choice—select the best answer.

29. Which of the following is *not* an example of connective tissue?
    a. transitional
    b. reticular
    c. blood
    d. bone

30. Which of the following fibers is *not* found in connective tissue matrix?
    a. collagenous
    b. elastic
    c. fibroblastic
    d. reticular

31. Fibroblasts are usually present in the greatest numbers in which type of connective tissue?
    a. adipose
    b. loose fibrous
    c. reticular
    d. dense

32. Adipose tissue performs which of the following functions?
    a. insulation
    b. protection
    c. support
    d. all of the above

33. Which of the following connective tissue types forms the framework of the spleen, lymph nodes, and bone marrow?
    a. loose
    b. adipose
    c. reticular
    d. areolar

34. The mature cells of bone are called:
    a. fibroblasts.
    b. osteoclasts.
    c. osteoblasts.
    d. osteocytes.

35. The basic structural unit of bone is the microscopic:
    a. osteon.
    b. lacunae.
    c. lamellae.
    d. canaliculi.

36. Mature bone grows and is reshaped by the simultaneous activity of which two cells?
    a. osteoblasts and osteocytes
    b. osteoblasts and osteoclasts
    c. osteocytes and osteoclasts
    d. none of the above

37. The most prevalent type of cartilage is:
    a. hyaline cartilage.
    b. fibrous cartilage.
    c. elastic cartilage.
    d. none of the above.

38. When mast cells encounter an allergen, they release the chemical:
    a. benedryl.
    b. allergra.
    c. zyflo.
    d. histamine.

True or false

39. _____ The most prevalent types of cells in areolar connective tissue are fibroblasts and macrophages.

40. _____ The terms *osteon* and *Haversian system* are synonymous.

41. _____ The long bones of the body are formed through the process of intramembranous ossification.

42. _____ Cartilage is perhaps the most vascular tissue in the human body.

43. _____ Many researchers believe that one of the most basic factors in the aging process is the change in the molecular structure of collagen.

44. _____ The greater a person's weight while immersed, the higher the body-fat percentage.

Labeling—label the following images and identify the principal tissue type of each. Be as specific as possible. Consult your textbook if you need assistance.

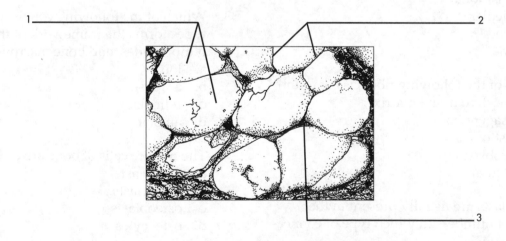

Tissue type: _____

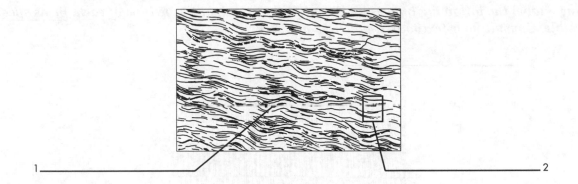

1 _____ 2

Tissue type: _____

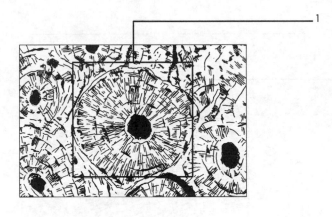

1

Tissue type: _____

▶ *If you had difficulty with this section, review pages 143-152.*

IV—MUSCLE TISSUE

Matching—identify the type of muscle tissue with its corresponding definition.

a. cardiac muscle
b. skeletal muscle
c. smooth muscle

45. _____ cylindrical, striated, voluntary cells

46. _____ nonstriated, involuntary, narrow fibers with only one nucleus per fiber

47. _____ striated, branching, involuntary cells with intercalated disks

48. _____ responsible for willed body movements

49. _____ also called *visceral muscle*

50. _____ found in the walls of hollow internal organs

Labeling—label the following images and identify the principal tissue type of each. Be as specific as possible. Consult your textbook if you need assistance.

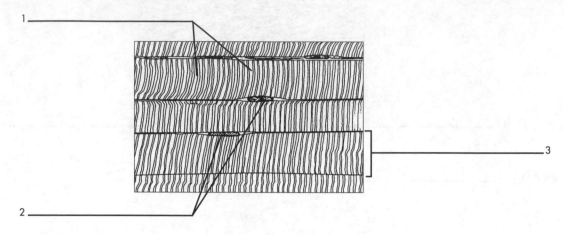

Tissue type: _____

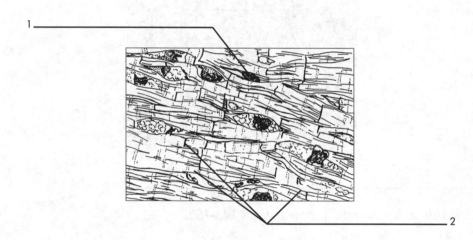

Tissue type: _____

▶ *If you had difficulty with this section, review pages 152-154.*

V—NERVOUS TISSUE

Matching—match each term with its corresponding description.

a. neuron
b. neuroglia
c. axon
d. soma
e. dendrite

51. _____ the cell body of the neuron

52. _____ supportive cells

53. _____ cell process that transmits nerve impulses away from the cell body

54. _____ the conducting cells of the nervous system

55. _____ cell process that carries nerve impulses toward the cell body

Labeling—label the following image and identify the principal tissue type. Be as specific as possible. Consult your textbook if you need assistance.

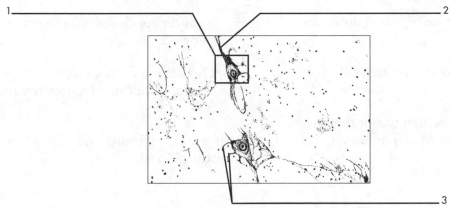

Tissue type: _____

▶ *If you had difficulty with this section, review page 154.*

VI—TISSUE REPAIR

Fill in the blanks.

56. _____ is the growth of new tissue (as opposed to scarring).

57. A _____ is an unusually thick scar.

58. Tissues usually repair themselves by allowing _____ cells to remove dead or injured cells.

59. Epithelial and _____ tissues have the greatest capacity to regenerate.

60. Like muscle tissue, _____ tissue has a very limited capacity to regenerate.

▶ *If you had difficulty with this section, review pages 154-155.*

VII—BODY MEMBRANES

Multiple Choice—select the best answer.

61. Which of the following is *not* an example of epithelial membrane?
    a. synovial membrane
    b. cutaneous membrane
    c. serous membrane
    d. mucous membrane

62. Pleurisy is a condition that affects which membrane?
    a. cutaneous membrane
    b. serous membrane
    c. mucous membrane
    d. none of the above

True or false

63. _____ Parietal membranes cover the surface of organs.

64. _____ Synovial membrane is an example of connective tissue membrane.

▶ *If you had difficulty with this section, review pages 155-158.*

VIII—TUMORS AND CANCER

Circle the correct answer.

65. Benign tumors usually grow (slowly or quickly).

66. Malignant tumors (are or are not) encapsulated.

67. An example of a benign tumor that arises from epithelial tissue is (papilloma or lipoma).

68. Malignant tumors that arise from connective tissues are generally called (melanoma or sarcoma).

69. A cancer specialist is an (osteologist or oncologist).

70. Chemotherapy uses (cytotoxic or cachexic) compounds to destroy malignant cells.

▶ *If you had difficulty with this section, review pages 158-160.*

Crossword Puzzle

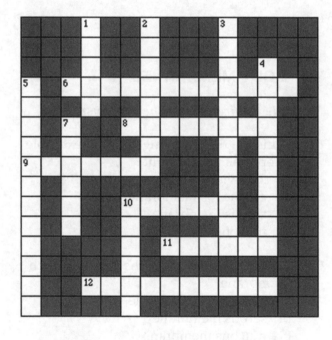

Across
6. Response to a tissue irritant
8. Provides strength for connective tissue
9. Tissue that contains neurons and neuroglia
10. Membrane that lines surfaces that lead to the exterior
11. Cells that perform a common function
12. Tissue that includes glandular

Down
1. Exocrine
2. "Scaly"
3. Process of primary germ layer's tissue development
4. Tissue that includes adipose
5. Growth of new tissue
7. Membrane that lines body cavities
10. Nonliving intercellular material

 APPLYING WHAT YOU KNOW

71. Holly is a bodybuilder who is obsessed with her physique. She exercises daily and eats a very low-fat diet. A personal fitness trainer has assessed her body fat at 12%. Determine whether she is too lean or too fat. Explain the relationship between her body-fat percentage and lifestyle.

72. Bruce is a sedentary, cigarette smoking, middle-aged man who is complaining of chest pain. Ultimately, he is diagnosed with lung cancer. What tests may have been utilized to determine his diagnosis? Which type of tissues would be involved?

DID YOU KNOW

- As many as 500,000 Americans die from cancer each year. That's more than all the lives lost in the past 100 years by the U.S. military forces. Half of all cancers are diagnosed in people under the age of 67.

ONE LAST QUICK CHECK

Labeling—label the following images and identify the principal tissue type of each. Be as specific as possible. Consult your textbook if you need assistance.

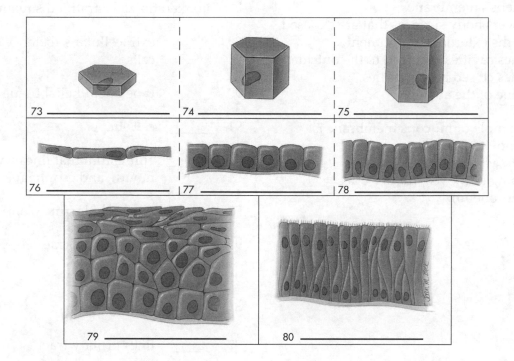

73 _____ 74 _____ 75 _____

76 _____ 77 _____ 78 _____

79 _____ 80 _____

Multiple Choice—select the best answer.

81. Which of the following is *not* an example of connective tissue?
    a. glands
    b. blood
    c. fat
    d. bone

82. Stratified squamous (nonkeratinized) epithelium can be found in all of the following *except*:
    a. vagina.
    b. mouth.
    c. esophagus.
    d. skin.

83. The most abundant and widespread tissue is:
    a. epithelial.
    b. connective.
    c. muscle.
    d. nervous.

84. Loose connective tissue is also known as:
    a. voluntary.
    b. hyaline.
    c. areolar.
    d. visceral.

85. Tissue that insulates to conserve body heat is:
    a. reticular.
    b. fibrous.
    c. adipose.
    d. osseous.

86. What statement regarding blood is true?
    a. Erythrocytes are white blood cells.
    b. Thrombocytes are also known as *platelets*.
    c. Leukocytes are red blood cells.
    d. Formed elements are known as *plasma*.

87. Cutaneous membrane:
    a. covers body surfaces that are exposed to the external environment.
    b. lines cavities that lead to the outside.
    c. lines closed body cavities.
    d. none of the above.

88. An example of mucous membrane is:
    a. synovial fluid.
    b. bursae.
    c. lining of the respiratory tract.
    d. peritoneum.

Matching—match the term with the corresponding description.

a. sebaceous
b. synovial fluid
c. matrix
d. papilloma
e. squamous
f. metastasis
g. membranous
h. erythrocytes
i. adipocytes
j. bone
k. mucous membrane
l. nonkeratinized stratified squamous

89. _____ extracellular substance of tissue cells

90. _____ type of epithelial tissue

91. _____ cell shape

92. _____ epithelium that lines vagina, mouth, and esophagus

93. _____ type of holocrine gland

94. _____ connective tissue

95. _____ fat cell

96. _____ red blood cell

97. _____ lines urinary tract

98. _____ lubricates joints

99. _____ a manner of spreading in disease

100. _____ wart

CHAPTER 7

Skin and Its Appendages

More of our time, attention, and money are spent on this system than any other. Every time we look into a mirror we become aware of the integumentary system, as we observe our skin, hair, nails, and the appendages that give luster and comfort to this system. The discussion of the skin begins with the structure and function of the two primary layers called the *epidermis* and *dermis*. It continues with an examination of the appendages of the skin, which include the hair, receptors, nails, sebaceous glands, and sudoriferous glands.

Your study of the skin concludes with a review of one of the most serious and frequent threats to the skin—burns. An understanding of the integumentary system provides you with an appreciation of the danger that severe burns or trauma can pose to this system.

I—SKIN FUNCTION AND STRUCTURE

Multiple Choice—select the best answer.

1. Beneath the dermis lies a loose layer of skin rich in fat and areolar tissue called the:
   a. dermo-epidermal junction.
   b. hypodermis.
   c. epidermis.
   d. none of the above.

2. The most important cells in the epidermis are the:
   a. keratinocytes.
   b. melanocytes.
   c. Langerhans cells.
   d. dermal papillae.

3. The order of the cells of the epidermis, from superficial to deep, are:
   a. stratum corneum, stratum lucidum, stratum spinosum, stratum granulosum, stratum basale.
   b. stratum corneum, stratum spinosum, stratum lucidum, stratum granulosum, stratum basale.
   c. stratum basale, stratum corneum, stratum lucidum, stratum spinosum, stratum granulosum.
   d. stratum corneum, stratum lucidum, stratum granulosum, stratum spinosum, stratum basale.

4. In which area of the body would you expect to find an especially thick stratum?
   a. back of the hand
   b. thigh
   c. abdomen
   d. sole of the foot

5. In which layer of the skin do cells divide by mitosis to replace cells lost from the outermost surface of the body?
   a. stratum basale
   b. stratum corneum
   c. stratum lucidum
   d. stratum spinosum

6. Smooth muscles that produce "goose bumps" when they contract are:
   a. papillary muscles.
   b. hair muscles.
   c. follicular muscles.
   d. arrector pili muscles.

7. Keratin is found in which layer of the skin?
   a. dermis
   b. epidermis
   c. subcutaneous
   d. serous

8. Meissner's corpuscles are specialized nerve endings that make it possible for skin to detect:
   a. heat.
   b. cold.
   c. light touch.
   d. deep pressure.

9. The basic determinant of skin color is the quantity of:
   a. keratin.
   b. melanin.
   c. albinin.
   d. none of the above.

10. Which of the following is *not* a contributing factor to skin color?
    a. exposure to sunlight
    b. genetics
    c. place of birth
    d. volume of blood in skin capillaries

True or false

11. _____ Most of the body is covered by thick skin.

12. _____ A surgeon would most likely prefer to make an incision parallel to Langer cleavage lines.

13. _____ If the enzyme tyrosinase is absent from birth because of a congenital defect, a condition called *albinism* results.

14. _____ The epidermis is the "true skin" and is composed of two layers.

15. _____ *Subcutaneous layer* and *hypodermis* are synonymous terms.

Labeling—match each term with its corresponding number on the following diagram of a cross-section of skin. Terms may be used more than once.

_____ dermal papillae

_____ shaft of hair

_____ root of hair

_____ friction ridge

_____ sulcus

_____ ridges of dermal papillae

_____ subcutaneous adipose tissue

_____ blood vessels

_____ dermis

_____ dermo-epidermal junction

_____ sweat duct

_____ opening of sweat duct

_____ epidermis

_____ reticular layer of dermis

_____ papillary layer of dermis

_____ hypodermis

_____ sweat gland

_____ lamellar (Pacini) corpuscle

_____ arrector pili muscle

_____ hair follicle

_____ sebaceous gland

_____ nerve fibers

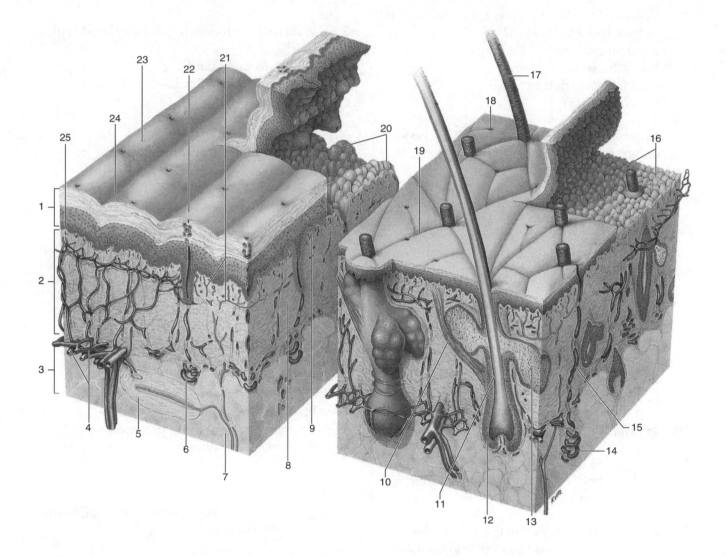

▶ *If you had difficulty with this section, review pages 169-181.*

II—FUNCTIONS OF THE SKIN

Multiple Choice—select the best answer.

16. Which of the following is *not* a function of the skin?
    a. sensation
    b. excretion
    c. immunity
    d. all of the above are skin functions

17. Which of the following vitamins is synthesized by the skin?
    a. vitamin A
    b. vitamin B
    c. vitamin C
    d. vitamin D

18. Which of the following is *not* a mechanism of heat loss by the skin?
    a. evaporation
    b. radiation
    c. vasoconstriction
    d. convection

19. Vitamin D fulfills the requirements necessary for a substance to be classified as a(n):
    a. hormone
    b. mineral
    c. nucleic acid
    d. enzyme

20. Which structure compares actual body temperature with set point temperature and then sends out appropriate correction signals to effectors?
    a. pituitary
    b. hypothalamus
    c. thalamus
    d. none of the above

True or false

21. _____ Skin is a minor factor in the body's thermoregulatory mechanism.

22. _____ Skin plays a major role in the overall excretion of body wastes.

23. _____ To help dissipate heat during exercise, sweat production can reach as much as 3 liters per hour.

▶ *If you had difficulty with this section, review pages 181-185.*

III—APPENDAGES OF THE SKIN

Multiple Choice—select the best answer.

24. The developing fetus is covered by an extremely fine, soft hair coat called:
    a. vellus.
    b. lanugo.
    c. fatalis follicle.
    d. none of the above.

25. Which of the following is associated with hair?
    a. sebaceous glands
    b. ceruminous glands
    c. eccrine glands
    d. none of the above

26. Ceruminous glands are found in the:
    a. axillae.
    b. soles of feet.
    c. ear canal.
    d. none of the above.

27. The most numerous, important, and widespread sweat glands in the body are:
    a. apocrine.
    b. eccrine.
    c. ceruminous.
    d. sebaceous.

28. Hair growth is stimulated by:
    a. cutting it frequently.
    b. shaving.
    c. increasing melanin production.
    d. none of the above.

True or false

29. _____ The visible portion of a hair is the shaft.

30. _____ The inner core of the hair is called the *cortex*.

31. _____ Sweat, or sudoriferous, glands are the most numerous of the skin glands.

32. _____ One of the factors associated with male pattern baldness is androgens.

33. _____ Growth of nails is due to mitosis in the stratum basale.

▶ *If you had difficulty with this section, review pages 185-189.*

IV—MECHANISMS OF DISEASE

Matching—identify the term with the corresponding description.

a. papilloma
b. furuncle
c. ringworm
d. hard skin
e. symptom of underlying condition
f. staph or strep infection
g. bedsores
h. hives

34. _____ impetigo

35. _____ tinea

36. _____ warts

37. _____ boils

38. _____ decubitus ulcers

39. _____ urticaria

40. _____ scleroderma

41. _____ eczema

Fill in the blanks.

42. _____ is the term associated with an unusually high body temperature.

43. _____ _____ occurs when the body loses a large amount of fluid resulting from heat-loss mechanisms.

44. _____ _____ is also known as *sunstroke.*

45. Local damage caused by extremely low temperatures is referred to as _____.

▶ *If you had difficulty with this section, review pages 189-192.*

V—BURNS

Multiple Choice—select the best answer.

46. The "rule of palms" assumes that the palm size of a burn victim equals about ____ of total body surface area.
    a. 1%
    b. 2%
    c. 5%
    d. none of the above

47. Blisters, severe pain, and generalized swelling are characteristic of which type of burn?
    a. first-degree burns
    b. second-degree burns
    c. third-degree burns
    d. none of the above

True or false

48. _____ According to the "rule of nines," the body is divided into nine areas of 9%.

49. _____ Immediately after injury, third-degree burns hurt less than second-degree burns.

Matching—identify each term with its corresponding description.

a.   first-degree burn
b.   second-degree burn
c.   third-degree burn
d.   partial-thickness burn
e.   full-thickness burn

50. _____ destroys both epidermis and dermis and may involve underlying tissue

51. _____ involves only the epidermis

52. _____ another name for first- and second-degree burns

53. _____ damage to epidermis and upper layers of dermis with blisters

54. _____ another name for third-degree burn

Labeling—using the "rule of nines" method, label the following diagram to estimate the amount of skin surface for each area.

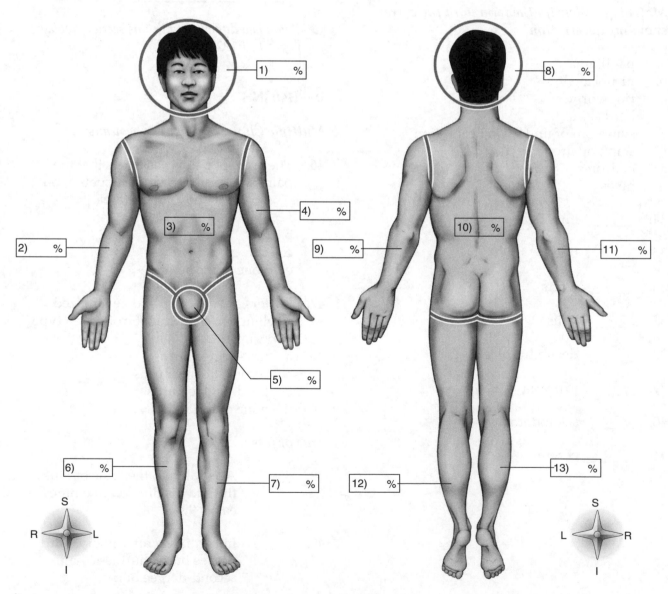

▶ *If you had difficulty with this section, review pages 192-194.*

Crossword Puzzle

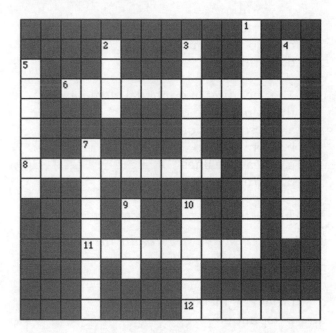

Across

6. Tube that contains the hair root (two words)
8. Skin
11. Outer layer of skin
12. "Layer"

Down

1. Layer beneath the dermis
2. Appendage of skin
3. Determines skin color
4. Sudoriferous gland (two words)
5. Water-repellent protein
7. Gland that secretes oil
9. Keratinized epithelial cells form this structure
10. Inner layer of skin

APPLYING WHAT YOU KNOW

55. Mr. Ziven was admitted to the hospital with second- and third-degree burns. Both arms, the anterior trunk, right anterior leg, and genital region were affected by the burns. The doctor quickly estimated that _____% of Mr. Ziven's body had been burned.

56. After investigating the scene of the crime, Officer Gorski announced that dermal papillae were found that would help solve the case. What did he mean?

57. Bernie is 65 and was recently diagnosed with melanoma. He finds this diagnosis difficult to believe because has lived in Alaska for the past 20 years and gets very little exposure to sun. Can you suggest a possible explanation for his diagnosis?

DID YOU KNOW

- Because the dead cells of the epidermis are constantly being worn and washed away, we get a new outer skin layer every 27 days.

- The average person sheds 40 pounds of skin in a lifetime.

ONE LAST QUICK CHECK

Multiple Choice—select the best answer.

58. Which of the following statements about hair follicles is true?
    a. Arrector pili muscles are associated with them.
    b. Sudoriferous glands empty into them.
    c. They arise directly from the epidermal layer of skin.
    d. All of the above are true.

59. Which of the following statements about apocrine glands is true?
    a. They can be classified as sudoriferous.
    b. They can be found primarily in the armpit area, the areolae of the breasts, and around the anus.
    c. They enlarge and begin to function at puberty.
    d. All of the above are true.

60. Which of the following, if any, is *not* found in the epidermal layer of the skin?
    a. nerves
    b. melanin
    c. blood vessels
    d. all of the above are found in the dermis

61. What characterizes second-degree burns?
    a. blisters
    b. swelling
    c. severe pain
    d. all of the above

62. Blackheads can result from the blockage of which of the following glands?
    a. lacrimal
    b. sebaceous
    c. ceruminous
    d. sudoriferous

63. A common type of skin cancer is:
    a. malignant melanoma.
    b. vitiligo.
    c. basal cell carcinoma.
    d. Kaposi sarcoma.

64. What is the fold of skin that hides the root of a nail called?
    a. lunula
    b. body
    c. cuticle
    d. papillae

65. Which of the following is *not* an important function of the skin?
    a. sense organ activity
    b. absorption
    c. protection
    d. temperature

66. Another name for the dermis is:
    a. corium.
    b. strata.
    c. subcutaneous.
    d. lunula.

67. The shedding of epithelial elements from the skin surface is called:
    a. desquamation.
    b. convection.
    c. cleavage lines.
    d. turnover.

Matching—identify the correct answer for each item.

a. fingerprint
b. pressure
c. brown pigment
d. perspiration
e. oil
f. follicle
g. little moon
h. axilla sweat glands
i. fungal infection
j. genetic inflammatory skin disorder

68. _____ melanin
69. _____ Pacini corpuscle
70. _____ sebaceous
71. _____ hair
72. _____ lunula
73. _____ dermal papillae
74. _____ sudoriferous
75. _____ apocrine
76. _____ tinea
77. _____ psoriasis

CHAPTER 8

Skeletal Tissues

How strange we would look without our skeleton! It is the skeleton that provides the rigid, supportive framework that gives shape to our bodies. But this is just the beginning, because the skeleton also protects the organs beneath it, maintains homeostasis of blood calcium, produces blood cells, and assists the muscular system in providing movement for us.

After reviewing the microscopic structure of bone and cartilage, you will understand how skeletal tissues are formed, their differences, and their importance in the human body. Your microscopic investigation will make the study of this system easier as you logically progress from this view to macroscopic bone formation and growth and visualize the structure of long bones.

Bones are classified structurally by their shape: long bones, short bones, flat bones, irregular bones, and sesamoid bones. They are also classified by the types of cells that form the bone: compact bone and cancellous, or spongy, bone. Throughout life, bone formation (ossification) and bone destruction (resorption) occur concurrently to assure a firm and comfortable framework for our bodies.

I—TYPES OF BONES

Matching—identify each structure with its corresponding description.

a. epiphysis
b. medullary cavity
c. carpal
d. articular cartilage
e. femur
f. endosteum
g. vertebra
h. diaphysis
i. patella
j. periosteum
k. sternum

1. _____ the thin membrane that lines the medullary cavity

2. _____ an example of a flat bone

3. _____ the shaft of the long bone

4. _____ an example of a long bone

5. _____ the thin layer that cushions jolts and blows

6. _____ an example of a sesamoid bone

7. _____ an attachment for muscle fibers

8. _____ an example of a short bone

9. _____ the end of a long bone

10. _____ the tubelike, hollow space in the diaphysis of long bones

11. _____ an example of an irregular bone

▶ *If you had difficulty with this section, review pages 199-203.*

II—BONE TISSUE STRUCTURE, BONE MARROW, AND REGULATION OF BLOOD CALCIUM LEVELS

Multiple Choice—select the best answer.

12. Which of the following is *not* a component of bone matrix?
    a. inorganic salts
    b. organic matrix
    c. collagenous fibers
    d. all of the above are components of bone matrix

13. Small spaces in which bone cells lie are called:
    a. lamellae.
    b. lacunae.
    c. canaliculi.
    d. interstitial lamellae.

14. The basic structural unit of compact bone is:
    a. trabeculae.
    b. cancellous bone.
    c. osteon.
    d. none of the above.

15. The cells that produce the organic matrix in bone are:
    a. chondrocytes.
    b. osteoblasts.
    c. osteocytes.
    d. osteoclasts.

16. The bones in an adult that contain red marrow include all of the following *except*:
    a. ribs.
    b. tarsals.
    c. pelvis.
    d. femur.

17. Low blood calcium evokes a response from:
    a. calcitonin.
    b. the thyroid.
    c. parathyroid hormone.
    d. none of the above.

True or false

18. _____ Haversian canals run lengthwise, whereas Volkmann's canals run transverse to the bone.

19. _____ Giant, multinucleate cells that are responsible for bone resorption are called *osteocytes*.

20. _____ Bone marrow is found not only in the medullary cavities of certain long bones but also in the spaces of cancellous bone.

21. _____ Calcitonin functions to stimulate osteoblasts and inhibit osteoclasts.

22. _____ *Hematopoiesis* is a term referring to the formation of new Haversian systems.

23. _____ Yellow marrow is found in almost all of the bones of an infant's body.

▶ *If you had difficulty with this section, review page 200 and pages 203-209.*

III—BONE DEVELOPMENT, REMODELING, AND REPAIR

Multiple Choice—select the best answer.

24. The primary ossification center is located at the:
    a. epiphysis.
    b. diaphysis.
    c. articular cartilage.
    d. none of the above.

25. The primary purpose of the epiphyseal plate is:
    a. mending fractures.
    b. enlarging the epiphysis.
    c. providing bone strength.
    d. lengthening long bones.

26. The epiphyseal plate is composed mostly of:
    a. chondrocytes.
    b. osteocytes.
    c. osteoclasts.
    d. none of the above.

27. Bone loss normally begins to exceed bone gain between the ages of:
    a. 30 and 35 years.
    b. 35 and 40 years.
    c. 55 and 60 years.
    d. 65 and 70 years.

28. The first step to healing a bone fracture is:
    a. callus formation.
    b. fracture hematoma formation.
    c. alignment of the fracture.
    d. collar formation.

True or false

29. _____ The addition of bone to its outer surface resulting in growth in diameter is called *appositional growth*.

30. _____ Most bones of the body are formed by intramembranous ossification.

31. _____ Once an individual reaches skeletal maturity, the bones undergo years of metabolic rest.

32. _____ Lack of exercise tends to weaken bones through decreased collagen formation and excessive calcium withdrawal.

33. _____ When bones reach their full length, the epiphyseal plate disappears.

▶ *If you had difficulty with this section, review pages 209-214.*

IV—CARTILAGE

Multiple Choice—select the best answer.

34. The fibrous covering of cartilage is:
    a. periosteum.
    b. perichondrium.
    c. chondroclast.
    d. none of the above.

35. The external ear, epiglottis, and the auditory tube are composed of:
    a. hyaline cartilage.
    b. fibrocartilage.
    c. elastic cartilage.
    d. none of the above.

36. Vitamin D deficiency can result in:
    a. scurvy.
    b. rickets.
    c. osteochondroma.
    d. none of the above.

True or false

37. _____ Both bone and cartilage are well-vascularized.

38. _____ The intervertebral discs are composed of fibrocartilage.

39. _____ The growth of cartilage occurs by both appositional and interstitial growth.

Labeling—label the following diagrams.

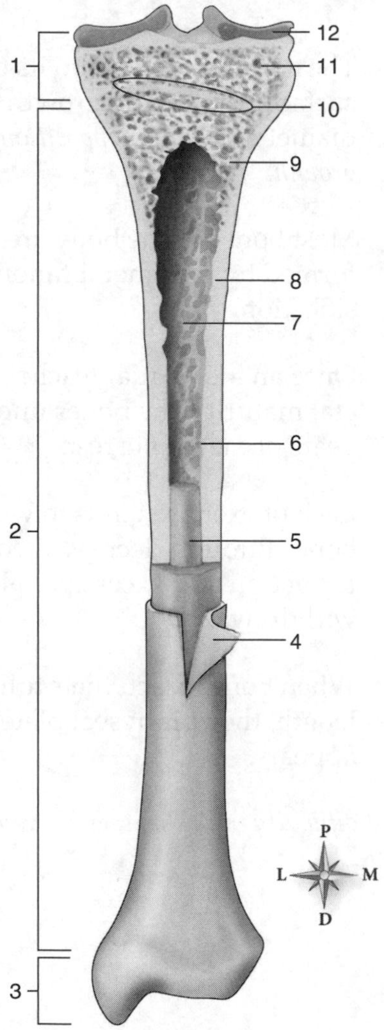

Long bone.

1 _____

2 _____

3 _____

4 _____

5 _____

6 _____

7 _____

8 _____

9 _____

10 _____

11 _____

12 _____

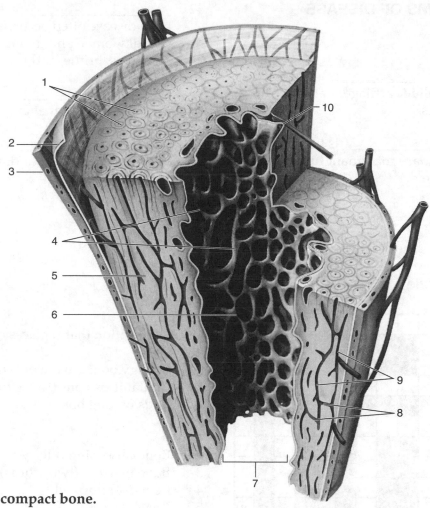

Cancellous and compact bone.

1 _____

2 _____

3 _____

4 _____

5 _____

6 _____

7 _____

8 _____

9 _____

10 _____

▶ *If you had difficulty with this section, review pages 214-216.*

V—MECHANISMS OF DISEASE

Fill in the blanks.

40. _____ is a malignant tumor of hyaline cartilage that arises from chondroblasts.

41. _____ is the most common primary malignant tumor of skeletal tissue.

42. _____ is a common bone disease often occurring in postmenopausal women and manifesting symptoms of porous, brittle, and fragile bones.

43. _____ _____ is also known as *osteitis deformans*.

44. _____ is a bacterial infection of the bone and marrow tissue.

▶ *If you had difficulty with this section, review pages 216-218.*

Crossword Puzzle

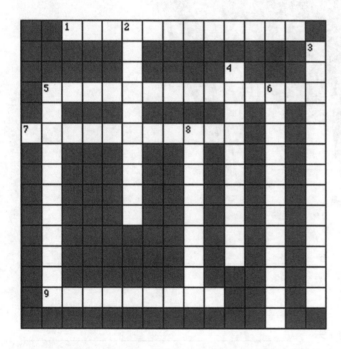

Across
1. Ossification that replaces cartilage with bone
5. Spongy bone (two words)
7. Contains osteons (two words)
9. Ends of long bone

Down
2. Bone-absorbing cell
3. Bone marrow (two words)
4. Bone-forming cell
5. Cartilage cell
6. Bone formation
8. Bone cell

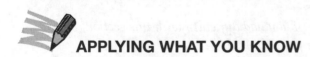

APPLYING WHAT YOU KNOW

45. Mrs. Harris is a 60-year-old white woman. She has noticed in recent years that her height has slightly decreased. Recently, she fractured her wrist in a slight fall. Which skeletal system disorder might she be suffering from? What techniques could be used to diagnose her condition? What treatments are available?

46. Mrs. Wiedeke had advanced cancer of the bone. As the disease progressed, Mrs. Wiedeke required several blood transfusions throughout her therapy. She asked the doctor one day to explain the necessity for the transfusions. What explanation might the doctor give to Mrs. Wiedeke?

47. Dr. Kennedy, an orthopedic surgeon, called the admissions office of the hospital and advised them that he would be admitting a patient in the next hour with an epiphyseal fracture. Without any other information, the patient is assigned to the pediatric ward. What prompted this assignment?

48. Ms. Strickland was in an auto accident. When the surgeon described the details of the surgery to her family, he stated that he was able to "patch" her fractures. Explain what he might have meant by "patching" the fractures.

DID YOU KNOW

- Approximately 25 million Americans have osteoporosis. Four out of five are women.

ONE LAST QUICK CHECK

Fill in the blanks.

49. Functions of bones include:

_____,
_____,
_____,
_____, and
_____.

50. The _____ _____ is the hollow area inside the diaphysis of a bone.

51. A thin layer of cartilage covering each epiphysis is the _____ _____.

52. The _____ lines the medullary cavity of long bones.

53. _____ is used to describe the process of blood cell formation.

54. Blood cell formation is a vital process carried on in _____ _____ _____.

55. The _____ is a strong fibrous membrane that covers a long bone except at joint surfaces.

56. Bones may be classified by shape. Those shapes include _____, _____, _____, _____, and _____.

57. Bones serve as the major reservoir for _____, a vital substance required for normal nerve and muscle function.

58. _____ is the most abundant type of cartilage.

Matching—identify the term with the proper selection.

a.   outer covering of bone
b.   dense bone tissue
c.   fibers embedded in a firm gel
d.   criss-crossing bony branches of spongy bone
e.   ends of long bones
f.   connect lacunae
g.   cartilage cells
h.   structural unit of compact bone
i.   mature bone cells
j.   ring of bone

59. _____ trabeculae

60. _____ compact

61. _____ spongy

62. _____ periosteum

63. _____ cartilage

64. _____ osteocytes

65. _____ canaliculi

66. _____ lamellae

67. _____ chondrocytes

68. _____ Haversian system

CHAPTER 9

Skeletal System

The skeletal system may be compared to a large 206-piece puzzle. Each bone, as with each puzzle piece, is unique in size and shape. And again, just like with a puzzle, pieces or bones are not interchangeable. They have a lock-and-key concept that allows them to fit in only one area of the skeletal frame and perform functions necessary for that location.

The skeleton is divided into two main areas: the axial skeleton and the appendicular skeleton. All of the 206 bones of the human body may be classified into one of these two areas. And although we can divide them neatly by this system, there are subtle differences that exist between a man's and a woman's skeleton that provide us with insight to the functional differences between the sexes. An understanding of the skeletal system gives us an appreciation of the complex and interdependent functions that make this system essential for maintenance of homeostasis and sustaining life.

I—DIVISIONS OF THE SKELETON

Matching—identify each term with its associated division of the skeleton.

a. axial skeleton   b.   appendicular skeleton

1. _____ coccyx

2. _____ 80 bones

3. _____ 126 bones

4. _____ spinal column

5. _____ carpals

6. _____ scapulae

7. _____ auditory ossicles (ear bones)

8. _____ shoulder girdle

9. _____ skull

10. _____ clavicles

▶ *If you had difficulty with this section, review pages 223-226.*

II—THE SKULL

Multiple Choice—select the best answer.

11. The squamous suture connects which two bones?
    a. frontal and parietal
    b. parietal and temporal
    c. temporal and sphenoid
    d. sphenoid and frontal

12. The mastoid sinuses are found in which bone?
    a. frontal
    b. sphenoid
    c. parietal
    d. temporal

13. The skull bone that articulates with the first cervical vertebrae is the:
    a. occipital.
    b. sphenoid.
    c. ethmoid.
    d. none of the above.

14. A *meatus* can be described as a:
    a. large bony prominence.
    b. shallow groove.
    c. tubelike opening or channel.
    d. raised, rough area.

15. Separation of the nasal and cranial cavities is achieved by the:
    a. cribriform plate of the ethmoid bone.
    b. sella turcica of the sphenoid bone.
    c. foramen magnum of the occipital bone.
    d. palatine process of the maxilla.

16. Which of the following is *not* a bone of the orbit?
    a. ethmoid
    b. nasal
    c. lacrimal
    d. frontal

True or false

17. _____ The sphenoid is a bone of the face.

18. _____ A specialized adaptation of the infant skull is called a *fontanel.*

19. _____ The cheek is shaped by the zygomatic, or malar, bone.

20. _____ The hyoid is one of several bones that do not articulate with any other bones.

21. _____ The external auditory meatus is located within the temporal bone.

Labeling—using the terms provided, label the following diagrams.

optic foramen of sphenoid bone
sphenoid bone
perpendicular plate of ethmoid bone
vomer
frontal bone
nasal bone

glabella
maxilla
mental foramen of mandible
ethmoid bone
parietal bone
mandible

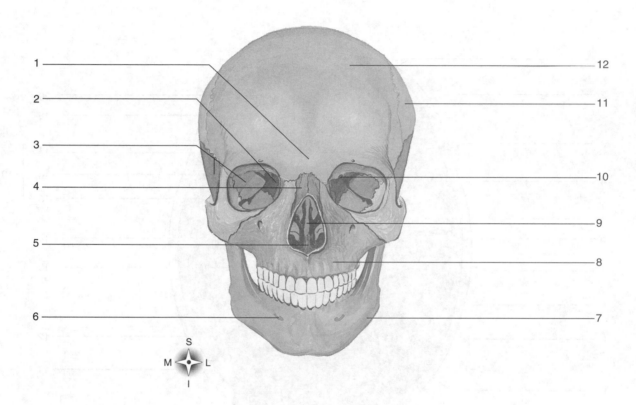

Anterior view of the skull.

foramen spinosum
jugular foramen
occipital bone
superior orbital fissure
foramen magnum
greater wing
foramen lacerum
petrous part of temporal bone
crista galli of ethmoid bone
optic foramen

sella turcica
sphenoid bone
foramen ovale
internal acoustic meatus
parietal bone
temporal bone
lesser wing
ethmoid bone
cribriform plate
frontal bone

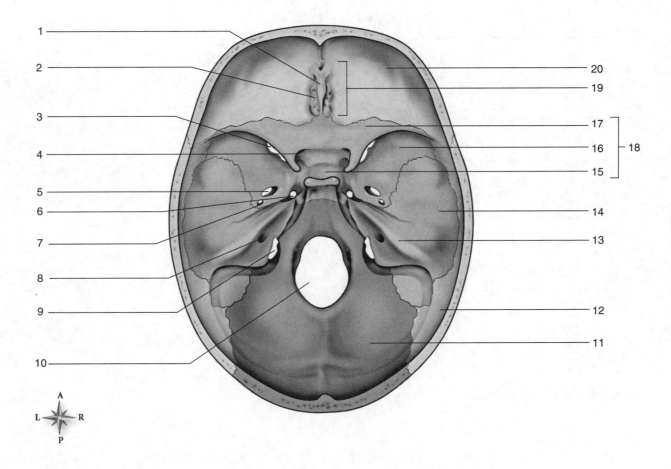

Floor of the cranial cavity viewed from above.

mastoid process
foramen lacerum
incisive foramen of maxilla
temporal bone
medial pterygoid plate of sphenoid
zygomatic arch
foramen magnum
occipital condyle
zygomatic process of temporal bone
horizontal plate of palatine bone
parietal bone
occipital bone

stylomastoid foramen
hard palate
styloid process
mastoid foramen
jugular foramen
vomer
palatine process of maxilla
foramen ovale
zygomatic process of maxilla
lateral pterygoid plate of sphenoid
temporal process of zygomatic bone
carotid canal

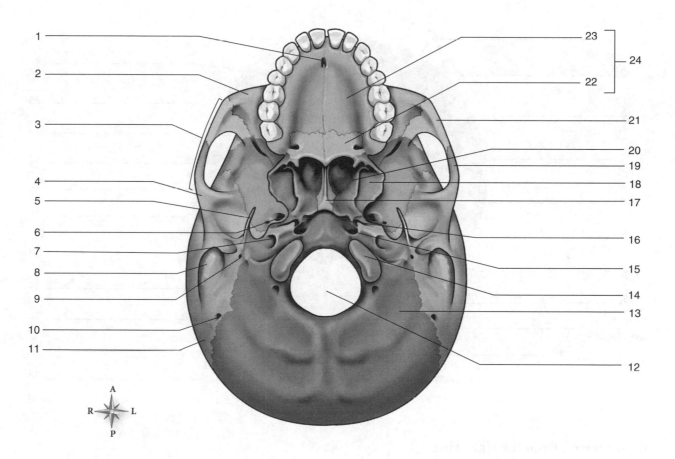

Skull viewed from below.

occipital bone
parietal bone
maxilla
sphenoid bone
lambdoid suture
external acoustic meatus of temporal bone
mental foramen of mandible
mastoid process of temporal bone
lacrimal bone
zygomatic bone
condyloid process of mandible

squamous suture
coronal suture
ethmoid bone
coronoid process of mandible
pterygoid process of sphenoid bone
mandible
nasal bone
frontal bone
temporal bone
styloid process

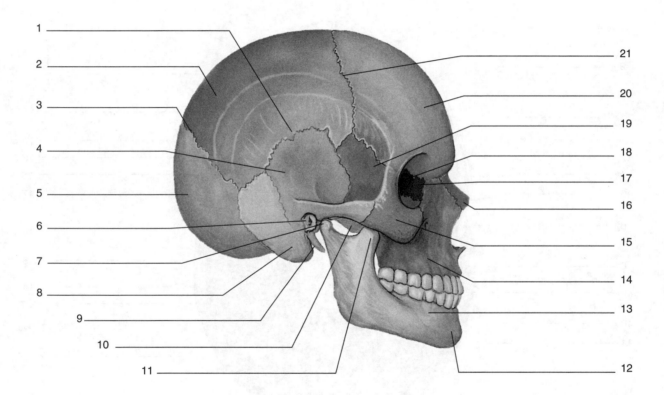

Skull viewed from the right side.

Labeling—label the following diagram.

Bones of left orbit.

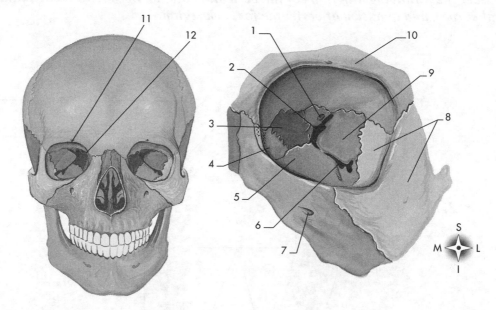

1 _____
2 _____
3 _____
4 _____
5 _____
6 _____

7 _____
8 _____
9 _____
10 _____
11 _____
12 _____

▶ *If you had difficulty with this section, review pages 226-243.*

III—VERTEBRAL COLUMN

Labeling—label the following diagrams of the vertebral column. Be sure to identify the spinal regions, spinal curves, and quantity of vertebrae for each region.

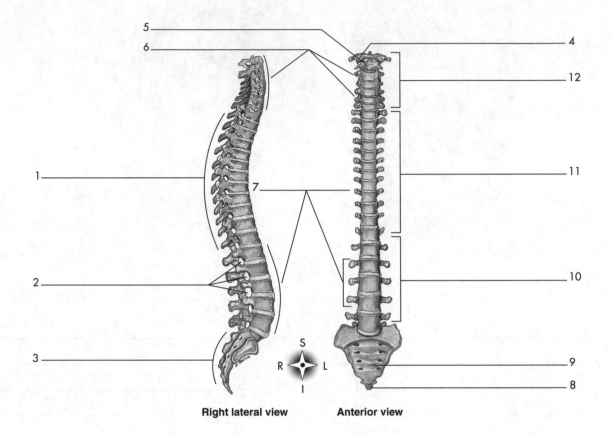

Right lateral view   **Anterior view**

Labeling—label the following images of vertebrae.

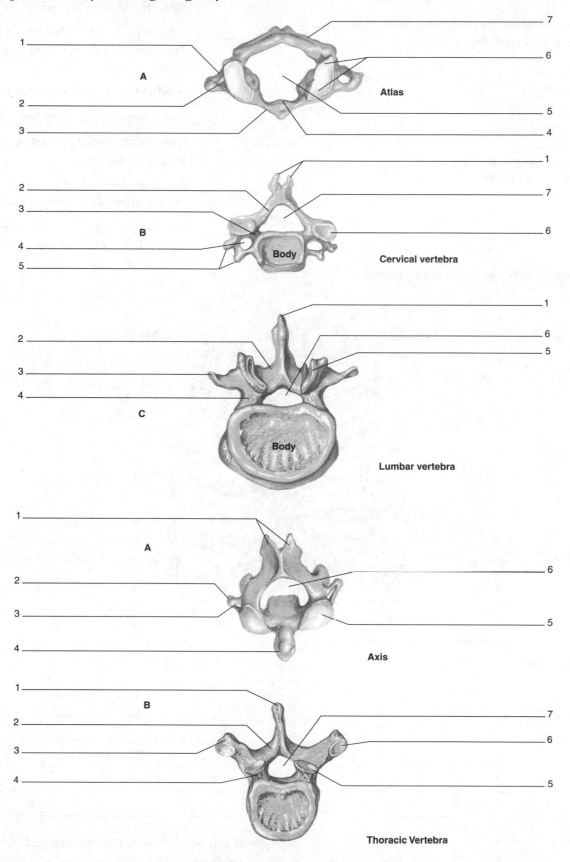

A

1
2
3

7
6
5
4

Atlas

B

2
3
4
5

Body

1
7
6

Cervical vertebra

C

2
3
4

Body

1
6
5

Lumbar vertebra

A

1
2
3
4

6

5

Axis

B

1
2
3
4

7

6

5

Thoracic Vertebra

▶ *If you had difficulty with this section, review pages 243-248.*

IV—STERNUM AND RIBS

Matching—identify each term with its corresponding description.

a. body
b. false ribs
c. floating ribs
d. manubrium
e. true ribs
f. xiphoid process
g. costal cartilage

22. _____ first seven pairs of ribs that attach directly to the sternum

23. _____ eleventh and twelfth ribs, which have no attachment to the sternum

24. _____ middle part of the sternum

25. _____ most superior part of the sternum

26. _____ the blunt, cartilaginous, lower tip of the sternum

27. _____ the five pairs of ribs that do not attach directly to the sternum

28. _____ tissue that attaches ribs directly or indirectly to the sternum

Labeling—label the following diagram.

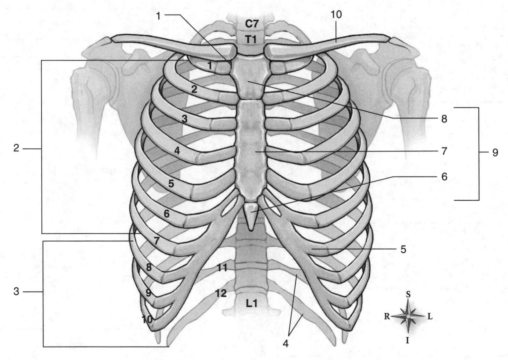

Thoracic cage.

1 _____

2 _____

3 _____

4 _____

5 _____

6 _____

7 _____

8 _____

9 _____

10 _____

▶ *If you had difficulty with this section, review pages 248-250.*

V—THE APPENDICULAR SKELETON/ UPPER EXTREMITY

Multiple Choice—select the best answer.

29. Which of the following is *not* part of the shoulder girdle?
    a. clavicle
    b. sternum
    c. scapula
    d. none of the above

30. The coronoid fossa is a:
    a. depression on the thumb.
    b. projection of the ulna.
    c. region on the spine.
    d. depression on the humerus.

31. The arm socket is the:
    a. coronoid fossa.
    b. olecranon fossa.
    c. coracoid process.
    d. glenoid cavity.

True or false

32. _____ The two bones that form the framework of the forearm are the radius and ulna.

33. _____ The wrist is composed of small bones called *metacarpals.*

34. _____ The medial forearm bone in the anatomical position is the ulna.

35. _____ The most evident carpal bone is the triquetrum.

Labeling—label the following diagrams.

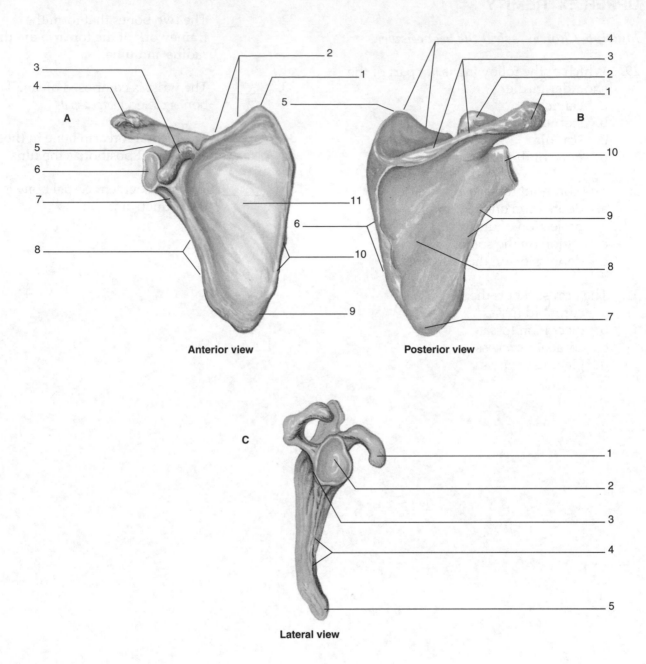

Anterior view

Posterior view

Lateral view

Scapula.

Labeling—match each term with its corresponding number on the following diagrams.

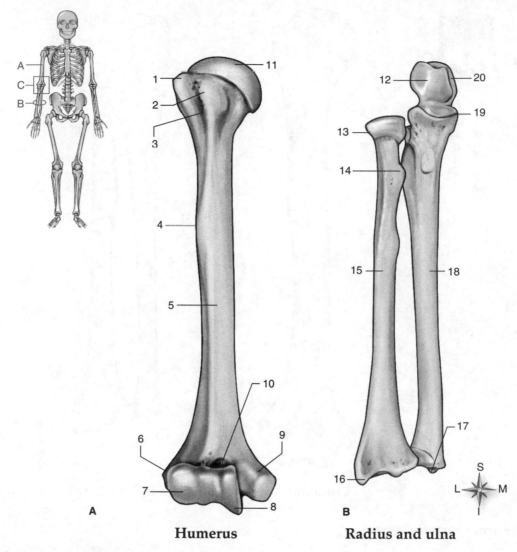

A

Humerus

B

Radius and ulna

Bones of the arm (anterior view).

_____ deltoid tuberosity	_____ lateral epicondyle
_____ capitulum	_____ greater tubercle
_____ coronoid fossa	_____ medial epicondyle
_____ radial tuberosity	_____ styloid process of ulna
_____ coronoid process	_____ trochlea
_____ intertubercular groove	_____ head
_____ humerus	_____ olecranon process
_____ radius	_____ trochlear notch
_____ head of radius	_____ styloid process of radius
_____ lesser tubercle	_____ ulna

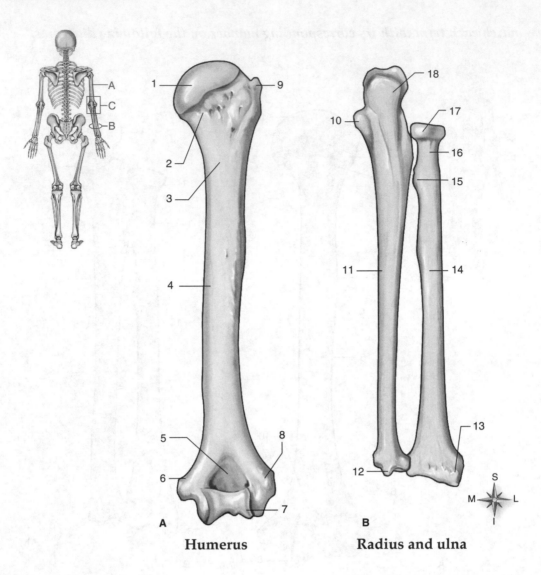

A

Humerus

B

Radius and ulna

Bones of the arm (posterior view).

_____ greater tubercle

_____ head of radius

_____ anatomical neck

_____ styloid process of ulna

_____ medial epicondyle

_____ trochlea

_____ surgical neck

_____ humerus

_____ radial tuberosity

_____ lateral epicondyle

_____ coronoid process

_____ ulna

_____ head

_____ olecranon fossa

_____ olecranon process

_____ radius

_____ neck

_____ styloid process of radius

Labeling—match each term with its corresponding number on the following diagrams. Some terms may be used more than once.

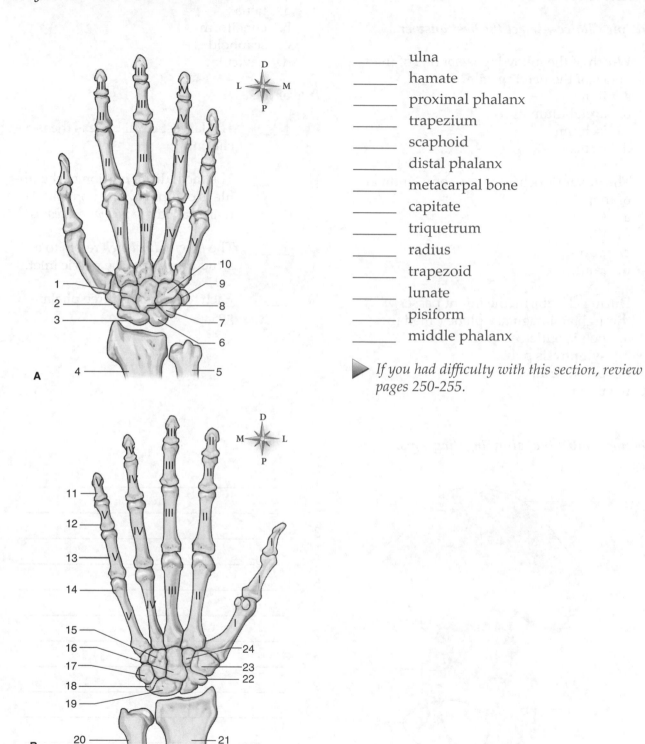

_____ ulna

_____ hamate

_____ proximal phalanx

_____ trapezium

_____ scaphoid

_____ distal phalanx

_____ metacarpal bone

_____ capitate

_____ triquetrum

_____ radius

_____ trapezoid

_____ lunate

_____ pisiform

_____ middle phalanx

▶ *If you had difficulty with this section, review pages 250-255.*

Bones of the hand and wrist.

VI—THE APPENDICULAR SKELETON/ LOWER EXTREMITY

Multiple Choice—select the best answer.

36. Which of the following is *not* one of the bones of the pelvic girdle?
    a. ilium
    b. acetabulum
    c. ischium
    d. pubis

37. The greater trochanter is a bony landmark of the:
    a. femur.
    b. tibia.
    c. pubis.
    d. ramus.

38. During childbirth, the infant passes through an imaginary plane called the:
    a. pelvic outlet.
    b. symphysis pubis.
    c. pelvic brim.
    d. ilium.

39. Which of the following is *not* a tarsal bone?
    a. talus
    b. cuneiform
    c. scaphoid
    d. navicular

True or false

40. _____ The largest coxal bone is the ischium.

41. _____ The most distal portion of the fibula is composed of a bony landmark called the *medial malleolus.*

42. _____ The *longitudinal arch* refers to a structure within the pelvic inlet.

43. _____ Each toe contains three phalanges.

Labeling—label the following diagrams.

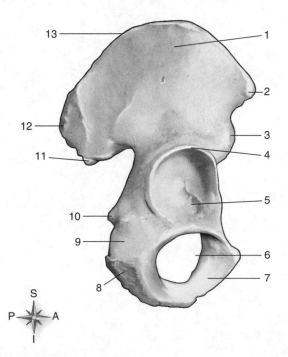

Coxal bone.

1 _____

2 _____

3 _____

4 _____

5 _____

6 _____

7 _____

8 _____

9 _____

10 _____

11 _____

12 _____

13 _____

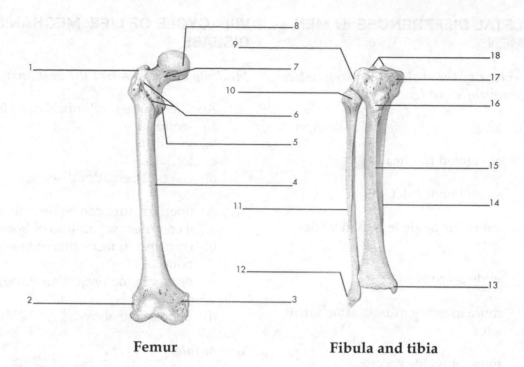

Femur   Fibula and tibia

Bones of the thigh and leg.

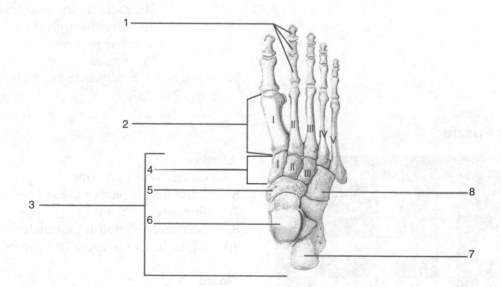

Bones of the foot.

If you had difficulty with this section, review pages 255-261.

VII—SKELETAL DIFFERENCES IN MEN AND WOMEN

Matching—identify the skeletal characteristics with the appropriate gender.

a.   male skeleton   b.   female skeleton

44. _____ elongated forehead

45. _____ small pelvic inlet

46. _____ subpubic angle less than 90 degrees

47. _____ wide sacrum

48. _____ more massive muscle attachment sites

49. _____ more movable coccyx

▶ *If you had difficulty with this section, review pages 261-262.*

VIII—CYCLE OF LIFE: MECHANISMS OF DISEASE

Multiple Choice—select the best answer.

50. Another name for "hunchback" is:
    a. scoliosis.
    b. kyphosis.
    c. lordosis.
    d. Osgood-Schlatter disease.

51. An open fracture can be described as:
    a. a complete separation of bones.
    b. fractures in more than one area of a bone.
    c. broken bone projecting through the skin.
    d. none of the above.

True or false

52. _____ *Swayback* and *kyphosis* are synonymous terms.

53. _____ Normal curvature of the spine is convex posteriorly through the thoracic region and concave posteriorly through the cervical and lumbar regions.

▶ *If you had difficulty with this section, review pages 262-267.*

Crossword Puzzle

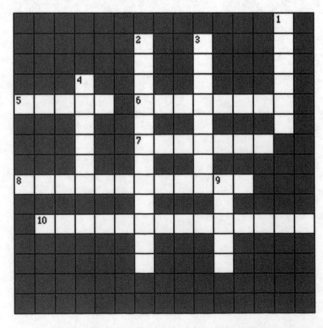

Across
5. Cavity within a bone
6. Bone that is part of the spinal column
7. Encases the brain
8. Section of skeleton that includes 126 bones
10. Clavicle and scapula (two words)

Down
1. Bony cage
2. Supports the trunk (two words)
3. "Soft spot"
4. Immovable joint in skull
9. Section of skeleton that includes 80 bones

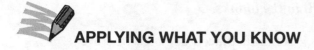

APPLYING WHAT YOU KNOW

54. While playing football, Bill was involved in a tackle that caused a forced hyperextension of his elbow joint. Which skeletal structures could he have injured?

55. Amanda loves to wear extremely high-heeled shoes. How does this affect the weight distribution onto the bones of her feet? Which skeletal structures are at risk of being damaged?

DID YOU KNOW

- The bones of the hands and feet make up more than half of the total 206 bones of the body.
- The bones of the middle ear are mature at birth.
- The skeleton of an average 160-pound body weighs about 29 pounds.

ONE LAST QUICK CHECK

Circle the one that does **not** *belong.*

56. cervical	thoracic	coxal	coccyx
57. pelvic girdle	ankle	wrist	axial
58. frontal	occipital	maxilla	sphenoid
59. scapula	pectoral girdle	ribs	clavicle
60. malleus	vomer	incus	stapes
61. ulna	ilium	ischium	pubis
62. carpal	phalanges	metacarpal	ethmoid
63. ethmoid	parietal	occipital	nasal
64. anvil	atlas	axis	cervical

Matching—identify the bone with its marking.
There may be more than one correct answer.

a. mastoid
b. pterygoid process
c. foramen magnum
d. sella turcica
e. mental foramen
f. conchae
g. xiphoid process
h. glenoid cavity
i. olecranon process
j. ischium
k. acetabulum
l. symphysis pubis
m. ilium
n. greater trochanter
o. medial malleolus
p. calcaneus
q. acromion process
r. frontal sinuses
s. coronoid process
t. tibial tuberosity

65. _____ occipital

66. _____ sternum

67. _____ coxal

68. _____ femur

69. _____ ulna

70. _____ temporal

71. _____ tarsals

72. _____ sphenoid

73. _____ ethmoid

74. _____ scapula

75. _____ tibia

76. _____ frontal

77. _____ mandible

Fill in the blanks.

78. A nondisplaced or *closed* fracture is also known as a _____ _____.

79. Prompt treatment of _____ _____ with antibiotics has made life-threatening cases of mastoiditis rare.

80. An abnormal side-to-side spinal curvature is called _____.

CHAPTER 10

Articulations

W e conclude our study of bones with a chapter on joints, or articulations. A joint, or articulation, is a point of contact between bones. Sitting, walking, and running are just a few examples of movements that would not be possible without the successful functioning of articulations. Joints also permit us to lift heavy objects and perform fine motor skills such as needlepoint. The unusual and unique shape and size of articulations are responsible for the variety and degree of motion that we expect from our body.

Joints may be classified according to structure (fibrous and cartilaginous) or according to function (synarthrosis—immovable; amphiarthrosis—slightly movable; diarthrosis—freely movable). Proper functioning of articulations is necessary for us to adapt to our environment with controlled, smooth, and pain-free movements.

I—CLASSIFICATION OF JOINTS

Multiple Choice—select the best answer.

1. The articulation between the root of a tooth and the alveolar process of the mandible or maxilla is called the:
   a. suture.
   b. gomphosis.
   c. synchondrosis.
   d. symphysis.

2. Immovable joints are called:
   a. synarthroses.
   b. amphiarthroses.
   c. diarthroses.
   d. none of the above.

3. The radioulnar articulation is classified as which type of articulation?
   a. syndesmosis
   b. synchondrosis
   c. symphysis
   d. diarthrosis

4. The most movable joints in the body are:
    a. symphyses.
    b. sutures.
    c. synovial joints.
    d. synchondroses.

5. An example of a symphysis is:
    a. the articulation between the pubic bones.
    b. the articulation between the bodies of adjacent vertebrae.
    c. both a and b.
    d. none of the above.

6. The inner surface of the joint capsule is lined with:
    a. bursae.
    b. a joint cavity.
    c. periosteum.
    d. synovial membrane.

7. The joint that allows for the widest range of movement is a _____ joint.
    a. gliding
    b. saddle
    c. ball-and-socket
    d. hinge

8. An example of a pivot joint is the:
    a. first metacarpal articulating with the trapezium.
    b. humerus articulating with the trapezium.
    c. interphalangeal joints.
    d. head of the radius articulating with the ulna.

True or false

9. _____ *Diarthrosis* and *synovial joint* refer to basically the same structure.

10. _____ The elbow joint is a ball-and-socket joint.

11. _____ The ability to oppose the fingers and thumb is achieved by a saddle joint.

12. _____ *Articulation* and *joint* are synonymous terms.

13. _____ Diarthrotic joints are the least common type of joint in the body.

14. _____ There are several examples of suture articulations throughout the entire body.

15. _____ Menisci are composed of hyaline cartilage.

16. _____ The shoulder joint is a ball-and-socket joint.

Matching—identify each joint or description with its corresponding classification.

a. amphiarthroses
b. diarthroses
c. synarthroses

17. _____ joint between bodies of vertebrae

18. _____ symphysis pubis

19. _____ hip joint

20. _____ fibrous joint

21. _____ immovable joint

22. _____ cartilaginous joint

23. _____ thumb

24. _____ joints between skull bones

25. _____ freely movable joint

26. _____ synovial joint

27. _____ slightly movable joint

28. _____ the most prevalent type of joint in the body

Matching—identify each joint with its corresponding functional classification.

a.   ball and socket
b.   condyloid
c.   gliding
d.   hinge
e.   pivot
f.   saddle

29. _____ elbow

30. _____ joints between facets of adjacent vertebrae

31. _____ ellipsoidal

32. _____ dens of axis/atlas joint

33. _____ knee joint

34. _____ least movable group of the synovial joints

35. _____ hip joint

36. _____ shoulder joint

37. _____ joint between first metacarpal and trapezium

Labeling—label the structures of the synovial joint on the following diagram.

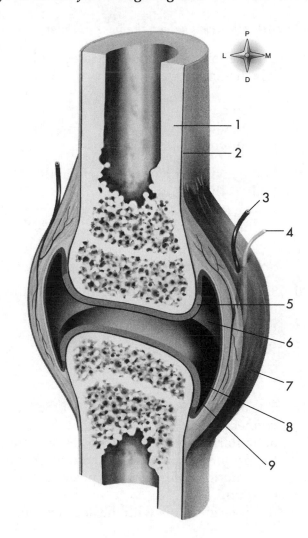

1 _____

2 _____

3 _____

4 _____

5 _____

6 _____

7 _____

8 _____

9 _____

▶ *If you had difficulty with this section, review pages 271-277.*

II—REPRESENTATIVE SYNOVIAL JOINTS

Multiple Choice—select the best answer.

38. The glenoid labrum is associated with which joint?
    a. hip
    b. knee
    c. shoulder
    d. vertebral

39. Perhaps the strongest ligament in the body is the:
    a. rotator cuff.
    b. iliofemoral.
    c. pubofemoral.
    d. intertrochanteric.

40. The largest and most complex joint of the body is the:
    a. shoulder.
    b. knee.
    c. hip.
    d. ankle.

41. The anterior cruciate ligament of the knee connects the:
    a. anterior tibia with the posterior femur.
    b. posterior tibia with the anterior femur.
    c. anterior fibula with the posterior femur.
    d. anterior fibula with the anterior femur.

42. Vertebral bodies are connected by:
    a. the anterior longitudinal ligament.
    b. the posterior longitudinal ligament.
    c. the ligamentum flavum.
    d. both a and b.

43. Protrusion of the nucleus pulposus through the annulus fibrosus results in:
    a. bursitis.
    b. housemaid's knee.
    c. herniated disk.
    d. none of the above.

44. The medial and lateral menisci are:
    a. ligaments.
    b. cartilage.
    c. bursae.
    d. none of the above.

45. "Joint mice" are structurally:
    a. impinged bursae.
    b. loose pieces of synovial membrane.
    c. loose pieces of articular cartilage.
    d. cracks in the articular cartilage.

Labeling—label the following diagrams of synovial joints.

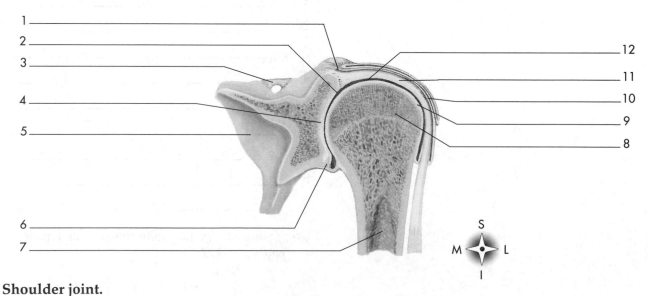

Shoulder joint.

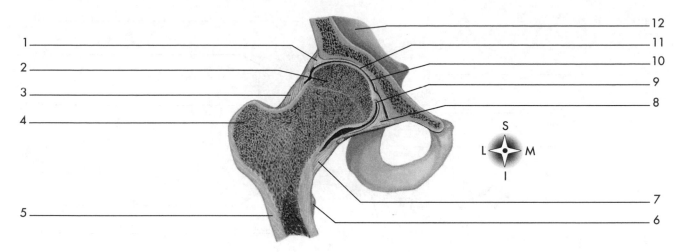

Hip joint.

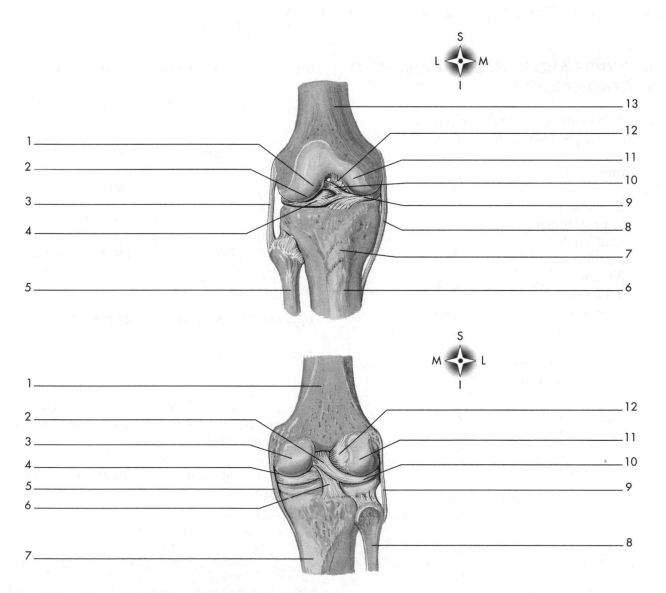

Knee joint. A, anterior view. **B,** posterior view.

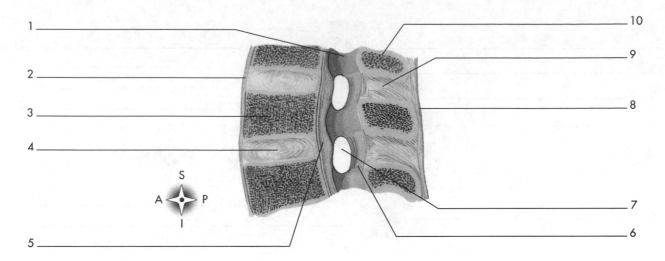

Vertebrae and their ligaments.

▶ *If you had difficulty with this section, review pages 277-286.*

III—TYPES AND RANGE OF MOVEMENT AT SYNOVIAL JOINTS

Matching—identify each term with its corresponding definition or description.

a.   plantar flexion
b.   extension
c.   abduction
d.   hyperextension
e.   goniometer
f.   rotation
g.   flexion
h.   inversion
i.   depression
j.   adduction

46. _____   instrument that measures range of motion

47. _____   lifting the arms away from the midline

48. _____   turning the head as to say "no"

49. _____   elbow movement, as when lifting weights during a "bicep curl"

50. _____   increasing joint angle

51. _____   moving beyond extension

52. _____   causes extension of the leg as a whole

53. _____   turning sole of foot inward

54. _____   opening your mouth

55. _____   bringing fingers together

▶ *If you had difficulty with this section, review pages 286-292.*

IV—MECHANISMS OF DISEASE

Fill in the blanks.

56. _____ is an imaging technique that allows a physician to examine the internal structure of a joint without the use of extensive surgery.

57. The most common noninflammatory joint disease is _____ or _____ _____ _____.

58. A general name for many different inflammatory joint diseases is
_____.

59. A metabolic type of inflammatory arthritis
is _____ _____.

60. An acute musculoskeletal injury to the
ligamentous structure surrounding a joint
and disrupting the continuity of the synovial membrane is a _____.

▶ *If you had difficulty with this section, review
pages 292-297.*

Crossword Puzzle

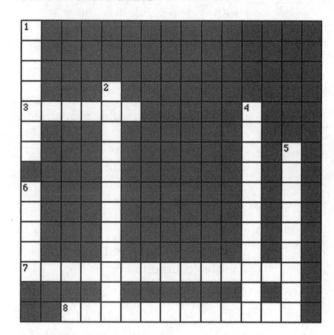

Across
3. Immovable joint in the skull
7. Cartilaginous joint
8. Fibrous joint

Down
1. Articular disks
2. Joint
4. Synovial joint
5. A joint where fibrocartilage connects two
bones
6. Pillowlike structure found between synovial joints

 APPLYING WHAT YOU KNOW

61. Lowell is afflicted with severely inflamed joints because of arthritis. If he is suffering from the
chronic systemic version of this disease, what symptoms would he be experiencing? Which
joints are most likely involved and what is the most likely cause?

62. Sam is suffering from a type of arthritis associated with excess blood levels of uric acid. What
type of arthritis is this? What symptoms might he experience, which joints would be affected,
and how is this form of arthritis treated?

 DID YOU KNOW

• The average person uses the leg joints to walk an average of 115,000 miles during his or her
lifetime.

ONE LAST QUICK CHECK

Circle the correct answer.

63. Freely movable joints are (amphiarthroses or diarthroses).

64. The sutures in the skull are (synarthrotic or amphiarthrotic).

65. All (diarthrotic or amphiarthrotic) joints have a joint capsule, a joint cavity, and a layer of cartilage over the ends of the two adjoining bones.

66. (Ligaments or tendons) grow out of periosteum and attach two bones together.

67. The (articular cartilage or epiphyseal cartilage) cushions surfaces of bones.

68. Gliding joints are the (least movable or most movable) of the diarthrotic joints.

69. The knee is the (largest or smallest) joint.

70. Hinge joints allow motion in (two or four) directions.

71. The saddle joint at the base of each of our thumbs allows for greater (strength or mobility).

72. When you rotate your head, you are using a (gliding or pivot) joint.

True or false

73. _____ A uniaxial joint is a synovial joint.

74. _____ Joints identified as synchondroses are synovial joints.

75. _____ Inflammation of the bursa is referred to as *pleurisy*.

76. _____ The main bursa of the shoulder joint is the subdeltoid bursa.

77. _____ Angular movements change the size of the angle between articulating bones.

78. _____ Pronation is a circular movement.

79. _____ Gliding movements are the most complex of movements.

80. _____ Protraction is an angular movement.

81. _____ Juvenile rheumatoid arthritis is more common in boys.

82. _____ The knee joint has a "baker's dozen," or 13, bursae, which serve as protective pads around it.

CHAPTER 11

Anatomy of the Muscular System

The muscular system is often referred to as the "power system," and rightfully so, because it is this system that provides the force necessary to move the body and perform organic functions. Just as an automobile relies on the engine to provide motion, the body depends on the muscular system to perform both voluntary and involuntary types of movements. The power of this system is impressive indeed, for if we were able to direct all of our muscles in one direction, it is estimated that we would have the power to move 25 tons.

Over 600 skeletal muscles constitute 40–50% of our body weight. They are attached snugly over the skeletal frame to shape and mold the contours of our body. And while memorizing the names and locations of skeletal muscles appears to be an overwhelming task, it is comforting to learn that muscles are named and categorized quite simply. Classification and identification are focused upon location, function, shape, direction of fibers, number of heads or divisions, or points of attachment. This chapter assists you in understanding the structure of skeletal muscles and the logical approach to muscle recognition.

I—SKELETAL MUSCLE STRUCTURE

Multiple Choice—select the best answer.

1. An entire skeletal muscle is covered by a coarse sheath called:
   a. endomysium.
   b. perimysium.
   c. epimysium.
   d. aponeurosis.

2. Muscles that are arranged like the feathers in a plume are described as:
   a. parallel.
   b. convergent.
   c. sphincter.
   d. pennate.

3. An aponeurosis is:
   a. broad and flat.
   b. tube-shaped.
   c. featherlike.
   d. none of the above.

4. Antagonists are muscles that:
   a. oppose prime movers.
   b. facilitate prime movers.
   c. stabilize muscles.
   d. directly perform movements.

5. A fixed point about which a rod moves is called a:
   a. lever.
   b. bone.
   c. belly.
   d. fulcrum.

6. In first-class levers, the:
   a. fulcrum is between the pull and the load.
   b. load is between the fulcrum and the force.
   c. force is between the fulcrum and the load.
   d. load and force are equal.

True or false

7. _____ The origin of a muscle is the point of attachment that moves when the muscle contracts.

8. _____ Skeletal muscles usually act in groups rather than individually.

9. _____ *Prime mover* and *agonist* are synonymous.

10. _____ The optimum angle of pull of a muscle is generally parallel to the long axis of the bone.

11. _____ Tipping the head back, as in looking up at the sky, is an example of a first-class lever.

▶ *If you had difficulty with this section, review pages 301-308.*

II—HOW MUSCLES ARE NAMED

Matching—identify each muscle with the appropriate characteristic.

a. location
b. function
c. shape
d. direction of fibers
e. number of heads
f. points of attachment
g. size of muscle

12. _____ deltoid

13. _____ brachialis

14. _____ sternocleidomastoid

15. _____ quadriceps

16. _____ gluteus maximus

17. _____ adductor

18. _____ rectus

▶ *If you had difficulty with this section, review pages 308-311.*

III—IMPORTANT SKELETAL MUSCLES: MUSCLES OF THE FACE AND NECK

Matching—identify each muscle with its appropriate body movement.

a. buccinator
b. corrugator supercilii
c. epicranius
d. orbicularis oculi
e. pterygoids
f. sternocleidomastoid

19. _____ wrinkling the forehead vertically

20. _____ grating the teeth during mastication

21. _____ smiling

22. _____ raising the eyebrows

23. _____ flexing the head

24. _____ closing the eyes

Labeling—label the following diagram.

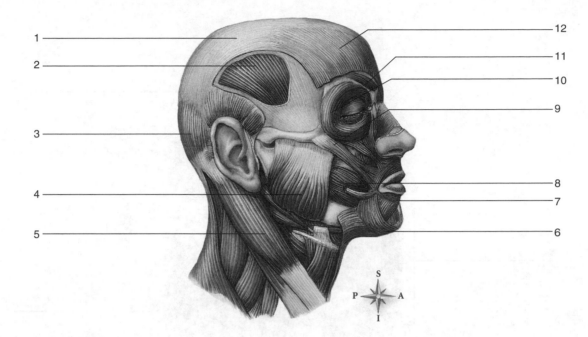

Facial muscles: lateral view.

▶ *If you had difficulty with this section, review pages 311-315.*

IV—TRUNK MUSCLES

True or false

25. _____ The external oblique compresses the abdomen.

26. _____ The rectus abdominis flexes the trunk.

27. _____ The levator ani closes the anal canal.

28. _____ The external intercostals function to elevate the ribs.

29. _____ The coccygeus muscles and levator ani form most of the pelvic floor.

Labeling—label the following diagrams.

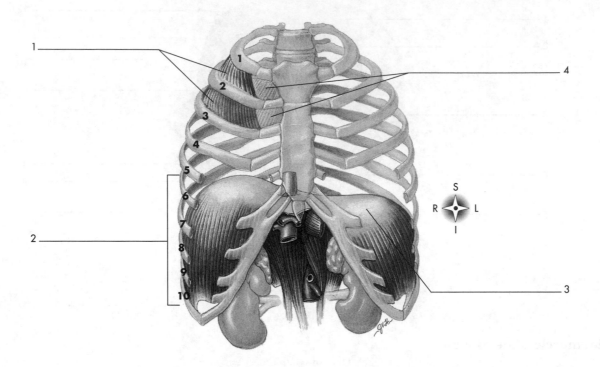

Muscles of the thorax.

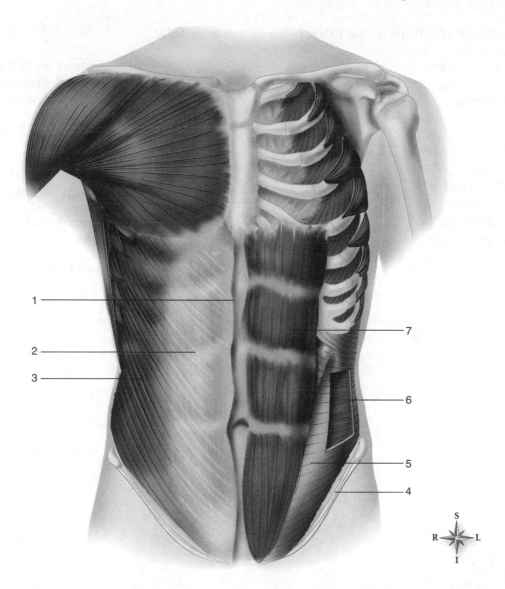

Muscles of the trunk and abdominal wall.

▶ *If you had difficulty with this section, review pages 315-322.*

V—UPPER LIMB MUSCLES

Multiple Choice—select the best answer.

30. All of the following are rotator cuff muscles *except:*
    a. deltoid.
    b. infraspinatus.
    c. supraspinatus.
    d. teres minor.

31. The muscle that shrugs the shoulders is the:
    a. sternocleidomastoid.
    b. deltoid.
    c. trapezius.
    d. pectoralis minor.

32. The posterior arm muscle that extends the forearm is the:
    a. triceps brachii.
    b. triceps surae.
    c. brachialis.
    d. biceps brachii.

33. The olecranon of the ulna is a site of insertion for the:
    a. biceps brachii.
    b. brachialis.
    c. brachioradialis.
    d. triceps brachii.

True or false

34. _____ Intrinsic muscles of the hand originate on the forearm and insert on the metacarpals.

35. _____ Carpal tunnel syndrome affects the median nerve.

36. _____ The deltoid is a good example of a multifunctional muscle.

37. _____ The pectoralis major flexes the upper arm.

38. _____ The biceps brachii is an extensor muscle.

Labeling—using the terms provided, label the following illustrations. Some terms may be used more than once.

levator scapulae
serratus anterior
rhomboid major
teres minor
seventh cervical vertebra
teres major (cut)
latissimus dorsi (cut)

rhomboid minor
trapezius
pectoralis minor (cut)
pectoralis minor
subscapularis
latissimus dorsi

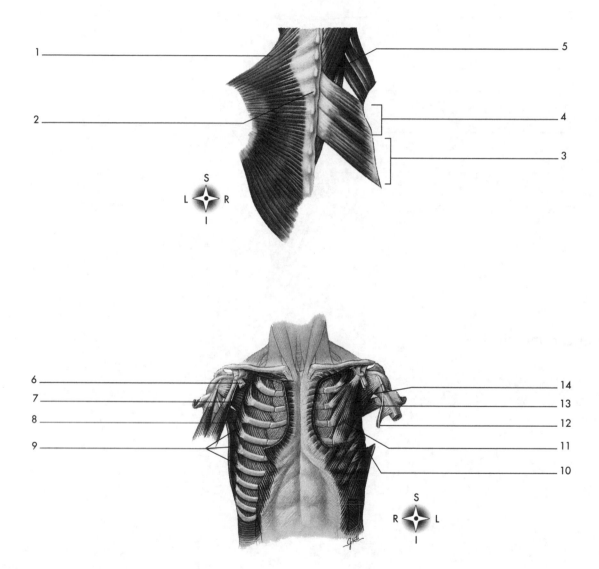

Muscles acting on the shoulder girdle.

Labeling—using the terms provided, label the following illustration.

subscapularis
acromion process
coracoid process
greater tubercle
intertubercular (bicipital) groove
teres minor

humerus
supraspinatus
lesser tubercle
infraspinatus
clavicle

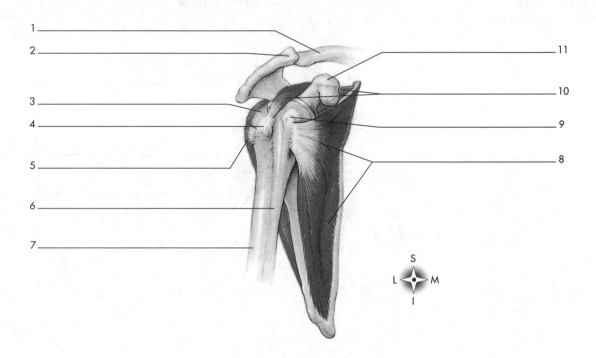

Rotator cuff muscles.

Labeling—label the following illustrations.

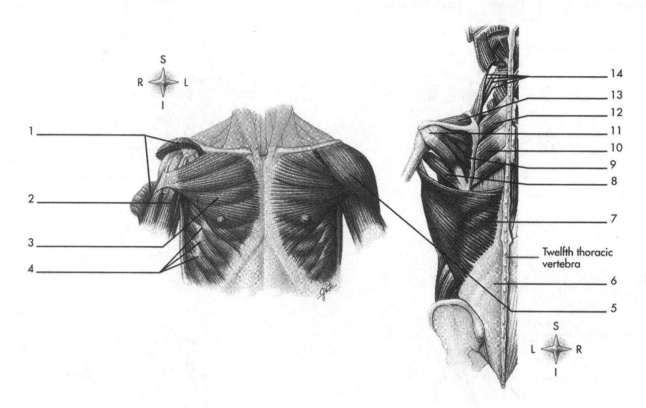

Muscles that move the upper arm.

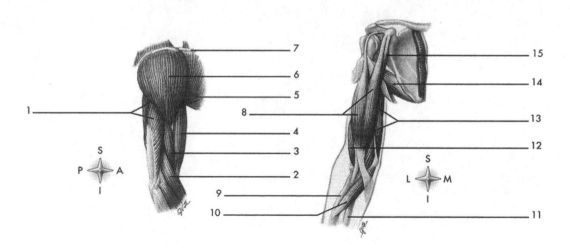

Muscles of the upper arm.

Labeling—on the following illustrations, label the muscles that act on the forearm. Also label the origin and insertion point of each muscle.

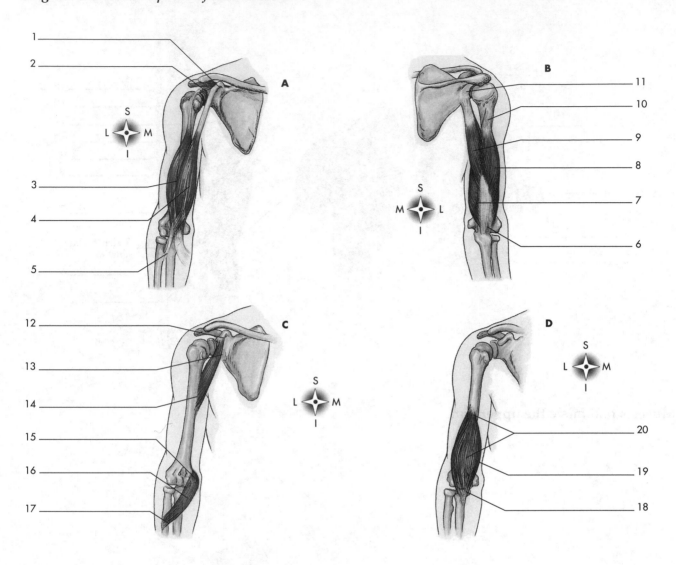

Muscles that act on the forearm.

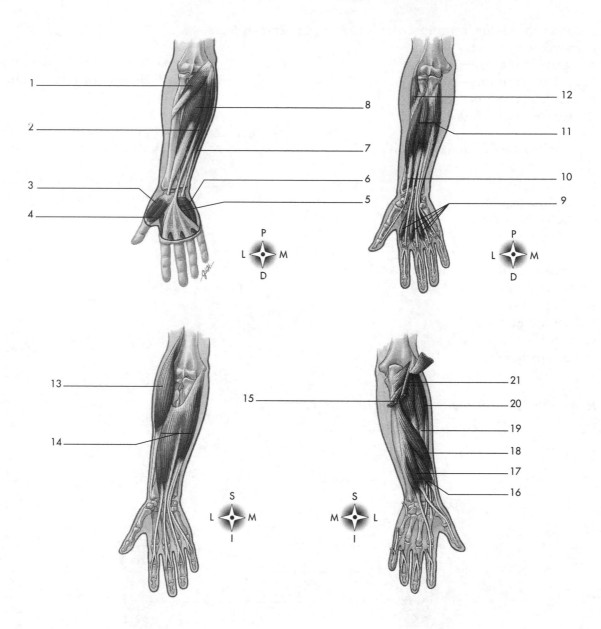

Muscles of the forearm.

▶ *If you had difficulty with this section, review pages 322-333.*

VI—LOWER LIMB MUSCLES

Multiple Choice—select the best answer.

39. The muscles of quadriceps femoris include all of the following *except:*
    a. vastus intermedius.
    b. vastus medialis.
    c. vastus lateralis.
    d. vastus femoris.

40. The anterior superior iliac spine is the site of origin for the:
    a. sartorius.
    b. rectus femoris.
    c. gracilis.
    d. iliacus.

41. A common site for intramuscular injections is the:
    a. gluteus maximus.
    b. gluteus minimus.
    c. gluteus medius.
    d. tensor fasciae latae.

42. Plantar flexion of the foot is achieved by the:
    a. tibialis anterior.
    b. tibialis posterior.
    c. peroneus brevis.
    d. soleus.

43. The muscles of the hamstrings include all of the following *except* the:
    a. iliopsoas.
    b. semitendinosus.
    c. semimembranosus.
    d. biceps femoris.

True or false

44. _____ The Achilles tendon is common to both the gastrocnemius and soleus.

45. _____ The iliopsoas is composed solely of the psoas major and the iliacus.

46. _____ The vastus intermedius originates on the posterior surface of the femur.

Labeling—label the following illustrations.

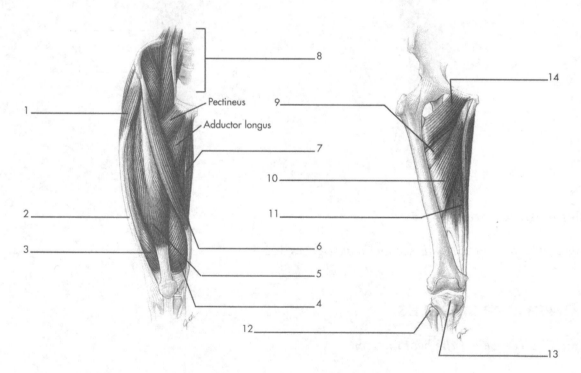

Pectineus

Adductor longus

Muscles of the thigh.

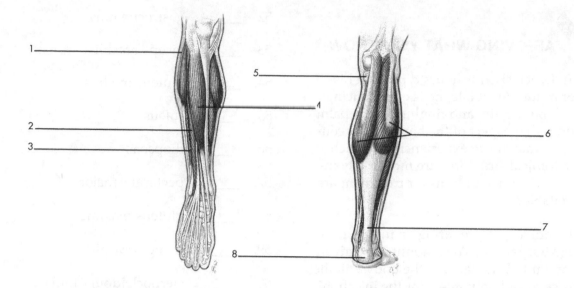

Muscles of the lower leg.

▶ *If you had difficulty with this section, review pages 333-344.*

Crossword Puzzle

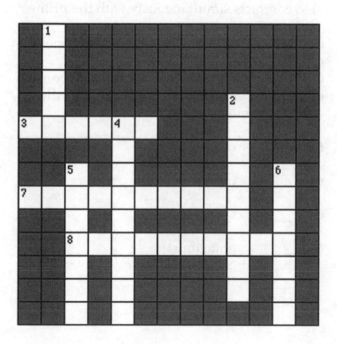

Across

3. Attachment that does not move
7. Agonist (two words)
8. Opposes prime mover

Down

1. Rigid bar free to turn about its fulcrum
2. Contracts at the same time as the prime mover
4. Attachment that moves
5. Joint stabilizer
6. Maintaining optimal body position

APPLYING WHAT YOU KNOW

47. Mr. Lynch spends hours typing on his computer. As of late, he is experiencing weakness, pain, and tingling in the palm and radial aspect of the hand. What condition may he be experiencing? Which anatomical structures are most likely involved? Which options for treatment are available?

48. The nurse was preparing an injection for Mrs. Tatakis. The amount to be given was 2 mL. What area of the body will the nurse most likely select for the injection?

49. Al is analyzing the musculature involved in the athletes he coaches. Today he is observing a basketball player executing a jump shot. Which muscles are involved at the hips, knees, and ankles as the athlete jumps? Which muscles are involved at the shoulders, elbows, and wrists as the athlete shoots the basketball?

DID YOU KNOW

- The muscles of the hand begin to grow rapidly between 6 and 7 years of age.

- A cat has 32 muscles in each ear.

ONE LAST QUICK CHECK

Matching—choose the proper function(s) for the muscles listed. Each may have more than one answer.

a. flexor
b. extensor
c. abductor
d. adductor
e. rotator
f. dorsiflexor or plantar flexor

50. _____ deltoid

51. _____ tibialis anterior

52. _____ gastrocnemius

53. _____ biceps brachii

54. _____ gluteus medius

55. _____ soleus

56. _____ iliopsoas

57. _____ pectoralis major

58. _____ gluteus maximus

59. _____ triceps brachii

60. _____ sternocleidomastoid

61. _____ trapezius

62. _____ gracilis

Matching—identify the term with the appropriate description.

a. contracts simultaneously with the prime mover
b. attachment to the more movable bone
c. functions as joint stabilizer
d. attachment to the more stationary bone
e. when contracting, directly opposes the prime mover

63. _____ origin

64. _____ insertion

65. _____ synergist

66. _____ antagonist

67. _____ fixator

CHAPTER 12

Physiology of the Muscular System

Although the muscular system has several functions, the primary purpose is to provide movement or power. Muscles produce power by contracting. The ability of a large muscle or muscle group to contract depends on the ability of microscopic muscle fibers to contract within the larger muscle. An understanding of these microscopic muscle fibers will assist you as your study progresses to the larger muscles and muscle groups.

Three types of muscles provide us with a variety of motions. When skeletal or voluntary muscles contract, they provide movement of bones, heat production, and posture. Smooth muscles are found throughout the viscera of our body and assist with involuntary functions such as peristalsis. Cardiac muscle is the third and final type of muscle. It makes up the wall of the heart and provides the pumping action necessary for life. Our muscles must be used to keep the body healthy and in good condition. Scientific evidence keeps pointing to the fact that the proper use and exercise of muscles may prolong life. An understanding of the structure and function of the muscular system may, therefore, add quality and quantity to our lives.

I—FUNCTION OF SKELETAL MUSCLE TISSUE

Multiple Choice—select the best answer.

1. Which of the following is *not* a general function of muscle tissue?
   a. movement
   b. protection
   c. heat production
   d. posture

2. The skeletal muscle fiber characteristic of excitability directly results in these cells being capable of:
   a. responding to nerve signals.
   b. shortening.
   c. returning to resting length after contracting.
   d. producing heat.

3. The correct order of arrangement of skeletal muscle cells, from largest to smallest, is:
   a. fiber, myofibril, myofilament.
   b. myofibril, myofilament, fiber.
   c. myofilament, myofibril, fiber.
   d. fiber, myofilament, myofibril.

4. Sarcoplasmic reticulum is:
   a. a system of transverse tubules that extend at a right angle to the long axis of the cell.
   b. a segment of the myofibril between two successive Z lines.
   c. a unique name for the plasma membrane of a muscle fiber.
   d. none of the above.

5. Which of the following are myofilament proteins?
   a. troponin
   b. tropomyosin
   c. a and b
   d. none of the above

6. The contractile unit of a myofibril is the:
   a. sarcomere.
   b. triad.
   c. sarcolemma.
   d. cross-bridge.

7. The chief function of the T tubule is to:
   a. provide nutrients to the muscle fiber.
   b. allow the fiber to contract.
   c. allow the electrical signal to move deep into the cell.
   d. allow the generation of new muscle fibers.

8. Myosin heads are also called:
   a. cross-bridges.
   b. motor endplates.
   c. synapses.
   d. motor neurons.

9. During muscle contraction, Ca^{++} is released from the:
   a. synaptic cleft.
   b. mitochondria.
   c. sarcoplasmic reticulum.
   d. sarcoplasm.

10. The region of a muscle fiber where a motor neuron connects to the muscle fiber is called the:
    a. synaptic vesicle.
    b. motor endplate.
    c. H band.
    d. none of the above.

True or false

11. _____ The thick myofilament is made up of myosin.

12. _____ Skeletal muscle has a poor ability to stretch.

13. _____ A T tubule sandwiched between sacs of sarcoplasmic reticulum is called a *codon.*

14. _____ Actin, troponin, and tropomyosin are present on the thin myofilament.

15. _____ The I band resides within a single sarcomere.

16. _____ Rigor mortis is caused by a lack of ATP to "turn off" muscle contraction.

17. _____ The cell membrane of a muscle fiber is called the *sarcoplasmic reticulum.*

18. _____ Anaerobic respiration is the first choice of the muscle cell for the production of ATP.

19. _____ During rest, excess oxygen molecules in the sarcoplasm are attracted to a large protein molecule called *myoglobin.*

20. _____ Anaerobic respiration results in the formation of an incompletely catabolized molecule called *lactic acid.*

Labeling—match each term with its corresponding number on the following diagram of the structure of skeletal muscle.

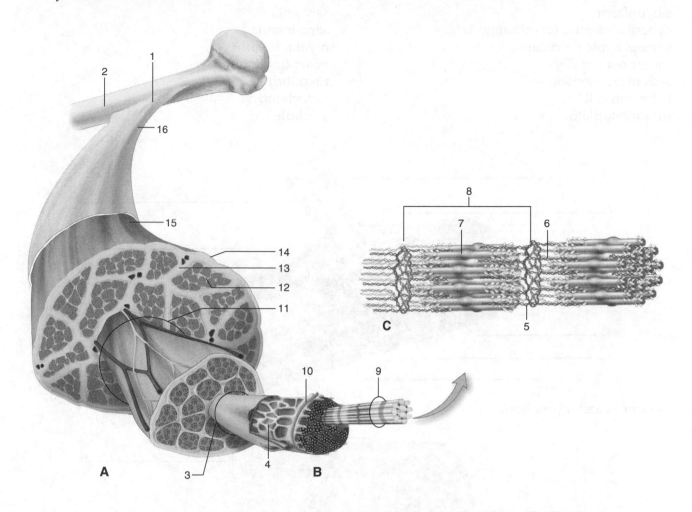

_____ sarcomere

_____ sarcoplasmic reticulum

_____ myofibril

_____ thin filament

_____ bone

_____ T tubule

_____ fascicle

_____ fascia

_____ muscle fiber (muscle cell)

_____ perimysium

_____ epimysium

_____ Z disk

_____ thick filament

_____ tendon

_____ endomysium

_____ muscle

Labeling—using the terms provided, label the following diagrams.

sarcoplasm

synaptic vesicles (continuing Ach)

sarcoplasmic reticulum

motor neuron fiber

Ach receptor sites

Schwann cell

motor endplate

sarcomere

sarcolemma

myelin sheath

synaptic cleft

myofibril

mitochondria

T tubule

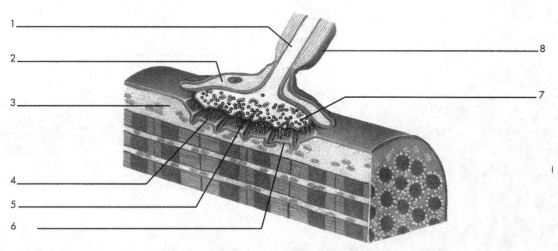

Neuromuscular junction.

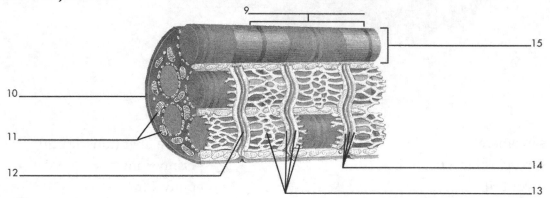

Skeletal muscle cell.

▶ *If you had difficulty with this section, review pages 347-360.*

II—FUNCTION OF SKELETAL MUSCLE ORGANS

Multiple Choice—select the best answer.

21. The principal component(s) of a motor unit is/are:
    a. one somatic motor neuron.
    b. the muscle fibers supplied by a somatic motor neuron.
    c. none of the above.
    d. both a and b.

22. The staircase phenomenon is also known as:
    a. tetanus.
    b. electromyography.
    c. wave summation.
    d. treppe.

23. Skeletal muscles are innervated by:
    a. somatic motor neurons.
    b. autonomic motor neurons.
    c. both a and b.
    d. internal stimulation.

24. Which of the following statements concerning isometric contractions is true?
    a. The length of the muscle changes.
    b. Muscle tension decreases.
    c. Joint movements are swift.
    d. Muscle length remains constant.

25. Physiologic muscle fatigue is caused by:
    a. relative lack of ATP.
    b. oxygen debt.
    c. lack of will.
    d. none of the above.

26. Increase in muscle size is called:
    a. hyperplasia.
    b. atrophy.
    c. hypertrophy.
    d. treppe.

27. Endurance training is also called:
    a. isometrics.
    b. hypertrophy.
    c. aerobic training.
    d. anaerobic training.

True or false

28. _____ A muscle contracts the instant it is stimulated.

29. _____ Isotonic contraction is one in which the tone or tension within a muscle remains the same, but the length of the muscle changes.

30. _____ One method of studying muscle contraction is called *myography*.

31. _____ Muscles with more tone than normal are described as *flaccid*.

Labeling—using the terms provided, label the following illustration of a motor unit.

myofibrils
neuromuscular junction
nucleus
motor neuron

myelin sheath
muscle fibers
Schwann cell

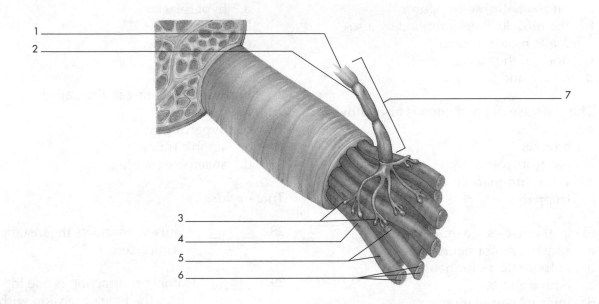

1 _____
2 _____

7 _____

3 _____
4 _____
5 _____
6 _____

▶ *If you had difficulty with this section, review pages 360-368.*

III—FUNCTION OF CARDIAC AND SMOOTH MUSCLE TISSUE

Matching—identify each muscle tissue with its corresponding characteristics.

a. cardiac muscle tissue
b. skeletal muscle tissue
c. smooth muscle tissue

32. _____ located in the walls of hollow organs

33. _____ contains many nuclei near the sarcolemma

34. _____ voluntary

35. _____ not striated

36. _____ striated; contains a single nucleus

37. _____ a principal function: peristalsis

38. _____ has larger-diameter T tubules that form diads with sarcoplasmic reticulum

39. _____ principal functions: movement of bones, heat production, and posture

40. _____ contains intercalated disks

41. _____ has loosely organized sarcoplasmic reticulum

Labeling—label the following diagram of a cardiac muscle fiber.

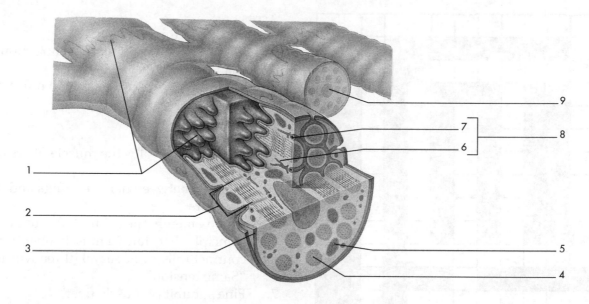

▶ *If you had difficulty with this section, review pages 368-372.*

IV—MECHANISMS OF DISEASE

Circle the correct answer.

42. Muscle strains are characterized by (myalgia or fibromyositis).

43. Crush injuries can cause (hemoglobin or myoglobin) to accumulate in the blood and result in kidney failure.

44. A viral infection of the nerves that control skeletal muscle movement is known as (poliomyelitis or muscular dystrophy).

45. (Muscular dystrophy or myasthenia gravis) is a group of genetic diseases characterized by atrophy of skeletal muscle tissues.

46. (Muscular dystrophy or myasthenia gravis) is an autoimmune disease in which the immune system attacks muscle cells at the neuromuscular junction.

▶ *If you had difficulty with this section, review pages 372-374.*

Crossword Puzzle

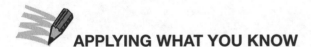

Across

1. Thick and thin
4. Smooth, sustained muscle contraction
8. "Same length"
9. Transverse structure unique to muscle cells (two words)

Down

1. Motor neuron plus the muscle fibers (two words)
2. Junction between nerve endings and muscle fibers
3. Plasma membrane of striated muscle fiber
5. Principle that states a muscle fiber will contract fully or not at all (three words)
6. "Same tension"
7. Fine subunit of muscle fiber

APPLYING WHAT YOU KNOW

47. Throughout Linda's life, she wanted to be a star in the 100-meter dash. However, no matter how hard she trained, she could never excel in this sport. On the other hand, she *did* achieve great success in much longer track events, especially the 10-kilometer race. Explain Linda's situation from the aspect of which skeletal muscle fiber type she may possess disproportionately by virtue of her genetics.

48. John is working in a hospital while he is studying to become a physician. One of his duties is to transport recently deceased patients to the morgue. While moving the patients onto the gurney, he is surprised to discover how stiff the bodies can be. Which physiologic phenomenon is responsible for this stiffness? Exactly why is it that these muscles can temporarily display stiffness?

DID YOU KNOW

*   The simple act of walking requires the use of 200 muscles in the human body.

*   People who are on bedrest or totally inactive lose approximately 1% of muscle strength per day.

ONE LAST QUICK CHECK

Multiple Choice—select the best answer.

49. When a muscle does not shorten and no movement results, the contraction is:
     a. isometric.
     b. isotonic.
     c. twitch.
     d. tetanic.

50. Pushing against a wall is an example of which type of contraction?
     a. isotonic
     b. isometric
     c. twitch
     d. tetanic

51. Prolonged inactivity causes muscles to shrink in mass, a condition called:
    a. hypertrophy.
    b. disuse atrophy.
    c. paralysis.
    d. muscle fatigue.

52. Muscle fibers usually contract to about _____% of their starting length.
    a. 50
    b. 60
    c. 70
    d. 80

53. Which statement is true of smooth muscle?
    a. It lines the walls of many hollow organs.
    b. It is striated.
    c. It is voluntary.
    d. There are many T tubules throughout smooth muscle.

54. What is a quick, jerky response of a given muscle to a single stimulus called?
    a. isometric
    b. lockjaw
    c. tetanus
    d. twitch

True or false

55. _____ The energy required for muscular contraction is obtained by hydrolysis of amino acids.

56. _____ A motor neuron together with the cells it innervates is called a *motor unit.*

57. _____ If muscle cells are stimulated repeatedly without adequate periods of rest, the strength of the muscle contraction will decrease, resulting in fatigue.

58. _____ The minimal level of stimulation required to cause a fiber to contract is called the *threshold stimulus.*

59. _____ Weakness of abdominal muscles can lead to a hernia.

60. _____ There are two types of smooth muscle: visceral and multiunit.

61. _____ Cardiac muscle is also known as *striated involuntary.*

62. _____ The length/tension relationship states that the maximal strength a muscle can develop is related to the length of the fibers.

63. _____ Skeletal muscles have little effect on body temperature.

CHAPTER 13

Nervous System Cells

The nervous system organizes and coordinates the millions of stimuli received each day to make communication with and enjoyment of our environment possible. The functioning unit of the nervous system is the neuron. Three types of neurons exist—sensory, motor, and interneurons—which are classified according to the direction in which they transmit impulses. Nerve impulses travel over routes made up of neurons and provide the rapid communication necessary for maintaining life.

Your study of the nervous system begins with the simplest concept of impulse conduction known as the *reflex arc*. It then progresses to the more complex pathways such as divergence/convergence. An understanding of the anatomy and physiology of the nervous system cells is necessary before you progress to the complexity of this system and its multiple divisions.

I—ORGANIZATION OF THE NERVOUS SYSTEM

Matching—identify each part of the nervous system with its definition.

a. afferent division
b. autonomic nervous system
c. central nervous system
d. efferent nervous system
e. parasympathetic division
f. peripheral nervous system
g. somatic nervous system
h. sympathetic division

1. _____ consists of the brain and spinal cord
2. _____ composed of nerves arising from the brain and spinal cord
3. _____ PNS subdivision that transmits incoming information from the sensory organs to the CNS
4. _____ produces the "fight or flight" response
5. _____ subdivision that carries information from the CNS to skeletal muscle
6. _____ subdivision of efferent division that transmits information to smooth muscle, cardiac muscle, and glands
7. _____ consists of all outgoing motor pathways
8. _____ coordinates the body's normal resting activities

▶ *If you had difficulty with this section, review pages 379-383.*

II—CELLS OF THE NERVOUS SYSTEM

Matching—identify each type of cell with its characteristics. Answers may be used more than once.

a.   astrocyte
b.   microglia
c.   oligodendrocyte
d.   Schwann cell

9.   _____   has the ability of phagocytosis

10.   _____   helps to form the blood-brain barrier

11.   _____   produces fatty myelin sheath in the PNS

12.   _____   largest and most numerous of the neuroglial cells

13.   _____   produces myelin sheath in the CNS

14.   _____   type of neuroglia that forms the neurilemma

15.   _____   "star cell"

16.   _____   disorder of this cell associated with multiple sclerosis

Multiple Choice—select the best answer.

17.   Which of the following is/are classified as nerve fibers?
a.   axon
b.   dendrites
c.   both a and c
d.   none of the above

18.   Which of the following conduct impulses toward the cell body?
a.   axons
b.   dendrites
c.   Nissl bodies
d.   none of the above

19.   A neuron with one axon and several dendrites is a:
a.   multipolar neuron.
b.   unipolar neuron.
c.   bipolar neuron.
d.   none of the above.

20.   Which type of neuron lies entirely within the CNS?
a.   afferent
b.   efferent
c.   interneuron
d.   none of the above

21.   Which sequence best represents the course of an impulse over a reflex arc?
a.   receptor, synapse, sensory neuron, motor neuron, effector
b.   effector, sensory neuron, synapse, motor neuron, receptor
c.   receptor, motor neuron, synapse, sensory neuron, effector
d.   receptor, sensory neuron, interneuron, motor neuron, effector

Labeling—label the following illustration showing the structure of a typical neuron.

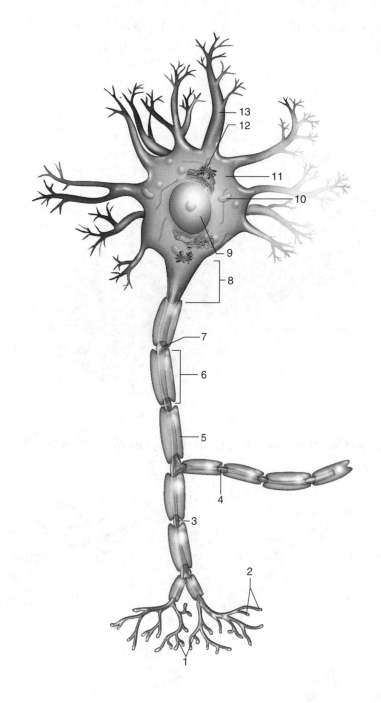

1	_____	8	_____
2	_____	9	_____
3	_____	10	_____
4	_____	11	_____
5	_____	12	_____
6	_____	13	_____
7	_____		

Labeling—using the terms provided, label the following illustration of a myelinated axon.

neurilemma (sheath of Schwann cell)   myelin sheath
plasma membrane of axon   node of Ranvier
nucleus of Schwann cell   neurofibrils, microfilaments, and microtubules

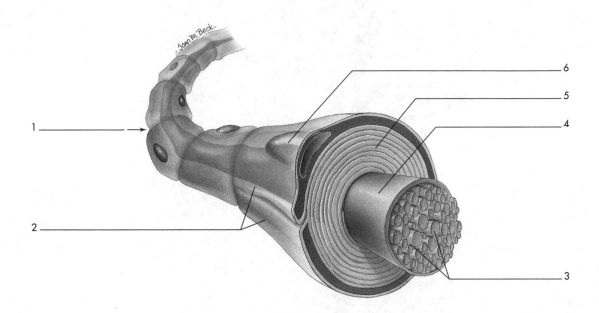

Labeling—identify the classification of each type of neuron in the following illustrations.

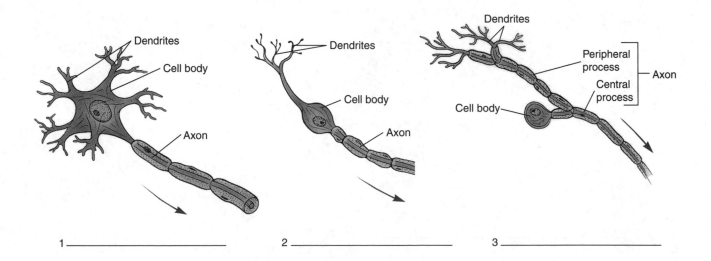

1 _____   2 _____   3 _____

Labeling—using the terms provided, label the following illustration of a reflex arc.

motor neuron axon
cell body
interneuron
dendrite
spinal nerve

sensory neuron axon
white matter
synapse
gray matter

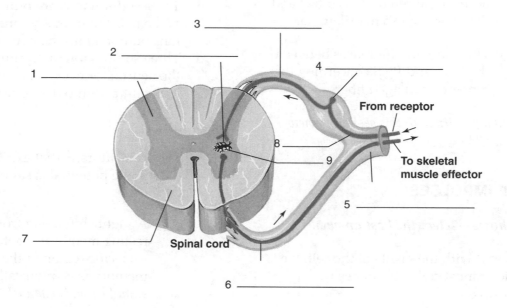

▶ *If you had difficulty with this section, review pages 383-392.*

III—NERVES AND TRACTS

Multiple Choice—select the best answer.

22. A complete nerve, consisting of numerous fascicles and their blood supply, is held together by a fibrous coat called the:
    a. endoneurium.
    b. perineurium.
    c. epineurium.
    d. fascicles.

23. Small, distinct regions of gray matter within the CNS are usually called:
    a. white matter.
    b. nuclei.
    c. ganglia.
    d. fascicles.

24. Nerves that contain mostly efferent fibers are called:
    a. sensory nerves.
    b. motor nerves.
    c. mixed nerves.
    d. Schwann nerves.

25. Gray matter in the CNS consists of:
    a. nerve fibers.
    b. neuroglia.
    c. axons.
    d. cell bodies.

26. Most nerves in the human nervous system are:
    a. sensory nerves.
    b. motor nerves.
    c. mixed nerves.
    d. reflex nerves.

▶ *If you had difficulty with this section, review page 392.*

IV—REPAIR OF NERVE FIBERS

True or false

27. _____   Evidence now indicates that neurons may be replaced.

28. _____   Regeneration of nerve fibers will occur if the cell body is intact and the fibers have a neurilemma.

29. _____   There are no differences between the CNS and PNS concerning the repair of damaged fibers.

▶ *If you had difficulty with this section, review pages 392-393.*

V—NERVE IMPULSES

Multiple Choice—select the best answer.

30. Compared with the inside of the cell, the outside of most cell membranes is:
    a. positive.
    b. negative.
    c. equal.
    d. none of the above.

31. The difference in electrical charge across a plasma membrane is called:
    a. depolarization.
    b. membrane potential.
    c. both a and b.
    d. none of the above.

32. A neuron's resting membrane potential is:
    a. 70 mV.
    b. –70 mV.
    c. 30 mV.
    d. –30 mV.

33. Which of the following statements is true concerning the sodium-potassium pump?
    a. Three sodium ions are pumped out of the neuron for every two potassium ions pumped into the neuron.
    b. Two sodium ions are pumped out of the neuron for every three potassium ions pumped into the neuron.
    c. Three sodium ions are pumped out of the neuron for every three chloride ions pumped into the neuron.
    d. Three sodium ions are pumped out of the neuron for every three potassium ions pumped into the neuron.

True or false

34. _____   A membrane that exhibits a membrane potential is said to be *polarized.*

35. _____   A slight shift away from the resting membrane potential in a specific region of the plasma membrane is often called a *stimulus-gated channel.*

36. _____   Chlorine ions (Cl^-) are the dominant extracellular cations.

▶ *If you had difficulty with this section, review pages 393-395.*

VI—ACTION POTENTIAL

Multiple Choice—select the best answer.

37. During a relative refractory period:
    a. an action potential is impossible.
    b. an action potential is possible only in response to a very strong stimuli.
    c. an action potential is occurring.
    d. none of the above.

38. Voltage-gated channels are:
    a. membrane channels that close during voltage fluctuations.
    b. ion channels that open in response to voltage fluctuations.
    c. membrane channels that are altered from an extremely high stimulus.
    d. none of the above.

39. When current leaps across an insulating myelin sheath from node of Ranvier to node of Ranvier, the type of impulse conduction is:
    a. repolarization.
    b. refraction.
    c. saltatory conduction.
    d. diffusion.

40. The larger the diameter of a nerve fiber:
    a. the slower the speed of conduction.
    b. the faster the speed of conduction.
    c. Fiber diameter does not influence speed of conduction.
    d. the more the speed fluctuates.

True or false

41. _____ *Action potential* and *nerve impulse* are synonymous.

42. _____ When repolarization has occurred, an impulse cannot be conducted.

43. _____ The action potential is an all-or-none response.

44. _____ Many anesthetics function by inhibiting the opening of sodium channels and thus blocking the initiation and conduction of nerve impulses.

▶ *If you had difficulty with this section, review pages 395-399.*

VII—SYNAPTIC TRANSMISSION

Multiple Choice—select the best answer.

45. Which of the following structures is *not* a main component of a chemical synapse?
    a. synaptic knob
    b. synaptic cleft
    c. synaptic process
    d. plasma membrane of postsynaptic neuron

46. A synaptic knob is located on the:
    a. synaptic cleft.
    b. axon.
    c. dendrite.
    d. cell body.

47. Which of the following is true of spatial summation?
    a. Neurotransmitters released simultaneously from several presynaptic knobs converge on one postsynaptic neuron.
    b. Simultaneous stimulation of more than one postsynaptic neuron occurs.
    c. Impulses are fired in a rapid succession by the same neuron.
    d. Speed of impulse transmission is increased when several neurotransmitters are released.

True or false

48. _____ In an adult, the nervous system is replete with both electrical synapses and chemical synapses.

49. _____ Rapid-succession stimulation of a postsynaptic neuron by a synaptic knob can have a cumulative effect over time that can result in an action potential.

50. _____ Ca^{++} ions cause the release of neurotransmitters across the synaptic cleft.

Labeling—match each term with its corresponding number on the following illustration of a chemical synapse.

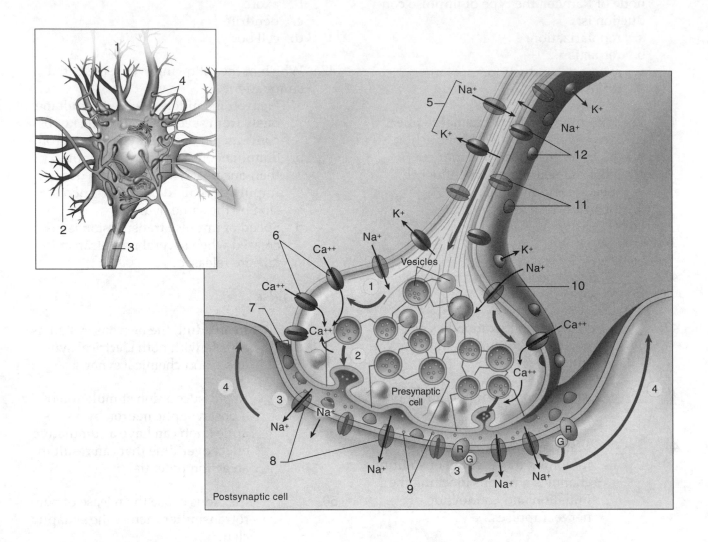

_____ axon of motor neuron

_____ synaptic knob

_____ stimulus-gated Na+ channels

_____ synaptic cleft

_____ action potential

_____ voltage-gated K+ channels

_____ axon of presynaptic neuron

_____ voltage-gated Ca++ channels

_____ neurotransmitters

_____ voltage-gated Na+ channels

_____ motor neuron cell body

_____ synaptic knobs

▶ *If you had difficulty with this section, review pages 399-404.*

VIII—NEUROTRANSMITTERS

Multiple Choice—select the best answer.

51. Neurotransmitters are released in a synapse and bind to:
    a. presynaptic terminals.
    b. the synaptic cleft.
    c. the base of the axon.
    d. receptors on the postsynaptic terminal.

52. The main chemical classes of neurotransmitters include all of the following *except:*
    a. acetylcholine.
    b. norepinephrine.
    c. amino acids.
    d. amines.

53. Which of the following is *not* an example of an amine neurotransmitter?
    a. serotonin
    b. histamine
    c. glycine
    d. dopamine

54. Severe depression can be caused by a deficit in which of the following neurotransmitters?
    a. acetylcholine
    b. amino acids
    c. amines
    d. neuropeptides

55. Which of the following is *not* a catecholamine?
    a. epinephrine
    b. norepinephrine
    c. dopamine
    d. serotonin

True or false

56. _____ Many biologists now believe that neuropeptides are the most common neurotransmitters in the CNS.

57. _____ Cocaine produces a temporary feeling of well-being by blocking the uptake of dopamine.

▶ *If you had difficulty with this section, review pages 404-411.*

IX—MECHANISMS OF DISEASE

Fill in the blanks.

58. _____ _____ is a disorder of the nervous system that involves the glia, rather than neurons.

59. _____ is a common type of brain tumor that is usually benign but may still be life-threatening.

60. A highly malignant form of astrocytic tumor is known as _____ _____.

61. An inherited glial disease characterized by numerous benign fibrous neuromas throughout the body is known as _____ _____.

62. Most disorders of the nervous system cells involve _____ rather than neurons.

▶ *If you had difficulty with this section, review pages 411-414.*

Crossword Puzzle

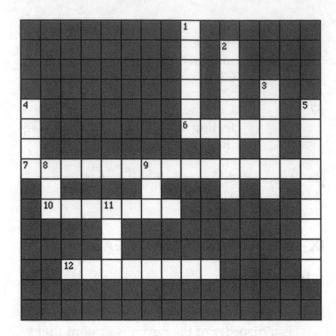

Across

6.   Bundle of peripheral nerve fibers
7.   Membrane potential of an active neuron (two words)
10. Place where signals are transmitted from one to another neuron
12. Transmits impulses toward the cell body

Down

1.   Consists of a cell body, an axon, and one or more dendrites
2.   _____ potential or difference in electrical charge across the plasma membrane
3.   White, fatty substance
4.   Supporting cell of the nervous system
5.   Signal conduction route to and from the CNS (two words)
8.   Center of entire nervous system (abbrev.)
9.   Nerves that lie in the "periphery" (abbrev.)
11. Transmits impulses away from the cell body

 APPLYING WHAT YOU KNOW

63. Jim is experiencing muscular weakness, loss of coordination, visual impairment, and speech disturbances. Which disease of the CNS could he be experiencing? Which nervous tissue cells are most likely involved? What specifically occurs to both the neurons and neuroglia of the CNS? What are the possible treatments and what are the theories as to the cause of this disease?

64. Lee Roy is a professional football player who, upon a severe compression blow to the head, lost the ability to move his lower body. He was rushed to the hospital where the doctors suspected crushing and bruising of the spinal cord. What are the chances of the damaged nervous tissue repairing itself?

 DID YOU KNOW

•   In the adult human body, there are 46 miles of nerves.

•   The longest cells in the human body are the motor neurons. They can be up to 4.5 feet (1.37 meters) long and run from the lower spinal cord to the big toe.

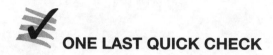

ONE LAST QUICK CHECK

Circle the correct answer.

65. A synaptic knob is a tiny bulge at the end of the (presynaptic or postsynaptic) neuron's axon.

66. Acetylcholine is an example of a (neurotransmitter or protein molecule receptor).

67. Neurotransmitters are chemicals that allow neurons to (communicate or reproduce) with one another.

68. Neurotransmitters are distributed (randomly or specifically) into groups of neurons.

69. Endorphins and enkephalins are neurotransmitters that inhibit conduction of (fear or pain).

70. Unipolar neurons are always (sensory or motor) neurons.

71. In the peripheral nervous system, small regions of gray matter are known as (nuclei or ganglia).

72. The distal tips of axons form branches called (telodendria or axon hillocks).

Matching—select the best choice for the following words and insert the correct letter in the blanks.

a.   neurons   b.   neuroglia

73. _____ axon

74. _____ supporting cells

75. _____ astrocytes

76. _____ sensory

77. _____ conduct impulses

78. _____ form the myelin sheath around central nerve fibers

79. _____ phagocytosis

80. _____ efferent

81. _____ multiple sclerosis

82. _____ multipolar

CHAPTER 14

Central Nervous System

Approximately one hundred billion neurons make up the brain. Everything we are and everything we hope to become are centered in this structure which is about the size of a small bowling ball. Our personality, communication skills, memory, and sensations depend upon the successful functioning of the brain. We are still in the infancy of our knowledge of this unique organ, as it still holds many mysteries for scientists to uncover. We are fascinated by the fact that although all pain is felt and interpreted in the brain, the brain itself has no pain sensation—even when cut! This simple example illustrates the complexity of the brain and some of the challenges ahead in identifying and understanding its capabilities for our body.

The central nervous system (CNS) is made up of the spinal cord and brain. The spinal cord provides access to and from the brain by means of ascending and descending tracts. In addition, the spinal cord functions as the primary reflex center of the body. The brain consists of the brain stem, cerebellum, diencephalon, and cerebrum. These areas provide the extraordinary network necessary to receive, interpret, and respond to most stimuli. Your study of the CNS will give you an appreciation of the complex mechanisms necessary to perform your daily tasks.

I—COVERINGS OF THE BRAIN AND SPINAL CORD

Multiple Choice—select the best answer.

1. From superficial to deep, which is the correct order of location of the meninges?
   a. dura mater, arachnoid membrane, pia mater
   b. pia mater, arachnoid membrane, dura mater
   c. arachnoid membrane, pia mater, dura mater
   d. dura mater, pia mater, arachnoid membrane

2. The falx cerebri separates the:
   a. two hemispheres of the cerebellum.
   b. cerebellum from the cerebrum.
   c. two hemispheres of the cerebrum.
   d. dura mater from the arachnoid.

3. The cerebrospinal fluid resides in the:
    a. epidural space.
    b. subarachnoid space.
    c. subdural space.
    d. piarachnoid space.

4. The layer of the meninges that serves as the inner periosteum of the cranial bones is the:
    a. pia mater.
    b. arachnoid membrane.
    c. dura mater.

Labeling—label the coverings of the brain on the following diagram.

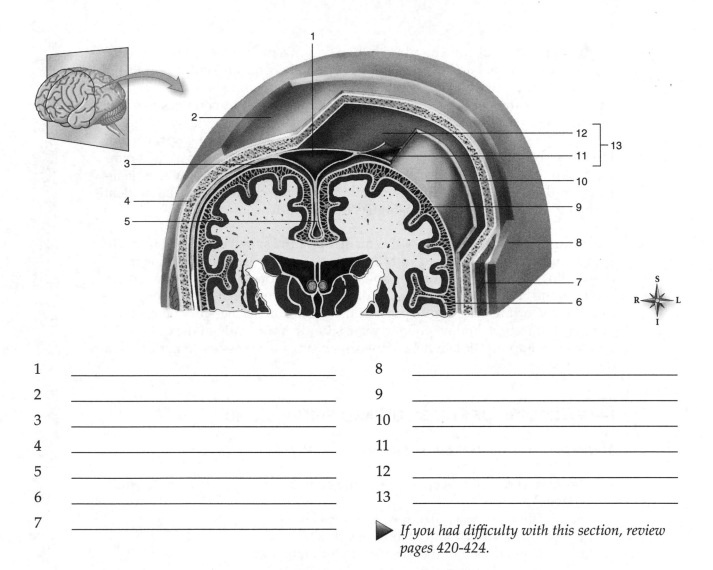

1	_____	8	_____
2	_____	9	_____
3	_____	10	_____
4	_____	11	_____
5	_____	12	_____
6	_____	13	_____
7	_____		

▶ *If you had difficulty with this section, review pages 420-424.*

II—CEREBROSPINAL FLUID

Multiple Choice—select the best answer.

5. Formation of the cerebrospinal fluid (CSF) occurs mainly in the:
   a. cerebral aqueduct.
   b. superior sagittal sinus.
   c. choroid plexuses.
   d. median foramen.

6. The lateral ventricles are located within the:
   a. cerebrum.
   b. cerebellum.
   c. spinal cord.
   d. none of the above.

7. CSF is absorbed into the venous blood via the:
   a. cisterna magna.
   b. choroid plexus.
   c. falx cerebri.
   d. arachnoid villus.

8. CSF is *not* found in the:
   a. central canal.
   b. subarachnoid space.
   c. third ventricle.
   d. subdural space.

True or false

9. ___I___ The four large, fluid-filled spaces within the brain are called *ventricles.*

10. ___F___ Interference of CSF circulation, causing the fluid to accumulate in the subarachnoid space, is referred to as *external hydrocephalus.*

Labeling—label the following illustration of the fluid spaces of the brain.

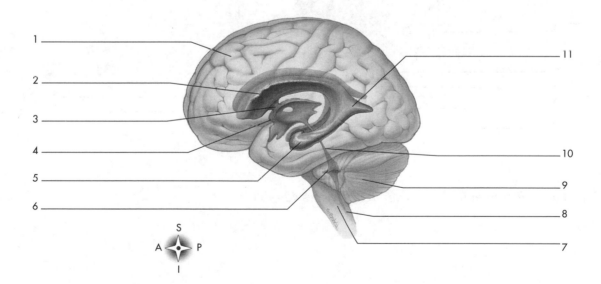

Labeling— using the terms provided, label the following illustrations depicting the flow of CSF and the layers of the brain.

cerebral aqueduct
cisterna magna
superior sagittal sinus (venous blood)
choroid plexus of third ventricle
subarachnoid space
falx cerebri (dura mater)
pia mater
choroid plexus of fourth ventricle
cerebral cortex

dura mater
arachnoid villus
choroid plexus of lateral ventricle
interventricular foramen
median foramen
central canal of spinal cord
lateral foramen
arachnoid layer

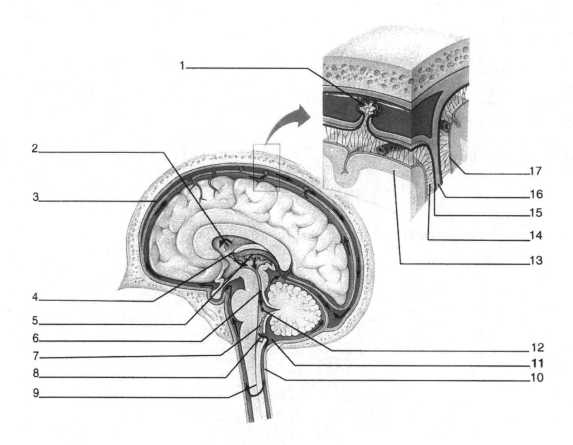

▶ *If you had difficulty with this section, review pages 424-426.*

III—THE SPINAL CORD

Matching—identify each ascending, or sensory, tract with its corresponding function.

a. lateral spinothalamic tract
b. anterior spinothalamic tract
c. fasciculi gracilis and cuneatus
d. spinocerebellar tract

11. _____ transmits impulses of crude touch and pressure

12. _____ transmits impulses of subconscious kinesthesia

13. _____ transmits impulses of crude touch, pain, and temperature

14. _____ transmits impulses of discriminating touch and kinesthesia

Matching—identify each descending, or motor, tract with its corresponding function.

a. lateral corticospinal tract
b. anterior corticospinal tract
c. reticulospinal tract
d. tectospinal tract
e. rubrospinal tract

15. _____ transmits impulses that control voluntary movement of muscles on the same side of the body

16. _____ facilitates head and neck movement related to visual reflexes

17. _____ helps maintain posture during skeletal muscle movements

18. _____ transmits impulses that control voluntary movement of muscles on the opposite side of the body

19. _____ transmits impulses that coordinate body movements and maintenance of posture

Labeling—match each spinal cord term with its corresponding number in the following illustration.

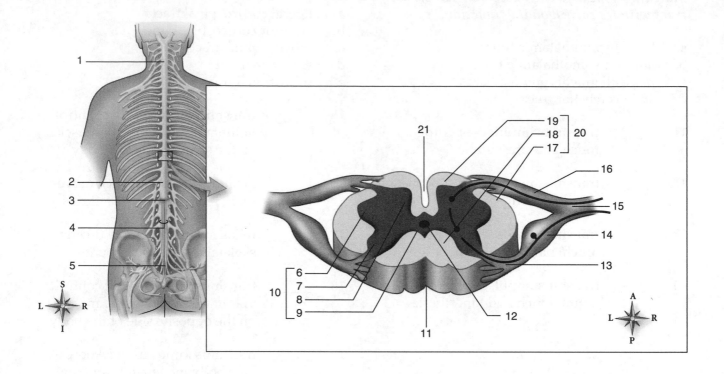

_____ white columns (funiculi)	_____ cervical enlargement
_____ anterior median fissure	_____ end of spinal cord
_____ cauda equina	_____ anterior column
_____ spinal nerve	_____ central canal
_____ posterior column	_____ dorsal (posterior) nerve root
_____ gray matter	_____ filum terminale
_____ lumbar enlargement	_____ lateral column
_____ posterior median sulcus	_____ gray commissure
_____ dorsal root ganglion	_____ ventral (anterior) nerve root
_____ lateral column	_____ anterior column
_____ posterior column	

Labeling—using the terms provided, label the major tracts of the spinal cord on the following diagram.

fasciculus gracilis
anterior spinothalamic
lateral spinothalamic
lateral corticospinal
anterior corticospinal
rubrospinal
reticulospinal

fasciculus cuneatus
posterior spinocerebellar
anterior spinocerebellar
spinotectal
vestibulospinal
tectospinal

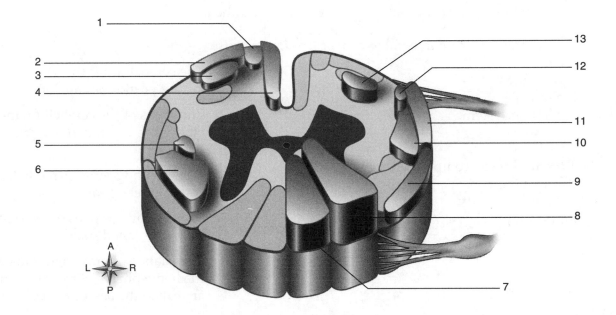

▶ *If you had difficulty with this section, review pages 426-429.*

IV—THE BRAIN

Multiple Choice—select the best answer.

20. Which of the following is *not* a part of the brain stem?
    a. medulla oblongata
    b. hypothalamus
    c. pons
    d. midbrain

21. Which of the following is *not* a component of the midbrain?
    a. cerebral peduncles
    b. corpora quadrigemina
    c. superior colliculi
    d. all of the above are parts of the midbrain

22. The internal white matter of the cerebellum is the:
    a. arbor vitae.
    b. vermis.
    c. peduncle.
    d. none of the above.

23. The part of the brain that secretes releasing hormones is the:
    a. thalamus.
    b. hypothalamus.
    c. medulla.
    d. pons.

24. Regulation of the body's biological clock and production of melatonin is performed by the:
    a. pons.
    b. thalamus.
    c. cerebellum.
    d. pineal body.

25. The central sulcus divides the:
    a. temporal lobe and parietal lobe.
    b. cerebrum into two hemispheres.
    c. frontal lobe and parietal lobe.
    d. occipital lobe and parietal lobe.

26. The part of the cerebrum integral to consciousness is:
    a. Broca's area.
    b. the reticular activating system.
    c. the limbic system.
    d. the insula.

27. Commissural tracts compose the:
    a. corpus callosum.
    b. mammillary body.
    c. hippocampus.
    d. central sulcus.

28. Emotions involve the functioning of the cerebrum's:
    a. Broca's area.
    b. limbic system.
    c. reticular activating system.
    d. caudate nucleus.

29. The type of brain wave associated with deep sleep is:
    a. delta.
    b. beta.
    c. alpha.
    d. theta.

True or false

30. _____ The cerebellum is the second largest portion of the brain.

31. _____ Functions of the cerebellum include language, memory, and emotions.

32. _____ The vomiting reflex is mediated by the cerebellum.

33. _____ The shallow grooves of the cerebrum are called *sulci*.

34. _____ The islands of gray matter inside the hemispheres of the cerebrum are called the *basal ganglia*.

Labeling—label the following illustration of the left hemisphere of the cerebrum.

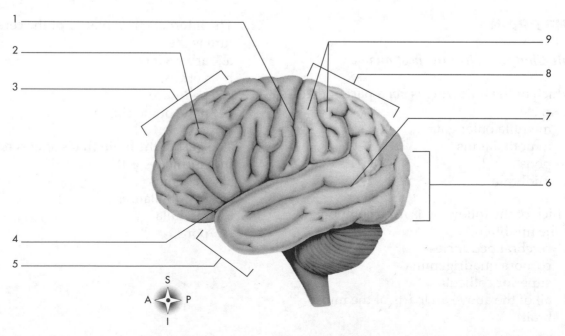

Labeling—label the functional areas of the cerebral cortex on the following illustration.

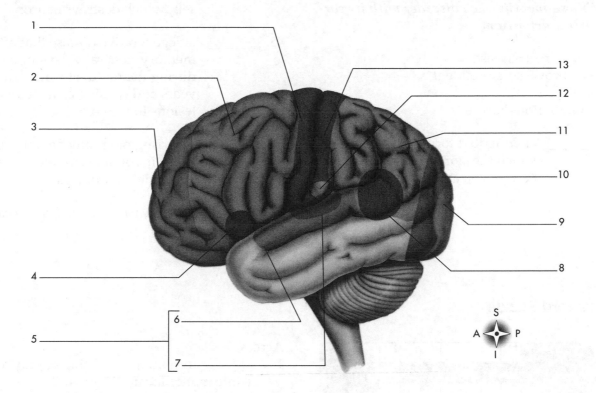

▶ *If you had difficulty with this section, review pages 429-448.*

V—SOMATIC SENSORY AND MOTOR PATHWAYS

Multiple Choice—select the best answer.

35. Which of the following is *not* a pathway that produces sensations of touch and pressure?
    a. medial lemniscal system
    b. spinothalamic pathway
    c. rubrospinal tract
    d. all of the above are pathways that produce sensations of touch and pressure.

36. Axons from the anterior gray horn of the spinal cord terminate in the:
    a. cerebral cortex.
    b. sensory receptors.
    c. skeletal muscle.
    d. none of the above.

37. Absence of reflexes is indicative of injury to:
    a. lower motor neurons.
    b. upper motor neurons.
    c. lower sensory neurons.
    d. upper sensory neurons.

True or false

38. _____ Poliomyelitis results in flaccid paralysis via destruction of anterior horn neurons.

39. _____ Extrapyramidal tracts are very simple pyramidal tracts.

▶ *If you had difficulty with this section, review pages 448-452.*

VI—MECHANISMS OF DISEASE

Matching—identify each disorder with its corresponding definition.

a. Alzheimer disease
b. cerebrovascular accident
c. epilepsy
d. Huntington disease

40. _____ an inherited form of dementia in which the symptoms first appear between 30 and 40 years of age

41. _____ a hemorrhage from or cessation of blood flow to the cerebral vessels, which destroys neurons

42. _____ a degenerative disease that affects memory, generally developing during the middle to late adult years and causing characteristic lesions in the cortex

43. _____ recurring or chronic seizure episodes involving sudden bursts of abnormal neuron activity

▶ If you had difficulty with this section, review pages 452-456.

Crossword Puzzle

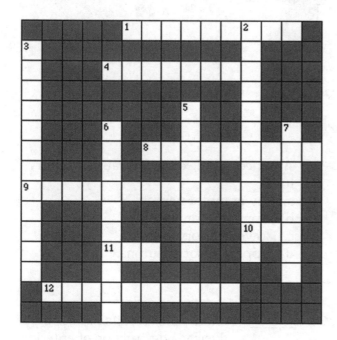

Across
1. _____ formation consisting of gray and white matter located in medulla
4. Largest division of the brain
8. Contains midbrain, pons, and medulla
9. Helps maintain normal body temperature
10. Electroencephalogram (abbrev.)
11. Cerebrospinal fluid (abbrev.)
12. Second largest part of the brain

Down
2. "Emotional brain" (two words)
3. "Between brain"
5. Part of diencephalon
6. Large, fluid-filled spaces within the brain
7. Membranous coverings of brain

APPLYING WHAT YOU KNOW

44. Baby Dania was born with an excessive accumulation of CSF in the ventricles. A catheter was placed in the ventricle and the fluid was drained by means of a shunt into the circulating bloodstream. What condition does this medical history describe?

45. Julius is exhibiting loss of memory, increasingly limited attention span, deteriorating motor control, and changes in his personality. What is the general term that can be used to describe his condition? What specific condition may he be suffering from?

DID YOU KNOW

- The short-term memory capacity for most people is between five and nine items or digits. This is one reason that phone numbers were kept to seven digits (not including the area code).

- The soft mass of the adult brain is motionless. Though it consumes up to 24% of the blood's oxygen supply, it does not grow, divide, or contract.

- The longest living cells in the body are brain cells which can live an entire lifetime.

ONE LAST QUICK CHECK

Multiple Choice—select the best answer.

46. The portion of the brain stem that joins the spinal cord to the brain is the:
    a. pons.
    b. cerebellum.
    c. diencephalon.
    d. hypothalamus.
    e. medulla.

47. Which one of the following is *not* a function of the brain stem?
    a. conducts sensory impulses from the spinal cord to the higher centers of the brain
    b. conducts motor impulses from the cerebrum to the spinal cord
    c. controls heartbeat, respiration, and blood vessel diameter
    d. contains centers for speech and memory

48. Which one of the following is *not* part of the diencephalon?
    a. cerebrum
    b. thalamus
    c. hypothalamus
    d. pineal gland

49. Which one of the following parts of the brain helps in the association of sensations with emotions, as well as aiding in the arousal or alerting mechanism?
    a. pons
    b. hypothalamus
    c. cerebellum
    d. thalamus
    e. none of the above is correct

50. Which one of the following is *not* a function of the cerebrum?
    a. language
    b. consciousness
    c. memory
    d. conscious awareness of sensations
    e. all of the above are functions of the cerebrum

51. The area of the cerebrum responsible for the perception of sound lies in the _____ lobe.
    a. frontal
    b. temporal
    c. occipital
    d. parietal

52. Visual perception is located in the _____ lobe.
    a. frontal
    b. temporal
    c. occipital
    d. parietal

53. Which one of the following is *not* a function of the cerebellum?
    a. maintains equilibrium
    b. helps produce smooth, coordinated movements
    c. helps maintain normal posture
    d. associates sensations with emotions

54. The largest section of the brain is the:
    a. cerebellum.
    b. pons.
    c. cerebrum.
    d. midbrain.

55. Which statement is *false*?
    a. The spinal cord performs two general functions.
    b. A lumbar puncture is performed to withdraw CSF.
    c. The cardiac, vasomotor, and respiratory control centers are called the *vital centers*.
    d. The meninges end at L1 in a tapered cone called the *cauda equina*.

56. Which of the following is *not* a function of the hypothalamus?
    a. major relay station between the cerebral cortex and lower autonomic centers
    b. serves as a higher autonomic center
    c. plays an essential role in maintaining the waking state
    d. regulates voluntary motor functions
    e. part of the mechanism for regulating appetite

CHAPTER 15

Peripheral Nervous System

Twelve pairs of cranial nerves attach to the ventral surface of the brain. The cranial nerves are identified by both name and number. The name indicates the structures innervated by the nerve (e.g., facial, optic) or may refer to the function of the nerve (e.g., oculomotor). The number is designated by Roman numerals. These numbers indicate the order of the nerves as they are positioned from anterior to posterior on the brain.

Cranial nerves may be further classified by function into three categories that are known as *mixed* cranial nerves, *sensory* cranial nerves, and *motor* cranial nerves. These distinctions refer to the bundles of axons that make up the nerves: mixed (axons of sensory and motor neurons), sensory (sensory axons only), and motor (mainly motor axons.)

Thirty-one pairs of spinal nerves are grouped into five regions of the vertebral column. They are the cervical, thoracic, lumbar, sacral, and coccygeal. Although they are not named individually, they are numbered according to the area of the vertebral column from which they emerge. Each spinal nerve is a mixed nerve consisting of both sensory and motor fibers. The fibers separate near the attachment of the nerve to the spinal cord, producing two "roots." The dorsal root is composed of the sensory fibers and is easily identified by a swelling known as the *dorsal root ganglion* (spinal ganglion). The ventral root is made up of motor fibers that carry information from the CNS towards effectors for appropriate response.

I—SPINAL NERVES

Multiple Choice—select the best answer.

1. Which of the following is an *incorrect* statement?
   a. There are 7 cervical nerve pairs.
   b. There are 12 thoracic nerve pairs.
   c. There are 5 lumbar nerve pairs
   d. All of the above are correct statements.

2. The spinal root that has a noticeable swelling is the:
   a. ventral root.
   b. anterior root.
   c. dorsal root.
   d. none of the above.

3. The dorsal root ganglion contains:
   a. sensory neuron cell bodies.
   b. motor neuron cell bodies.
   c. both sensory neuron and motor neuron cell bodies.
   d. motor neuron fibers.

4. The phrenic nerve innervates the:
   a. spleen.
   b. diaphragm.
   c. chest muscles.
   d. none of the above.

5. The femoral nerve arises from the:
   a. lumbar plexus.
   b. sacral plexus.
   c. coccygeal plexus.
   d. brachial plexus.

True or false

6. _____ The lower end of the spinal cord is called the *cauda equina*.

7. _____ There are 31 pairs of spinal nerves, all of which are composed of both motor and sensory fibers.

8. _____ Herpes zoster is a unique bacterial infection that almost always affects the skin of a single dermatome.

9. _____ *Dermatome* is a term referring to a skeletal muscle group innervated by motor neuron axons from a given spinal nerve.

10. _____ The brachial plexus is found deep within the shoulder.

Labeling—match each term with its corresponding number on the following illustration of spinal nerves.

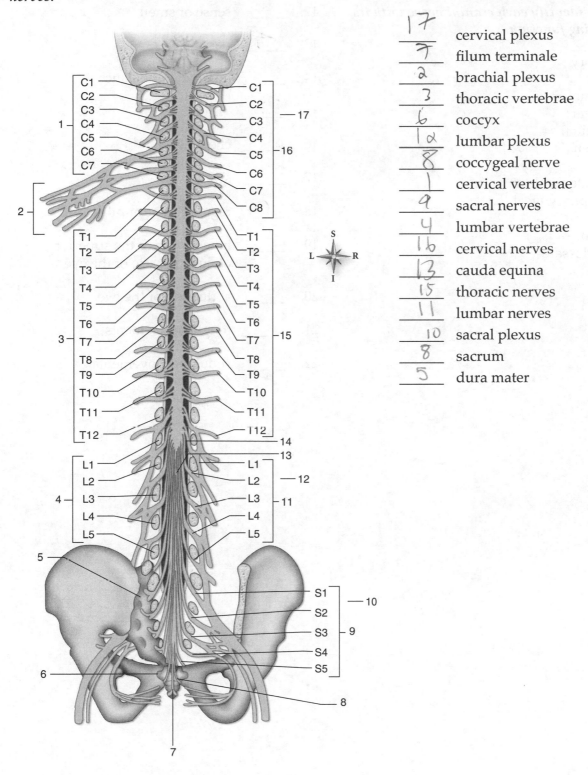

17	cervical plexus
7	filum terminale
2	brachial plexus
3	thoracic vertebrae
6	coccyx
12	lumbar plexus
8	coccygeal nerve
1	cervical vertebrae
9	sacral nerves
4	lumbar vertebrae
16	cervical nerves
13	cauda equina
15	thoracic nerves
11	lumbar nerves
10	sacral plexus
8	sacrum
5	dura mater

▶ *If you had difficulty with this section, review pages 463-473.*

II—CRANIAL NERVES

Matching—identify each cranial nerve with its corresponding function.

a.   olfactory
b.   optic
c.   oculomotor
d.   trochlear
e.   trigeminal
f.   abducens
g.   facial
h.   vestibulocochlear
i.   glossopharyngeal
j.   vagus
k.   accessory
l.   hypoglossal

11. __9__ facial expressions
12. __A__ sense of smell
13. __3__ peristalsis
14. __H__ hearing and balance
15. __b__ vision
16. __E__ chewing
17. __I__ swallowing
18. __C__ regulation of pupil size
19. __d__ innervation of the superior oblique muscle of the eye
20. __F__ abduction of the eye
21. __l__ tongue movements
22. __K__ shoulder movements

Labeling—identify the cranial nerves by matching each term with its corresponding number in the following illustration.

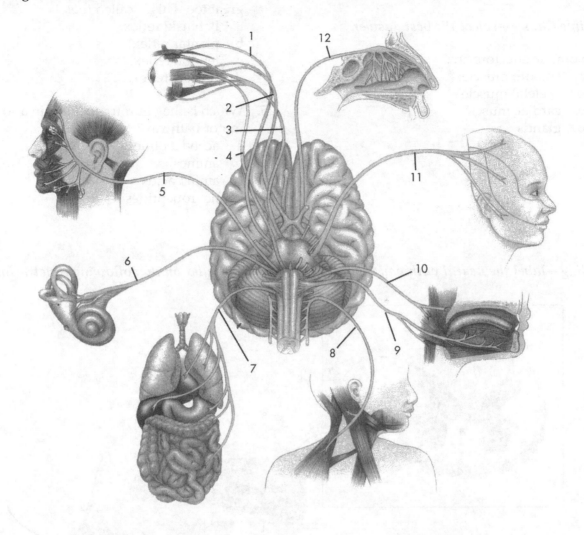

10 glossopharyngeal nerve (IX)	___ trigeminal nerve (V)
2 olfactory nerve (I)	3 oculomotor nerve (III)
4 abducens nerve (VI)	___ facial nerve (VII)
6 vestibulocochlear nerve (VIII)	1 trochlear nerve (IV)
___ vagus nerve (X)	9 accessory nerve (XI)
___ hypoglossal nerve (XII)	2 optic nerve (II)

▶ *If you had difficulty with this section, review pages 473-481.*

III—SOMATIC MOTOR NERVOUS SYSTEM

Multiple Choice—select the best answer.

23. Somatic effectors are:
    a. smooth muscle.
    b. skeletal muscle.
    c. cardiac muscle.
    d. glands.

24. When the outer sole of the foot is stimu-
    lated, a normal infant will extend the
    great toe. This is called the:
    a. Babinski reflex.
    b. plantar reflex.
    c. tendon reflex.
    d. corneal reflex.

25. Which is the neurotransmitter in a somatic
    motor pathway?
    a. acetylcholine
    b. amines
    c. amino acids
    d. neuropeptides

Labeling—label the neural pathway involved in the patellar reflex on the following illustration.

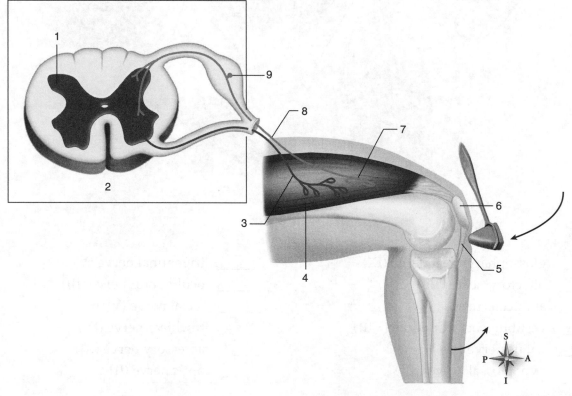

1 _____   6 _____

2 _____   7 _____

3 _____   8 _____

4 _____   9 _____

5 _____

▶ *If you had difficulty with this section, review
pages 481-484.*

Crossword Puzzle

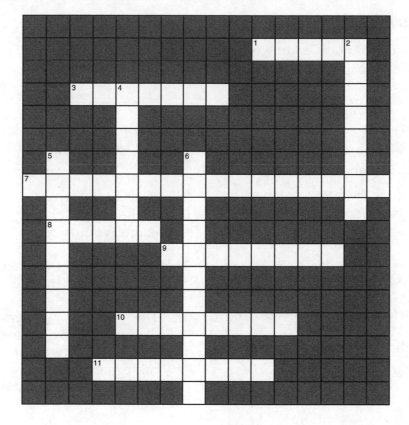

Across

1. Large branch of a spinal nerve as it emerges from the spinal cavity
3. Voluntary division of the peripheral nervous system that controls skeletal muscle
7. Acetylcholine
8. Cranial nerve that contains axons of sensory and motor neurons
9. Region of gray matter in peripheral nerves
10. Motor nerve that controls eye movements
11. Foot reflex present until 18 months of age

Down

2. Disease that often affects the skin of a single dermatome
4. Skeletal muscle or group of muscles that receives motor axons from a given spinal nerve
5. Skin surface area supplied by a specific spinal nerve
6. Horse's tail of spinal cord (two words)

 APPLYING WHAT YOU KNOW

26. Ethan had difficulty swallowing and he noticed his mouth was extremely dry. The doctor advised him that the problem may be related to a nerve. What two nerves might possibly be causing the problem? These nerves are mixed nerves. What is meant by that statement?

27. Mason is under great stress from trying to advance in his career, pursue graduate school, and raise two small children. After a particularly stressful event, he noticed a burning sensation in his axillary and pectoral regions. Days later he experienced an eruption of red swollen plaques in the same area. What condition is he experiencing? What is the name of the responsible pathogen? Why did he experience the symptoms that he did? What may be the reason that the pathogen was capable of breaching his immune system?

DID YOU KNOW

- The human brain continues sending out electrical wave signals for up to 37 hours after death.

- Your brain consists of approximately 100 billion neurons.

- There are no pain receptors in the brain, so the brain can feel no pain.

- The human brain is the fattest organ in the body and may consist of at least 60% fat.

ONE LAST QUICK CHECK

Multiple Choice—select the best answer.

28. Which one of the following doesn't have a sensory function?
    a. abducens
    b. trigeminal
    c. facial
    d. vagus

29. Which nerve is a mixed nerve that arises from the medulla and is distributed to numerous organs?
    a. trochlear
    b. accessory
    c. hypoglossal
    d. vagus

30. Parasympathetic innervation of the heart is assisted by the:
    a. vagus nerve.
    b. facial nerve.
    c. trigeminal nerve.
    d. glossopharyngeal nerve.

31. Which nerve is involved in smiling and frowning?
    a. vagus
    b. trigeminal
    c. facial
    d. glossopharyngeal

Fill in the blanks.

32. The _____ nerve assists with balance or equilibrium.

33. Tic douloureux is damage to the _____ nerve.

34. The most common cause of peripheral nerve damage in the United States and Europe is _____ _____.

35. The somatic motor nervous system includes all of the ___voluntary___ motor pathways outside the CNS.

36. Somatic reflexes are contractions of _____ muscle.

37. The _____ nerves supply the diaphragm. Any disease or injury to the spinal cord between the 3rd and 5th cervical segments may paralyze the _____ nerve, and therefore the diaphragm as well.

Matching—select the best choice for the following words and insert the correct letter in the answer blank.

a. cranial nerves   b. spinal nerves

38. __A__ 12 pairs

39. __B__ dermatome

40. __A__ vagus

41. __B__ shingles

42. __B__ 31 pairs

43. __A__ optic

44. __B__ C1

45. __B__ plexus

46. __B__ myotome

47. __A__ accessory

CHAPTER 16

Autonomic Nervous System

Wile you concentrate on this chapter, your body is performing a multitude of functions. Fortunately for us, the beating of the heart, digestion of food, breathing, and most of our day-to-day processes do not require our supervision or thought. They function automatically, and the division of the nervous system that regulates these functions is known as the *autonomic nervous system*.

The autonomic nervous system is a division of the peripheral nervous system (PNS). There are two functional divisions of the PNS—the afferent (sensory) division and the efferent (motor) division. The efferent division is divided into the somatic nervous system, responsible for voluntary motor responses, and the autonomic nervous system, responsible for involuntary motor responses. The autonomic nervous system consists of two divisions called the *sympathetic system* and the *parasympathetic system*. The sympathetic system functions as an emergency system and prepares us for "fight or flight." The parasympathetic system dominates control of many visceral effectors under normal everyday conditions. Together, these two divisions regulate the body's automatic functions in an effort to assist with the maintenance of homeostasis. Your understanding of this chapter will alert you to the functions and complexity of the peripheral nervous system and the "automatic pilot" of your body—the autonomic system.

I—STRUCTURES OF THE AUTONOMIC NERVOUS SYSTEM

Multiple Choice—select the best answer.

1. Somatic motor and autonomic pathways share all of the following *except:*
   a. direction of impulse conduction.
   b. effectors located outside the CNS.
   c. number of neurons between the CNS and effector.
   d. acetylcholine as a possible neurotransmitter.

2. Within the sympathetic chain ganglion, the preganglionic fiber may:
   a. synapse with a sympathetic postganglionic neuron.
   b. send an ascending branch through the sympathetic trunk.
   c. pass through chain ganglia and synapse in a collateral ganglion.
   d. all of the above.

3. Beta receptors bind with:
    a. acetylcholine.
    b. norepinephrine.
    c. toxin muscarine.
    d. none of the above.

4. Which of the following is *not* an example of sympathetic stimulation?
    a. decreased heart rate
    b. decreased secretion of the pancreas
    c. constriction of the urinary sphincters
    d. dilation of skeletal muscle blood vessels

5. "Fight or flight" physiologic changes include all of the following *except:*
    a. increased conversion of glycogen to glucose.
    b. constriction of respiratory airways.
    c. increased perspiration.
    d. dilation of blood vessels in skeletal muscles.

True or false

6. ___F___ Conduction of autonomic effectors requires only one efferent neuron.

7. ___T___ Many autonomic effectors are dually innervated.

8. ___T___ The sympathetic division is also called the *thoracolumbar division.*

9. ___F___ The sympathetic division is the dominant controller of the body at rest.

10. ___T___ Sympathetic responses are usually widespread, involving many organ systems at once.

Labeling—using the terms provided, label the following diagram of autonomic conduction paths.

sympathetic ganglion
postganglionic neuron's axon
collateral ganglion
axon of preganglionic sympathetic neuron
axon of somatic motor neuron

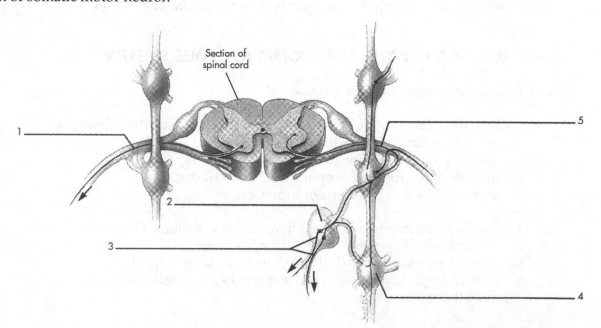

Fill in the blanks.

11. Each efferent autonomic pathway is made up of _Autonomic Nerves_, _ganglia_, and _plexuses_.

12. _Preganglionic_ neurons conduct impulses from the brain stem or spinal cord to an autonomic ganglion.

13. Sympathetic ganglia located a short distance from the spinal cord are known as _collateral_ ganglia.

14. Some postganglionic axons return to a spinal nerve by way of a short branch called the gray _____.

15. Axon terminals of autonomic neurons release either acetylcholine or _____.

Circle the correct answer.

16. In the sympathetic division, preganglionic neurons are relatively (short or long) and postganglionic neurons are relatively (short or long).

17. Norepinephrine affects visceral effectors by first binding to (cholinergic or adrenergic) receptors in their plasma membranes.

18. The effect of a neurotransmitter on any postsynaptic cell is determined by the (characteristics of the receptor or neurotransmitter).

19. A (nicotinic or beta) receptor is a main type of cholinergic receptor.

20. The action of acetylcholine is (slowly or quickly) terminated when hydrolyzed by the enzyme acetylcholinesterase.

▶ *If you had difficulty with this section, review pages 489-501.*

II—FUNCTIONS OF THE AUTONOMIC NERVOUS SYSTEM

True or false

21. _____ Both sympathetic and parasympathetic divisions are tonically active, meaning they continually conduct impulses to autonomic effectors.

22. __F__ Sympathetic impulses inhibit effectors and parasympathetic impulses stimulate effectors.

23. __T__ Autonomic centers function in a hierarchy in their control of the ANS with the highest ranking being the autonomic centers in the cerebral cortex.

24. __T__ The sympathetic system plays a crucial role in maintaining blood pressure.

25. __F__ The sympathetic system dominates during "rest and repair."

▶ *If you had difficulty with this section, review pages 498-502.*

Crossword Puzzle

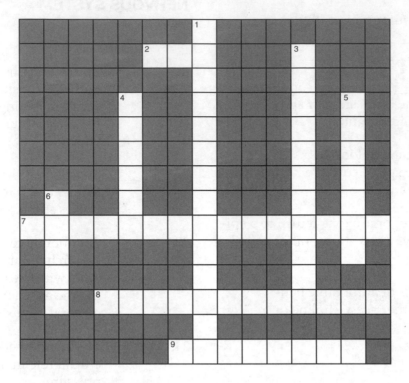

Across

2. Number of neurons between CNS and effector in an autonomic efferent pathway
7. Division that controls most autonomic effectors most of the time
8. Another name for the parasympathetic division
9. Ganglia in or near the effector in a parasympathetic pathway

Down

1. Released by axons known as *adrenergic fibers*
3. Division that serves as the "fight or flight" reaction
4. Complex network formed by ventral rami of most spinal nerves
5. Along with autonomic nerves and plexuses, these make up efferent autonomic pathways
6. Large branch of a spinal nerve as it emerges from the spinal cavity

 APPLYING WHAT YOU KNOW

26. Cara experiences great anxiety before her college final exams. As the professor distributes the exam, she experiences a classic "fight or flight" reaction. Which division of the autonomic nervous system is responsible for this phenomenon? Which body systems are affected and how do they respond? What is Cara's risk from chronic exposure to such stress?

27. Emma has periodic episodes of a "racing heart." Within minutes of an attack, she feels light-headed and extremely anxious. Her friend suggested that during an episode that she lie down on a bed, listen to soft, relaxing music, and periodically take her pulse to monitor her success in returning her heart to a normal rhythm. Emma has found the technique to be very helpful. What is this technique called?

DID YOU KNOW

- The brain uses less power than your refrigerator light.

- Even though the brain is very efficient, it is an energy hog. It is only 3% of the body's weight, but consumes 1/6 (17%) of the body's total energy.

- The brain begins to lose cells at a rate of 50,000 per day by age 30.

- Eighty percent of the average human brain is water.

ONE LAST QUICK CHECK

Matching—identify the term with the proper selection.

a. division of ANS
b. tissues to which autonomic neurons conduct impulses
c. voluntary actions
d. regulates body's involuntary effectors
e. efferent neurons that make up the ANS
f. conduct impulses between the spinal cord and a ganglion

28. __d__ autonomic nervous system

29. __E__ autonomic neurons

30. __f__ preganglionic neurons

31. __B__ visceral effectors

32. __A__ sympathetic system

33. __C__ somatic nervous system

Multiple Choice—select the best answer.

34. Dendrites and cell bodies of sympathetic preganglionic neurons are located in the:
    a. brain stem and sacral portion of the spinal cord.
    b. sympathetic ganglia.
    c. gray matter of the thoracic and upper lumbar segments of the spinal cord.
    d. ganglia close to effectors.

35. Which of the following is *not* correct?
    a. Sympathetic preganglionic neurons have their cell bodies located in the lateral gray column of certain parts of the spinal cord.
    b. Sympathetic preganglionic axons pass along the dorsal root of certain spinal nerves.
    c. There are synapses within sympathetic ganglia.
    d. Sympathetic responses are usually widespread, involving many organs.

36. Another name for the parasympathetic nervous system is:
    a. thoracolumbar.
    b. craniosacral.
    c. visceral.
    d. ANS.
    e. cholinergic.

37. Which statement is *not* correct?
    a. Sympathetic postganglionic neurons have their dendrites and cell bodies in sympathetic ganglion or collateral ganglia.
    b. Sympathetic ganglions are located in front of and at each side of the spinal column.
    c. Separate autonomic nerves distribute many sympathetic postganglionic axons to various internal organs.
    d. Very few sympathetic preganglionic axons synapse with postganglionic neurons.

Matching—select the correct response and insert the letter in the answer blank.

a.   sympathetic control
b.   parasympathetic control

38.   __B__   constricts pupils

39.   __A__   bronchial relaxation

40.   __A__   increases sweat secretion

41.   __B__   increases secretion of digestive juices and insulin

42.   __A__   constricts blood vessels

43.   __B__   slows heartbeat

44.   __A__   relaxes bladder

45.   __A__   increases epinephrine secretion

46.   __B__   increases peristalsis

47.   __B__   accommodates lens for near vision

CHAPTER 17

Sense Organs

Consider this scene for a moment. You are walking along a beautiful beach watching the sunset. You notice the various hues and are amazed at the multitude of shades that cover the sky. The waves are melodious as they splash along the shore and you wiggle your feet with delight as you sense the warm, soft sand trickling between your toes. You sip on a soda and then inhale the fresh salt air as you continue your stroll along the shore.

It is a memorable scene, but one that would not be possible without the assistance of your sense organs. The sense organs pick up messages that are sent over nerve pathways to specialized areas in the brain for interpretation. They make communication with and enjoyment of the environment possible. The visual, auditory, tactile, olfactory, and gustatory sense organs not only protect us from danger but also add an important dimension to our daily pleasures of life. Your study of this chapter will give you an understanding of another of the systems necessary for homeostasis and survival.

I—SENSORY RECEPTORS

Multiple Choice—select the best answer.

1. Which of the following is *not* a general sense?
    a. touch
    b. taste
    c. temperature
    d. pain

2. Which of the following is *not* a true statement?
    a. Mechanoreceptors are activated by stimuli that "deform" the receptor.
    b. Taste and smell are examples of chemoreceptors.
    c. Photoreceptors respond to light stimuli.
    d. Thermoreceptors are activated by pressure.

3. Which of the following structures is a disc-shaped nerve ending that is responsible for discerning light touch?
    a. Merkel disks
    b. pacinian corpuscles
    c. nociceptors
    d. Golgi tendon receptors

4. Which of the following is *not* a proprio-
    ceptor?
    a. muscle spindle
    b. root hair plexus
    c. Golgi tendon receptor
    d. all of the above are proprioceptors

5. Proprioceptors:
    a. function in relation to movements and
        body position.
    b. are superficial.
    c. are receptors for touch, pain, heat, and
        cold.
    d. are widely distributed throughout the
        skin.

True or false

6. _____ Mechanoreceptors are activated
    by a change in temperature.

7. _____ Free nerve endings are the sim-
    plest, most common, and most
    widely distributed sensory recep-
    tors.

8. _____ Somatic sense receptors located
    in muscles and joints are called
    visceroreceptors.

9. _____ Golgi tendon receptors are stimu-
    lated by excessive muscle con-
    traction.

10. _____ Exteroceptors are often called *cu-
    taneous receptors* because of their
    placement in the skin.

▶ *If you had difficulty with this section, review
pages 505-513.*

II—THE SENSE OF SMELL AND THE SENSE OF TASTE

Multiple Choice—select the best answer.

11. Olfactory receptors and taste buds are:
    a. thermoreceptors.
    b. chemoreceptors.
    c. nociceptors.
    d. mechanoreceptors.

12. Olfactory epithelium consists of:
    a. epithelial support cells.
    b. basal cells.
    c. cilia.
    d. all of the above.

13. All of the following are primary taste sen-
    sations *except*:
    a. sweet.
    b. sour.
    c. spicy.
    d. bitter.

14. Nerve impulses responsible for the sensa-
    tion of taste are carried in all of the follow-
    ing cranial nerves *except*:
    a. VII.
    b. VIII.
    c. IX.
    d. X.

True or false

15. _____ Olfaction requires the chemical
    response of a dissolved substance
    for a stimulus.

16. _____ The olfactory receptor cells lie in
    an excellent position functionally
    to smell delicate odors.

17. _____ The transmission pathway for
    olfactory sensations is as follows:
    olfactory cilia, olfactory bulb, ol-
    factory tract, thalamic and olfac-
    tory centers of the brain.

18. _____ The tip of the tongue reacts best
    to bitter taste.

Labeling—label the midsagittal section of the nasal area on the following illustration.

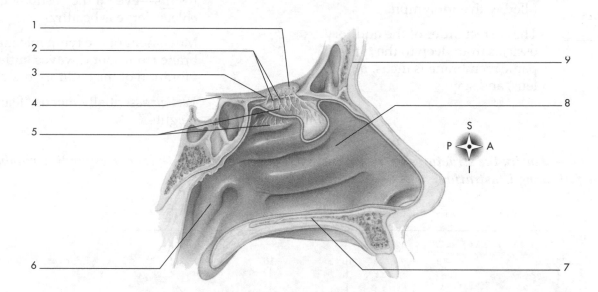

▶ *If you had difficulty with this section, review pages 513-517.*

III—SENSE OF HEARING AND BALANCE: THE EAR

Multiple Choice—select the best answer.

19. Which of the following is a structure of the middle ear?
    a. incus
    b. oval window
    c. cranial nerve VII
    d. vestibule

20. The auditory tube connects the:
    a. inner ear and cranial nerve VIII.
    b. middle ear and the auditory ossicles.
    c. middle ear and the nasopharynx.
    d. oval window and the round window.

21. The only structure of the inner ear concerned with hearing is the:
    a. utricle.
    b. saccule.
    c. semicircular canals.
    d. cochlear duct.

22. Dynamic equilibrium depends upon the functioning of the:
    a. organ of Corti.
    b. crista ampullaris.
    c. both a and b.
    d. none of the above.

23. The neuronal pathway of hearing begins at the:
    a. vestibular nerve.
    b. cochlear nerve.
    c. vestibulocochlear nerve.
    d. cranial nerve VII.

24. Dynamic equilibrium depends on the functioning of the:
    a. organ of Corti.
    b. crista ampullaris.
    c. macula.
    d. tectorial membrane.

25. The sense organ(s) responsible for the sense of balance is/are located in the:
    a. vestibule.
    b. cochlea.
    c. semicircular canals.
    d. both a and c.

True or false

26. ___T___ The membranous labyrinth is filled with endolymph.

27. ___F___ The correct order of the auditory ossicles from deep to the tympanic membrane is incus, malleus, and stapes.

28. ___T___ If the hairs of the organ of Corti are damaged, nerve deafness results—even if the vestibulocochlear nerve is healthy.

29. ___T___ Movement of the tympanic membrane from sound waves initiates vibration of the auditory ossicles.

30. ___F___ *Vertigo* essentially means "fear of heights."

Labeling—identify the structures of the ear by matching each term with its corresponding number on the following illustration.

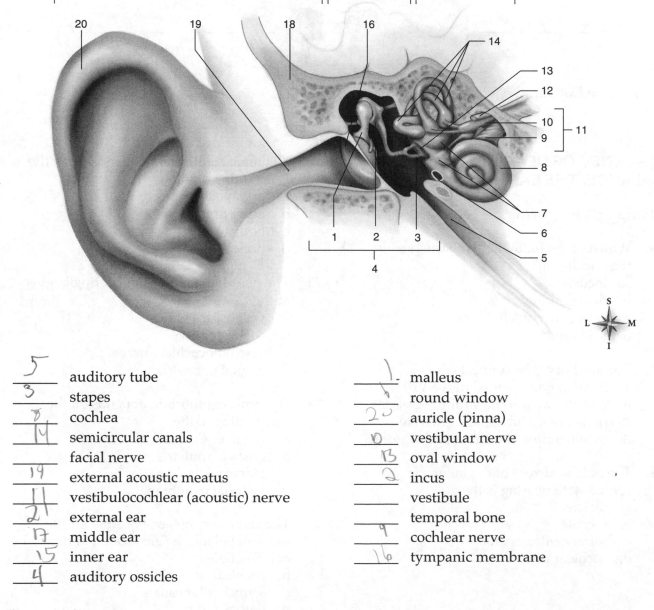

_5_	auditory tube	_1_	malleus
_3_	stapes	_6_	round window
_8_	cochlea	_20_	auricle (pinna)
_14_	semicircular canals	_10_	vestibular nerve
___	facial nerve	_13_	oval window
_19_	external acoustic meatus	_2_	incus
_11_	vestibulocochlear (acoustic) nerve	___	vestibule
_21_	external ear	___	temporal bone
_17_	middle ear	_9_	cochlear nerve
_15_	inner ear	_16_	tympanic membrane
_4_	auditory ossicles		

▶ *If you had difficulty with this section, review pages 517-524.*

IV—VISION: THE EYE

Multiple Choice—select the best answer.

31. From superficial to deep, the three layers of tissue that compose the eyeball are:
    a. sclera, retina, choroid.
    b. choroid, sclera, retina.
    c. sclera, choroid, retina.
    d. retina, choroid, sclera.

32. The anterior portion of the sclera is called the:
    a. cornea.
    b. iris.
    c. lens.
    d. conjunctiva.

33. The neurons of the retina—in the order in which they conduct impulses—are:
    a. photoreceptor neurons, bipolar neurons, ganglion neurons.
    b. photoreceptor neurons, ganglion neurons, bipolar neurons.
    c. bipolar neurons, photoreceptor neurons, ganglion neurons.
    d. bipolar neurons, ganglion neurons, photoreceptor neurons.

34. All of the axons of ganglion neurons extend back to an area of the posterior eyeball called the:
    a. fovea centralis.
    b. macula lutea.
    c. canal of Schlemm.
    d. optic disk.

35. Which of the following spaces contains the vitreous body?
    a. anterior chamber
    b. posterior chamber
    c. anterior cavity
    d. posterior cavity

36. The white of the eye is called the:
    a. sclera.
    b. choroid.
    c. retina.
    d. cornea.

37. The function of the lacrimal gland is to:
    a. secrete aqueous humor.
    b. secrete vitreous humor.
    c. secrete tears.
    d. none of the above.

38. Accommodation of the lens for near vision necessitates:
    a. increased curvature of the lens.
    b. relaxation of the ciliary muscle.
    c. contraction of the suspensory ligament.
    d. dilation of the pupil.

39. People whose acuity is worse than 20/200 after correction are considered to be:
    a. nearsighted.
    b. farsighted.
    c. legally blind.
    d. none of the above.

40. An intrinsic eye muscle is the:
    a. iris.
    b. pupil.
    c. sclera.
    d. retina.

True or false

41. ____ Mucous membrane, called *canthus*, lines each eyelid.

42. __F__ All the muscles associated with the eye are smooth or involuntary.

43. ____ Conjunctivitis is a highly contagious infection.

44. ____ Corneal tissue is avascular.

45. __F__ Deficiency of the blue-sensitive photopigments is the most common form of color blindness.

46. ____ The opening and separation of opsin and retinal in the presence of light is called *bleaching*.

47. ___T___ The retina is the incomplete innermost coat of the eyeball in that it has no anterior portion.

48. ___T___ *Refraction* means "the deflection or bending of light rays."

49. ___F___ A person with a 20/100 vision can see objects at 100 feet that a person with normal vision can see at 20 feet.

50. ___F___ A person with strabismus usually has double vision.

Labeling—using the terms provided, label the horizontal section through the eyeball on the following illustration.

sclera
pupil
ciliary body
optic nerve
posterior chamber
optic disk
central artery and vein
fovea centralis
lens

cornea (transparent)
lacrimal caruncle
iris
macula
choroid
retina
lower (inferior) lid
anterior chamber

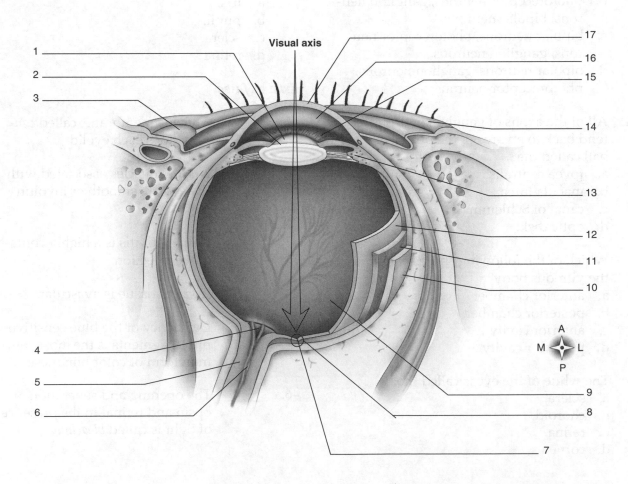

Labeling—label the extrinsic muscles of the right eye on the following illustration.

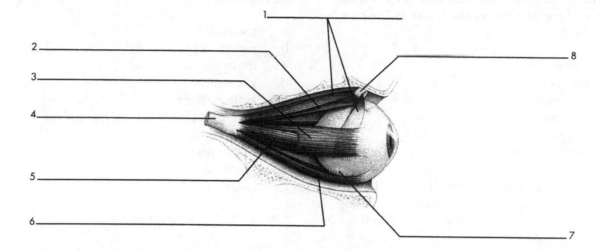

Labeling—label the structures of the lacrimal apparatus on the following illustration.

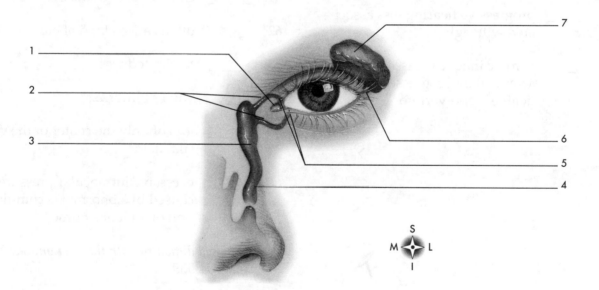

▶ *If you had difficulty with this section, review pages 524-534.*

V—MECHANISMS OF DISEASE

Matching—identify the best answer from the choices given and insert the letter in the answer blank.

a. tinnitus
b. presbycusis
c. otosclerosis
d. otitis media
e. vertigo
f. Ménière disease

51. ___c___ inherited bone disorder that impairs conduction by causing structural irregularities in the stapes

52. ___a___ "ringing in the ear"

53. ___d___ middle ear infection

54. ___e___ sensation of spinning

55. ___b___ progressive hearing loss associated with aging

56. ___f___ chronic inner ear disease characterized by progressive nerve deafness and vertigo

Matching—select the best answer from the choices given and insert the letter in the answer blank.

a. trachoma
b. retinopathy
c. myopia
d. glaucoma
e. astigmatism
f. conjunctivitis
g. nyctalopia
h. hyperopia
i. scotoma
j. cataracts

57. ___C___ nearsightedness

58. ___E___ an irregularity in the cornea

59. ___f___ "pink-eye"

60. ___A___ chlamydial conjunctivitis

61. ___j___ cloudy spots in the eye's lens

62. ___b___ often caused by diabetes mellitus

63. ___h___ farsightedness

64. ___g___ "night blindness"

65. ___i___ loss of only the center of the visual field

66. ___d___ excessive intraocular pressure caused by abnormal accumulation of aqueous humor

▶ *If you had difficulty with this section, review pages 534-539.*

Crossword Puzzle

Across

1. Photopigment in rods
4. "Snail"
8. Provides information related to head position or acceleration
10. Smell

Down

2. Pain receptor
3. Deflection of light rays
5. Inner ear
6. Crista _____; dynamic equilibrium
7. Taste
9. Innermost coat of eyeball

APPLYING WHAT YOU KNOW

67. Jada became ill repeatedly with throat infections during her first few years of school. Lately, however, she has noticed that whenever she has a throat infection, her ears become very sore also. What might be the cause of this additional problem?

68. Deb is a woman with unusually poor vision. Without glasses, she needs to stand 20 feet away from an object to see it, whereas a person with normal vision could see that same object from 400 feet. How would you quantify her visual acuity? What must she score in a visual acuity exam after correction with glasses to avoid being designated as legally blind? With which type of refraction disorder is she afflicted? What shape lenses would be required to focus a clear image on her retina?

DID YOU KNOW

- Synesthesia is a rare condition in which the senses are combined. Synesthetes see words, taste colors and shapes, and feel flavors.

- A human can taste one gram of salt in 500 liters of water (0.0001M).

- Men can read smaller print than women; women can hear better than men.

- The first sense to develop in utero is the sense of touch.

ONE LAST QUICK CHECK

Multiple Choice—select the best answer.

69. Where are the specialized mechanorecep-
    tors of hearing and balance located?
    a. inner ear
    b. malleus
    c. helix
    d. all of the above

70. The organ of Corti is the sense organ of
    what sense?
    a. sight
    b. hearing
    c. pressure
    d. taste

71. Where are taste sensations interpreted?
    a. cerebral cortex
    b. nasal cavity
    c. area of stimulation
    d. none of the above

72. An eye physician is an:
    a. oculist.
    b. optometrist.
    c. ophthalmologist.
    d. none of the above.

73. Which of the following statements about
    the sclera is true?
    a. It is a mucous membrane.
    b. It is called the *white of the eye*.
    c. It lies behind the iris.
    d. All of the above are true.

74. Which of the following are encapsulated
    nerve endings?
    a. gustatory receptors
    b. lamellar corpuscles
    c. olfactory receptors
    d. all of the above

75. The retina contains microscopic receptor
    cells called:
    a. mechanoreceptors.
    b. chemoreceptors.
    c. olfactory receptors.
    d. rods and cones.

76. Which two involuntary muscles make up
    the front part of the eye?
    a. malleus and incus
    b. iris and ciliary muscle
    c. retina and pacinian muscle
    d. sclera and iris

77. Which of the following statements about
    gustatory sense organs is true?
    a. They are called *taste buds*.
    b. The are innervated by cranial nerves
       VII and IX.
    c. They work together with the olfactory
       senses.
    d. All of the above are true.

78. The external ear consists of the:
    a. auricle and external acoustic meatus.
    b. labyrinth.
    c. organ of Corti and cochlea.
    d. none of the above.

True or false

79. _____ The tympanic membrane sepa-
    rates the middle ear from the ex-
    ternal ear.

80. ___F___ Glaucoma may result from a
    blockage of flow of the vitreous
    body.

81. _____ With the condition of presbyopia,
    the eye lens loses its elasticity.

82. ___F___ The crista ampullaris is located in
    the nasal cavity.

83. ___T___ Myopia occurs when images
    are focused in front of the retina
    rather than on it.

84. _____ Light enters through the pupil
    and the size of the pupil is regu-
    lated by the iris.

85. _____ The retina is the innermost layer
    of the eye and contains structures
    called *rods*.

86. ___T___ The olfactory receptors are chem-
    ical receptors.

87. ___T___ Meissner's corpuscle is a tactile
    corpuscle.

88. _____ The macula provides information
    related to head position or accel-
    eration.

CHAPTER 18

Endocrine Regulation

The endocrine system is a system of communication, regulation, and control. It differs from the nervous system in that hormones provide a slower, longer-lasting effect than do nerve stimuli and responses. It is a ductless system that releases hormones into the bloodstream to help regulate body functions. The pituitary gland stimulates many of the endocrine glands to secrete their powerful hormones. All hormones, whether stimulated in this manner or by other control mechanisms, are interdependent. A change in the level of one hormone may affect the level of many other hormones.

Hormones may be classified in many ways, but one of the most commonly accepted ways is simply as *steroid* or *nonsteroid* hormones. Steroid hormones are manufactured by endocrine cells from cholesterol and nonsteroid hormones are synthesized primarily from amino acids. Steroid hormones such as estrogen and testosterone enter target cells and directly interact with the DNA in the nucleus. Nonsteroid hormones such as adrenaline generally do not enter the target cell but instead bind to a receptor protein found on external cell membranes. This then causes a succession of metabolic effects.

In addition to the endocrine glands, prostaglandins, or "tissue hormones," are powerful substances similar to hormones that have been found in a variety of body tissues. These hormones are often produced in a tissue and diffuse only a short distance to act on cells within that area. Prostaglandins influence respiration, blood pressure, gastrointestinal secretions, and the reproductive system and may one day play an important role in the treatment of diseases such as hypertension, asthma, and ulcers.

As you review the endocrine system, you will be struck by the critical role that this system plays in our daily lives. Understanding the "system of hormones" will alert you to one of the mechanisms of our emotions, response to stress, growth, chemical balances, and many other body functions.

I—THE ENDOCRINE SYSTEM AND HORMONES

Multiple Choice—select the best answer.

1. The chemical messengers of the endocrine system are:
   a. hormones.
   b. neurotransmitters.
   c. target tissues.
   d. target organs.

2. Which of the following statements is true of the endocrine system?
   a. The cells secreting the chemical messengers are called *neurons*.
   b. The distance traveled by the chemical messengers is short (across a microscopic synapse).
   c. Its effects are slow to appear, yet long-lasting.
   d. None of the above.

3. Which of the following is *not* an endocrine gland?
   a. pineal
   b. placenta
   c. parathyroid
   d. intestines

4. The neuroendocrine system performs all of the following functions *except*:
   a. communication.
   b. control.
   c. conduction.
   d. integration.

5. The many hormones secreted by endocrine tissues can be classified simply as:
   a. steroid or nonsteroid hormones.
   b. anabolic or catabolic hormones.
   c. sex or nonsex hormones.
   d. tropic or hypotropic hormones.

6. Nonsteroid hormones include:
   a. proteins.
   b. peptides.
   c. glycoproteins.
   d. all of the above.

7. Anabolic hormones:
   a. target other endocrine glands and stimulate their growth and secretion.
   b. target reproductive tissue.
   c. stimulate anabolism in their target cells.
   d. stimulate catabolism in their target cells.

8. The second messenger often involved in nonsteroid hormone action is:
   a. cAMP.
   b. mRNA.
   c. ATP.
   d. GTP.

9. The control of hormone secretion is:
   a. usually part of a negative feedback loop.
   b. rarely part of a positive feedback loop.
   c. both a and b.
   d. none of the above.

10. When a small amount of hormone allows a second hormone to have its full effect on a target cell, the phenomenon is called:
    a. synergism.
    b. permissiveness.
    c. antagonism.
    d. combination.

True or false

11. __T__ The nervous system functions at a much greater speed than the endocrine system.

12. __T__ The most widely used method of hormone classification is by chemical structure.

13. __F__ Steroid hormone receptors are usually attached in the plasma membrane of a target cell.

14. __F__ Production of too much hormone of a diseased gland is termed *hyposecretion*.

15. __T__ Input from the nervous system influences secretion of hormones.

Labeling—label the locations of the major endocrine glands on the following illustration.

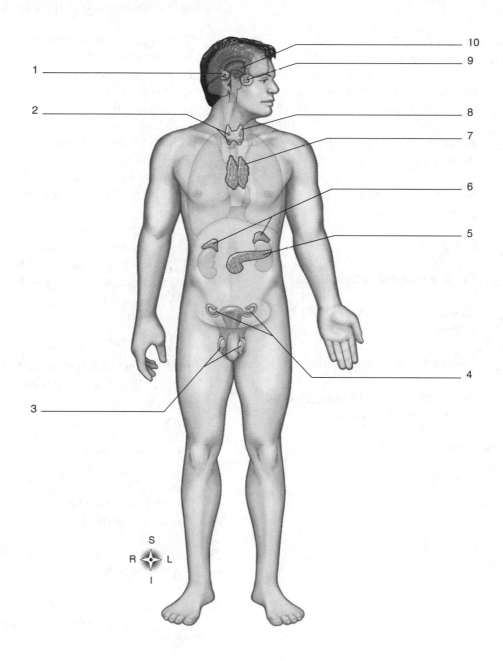

If you had difficulty with this section, review pages 545-555.

Matching—select the best choice for the following and insert the correct letter in the blanks.

a. Steroid hormone
b. Nonsteroid hormone

16. __B__ Binds to specific plasma membrane receptor

17. __A__ Response time is usually one hour to several days

18. __A__ Receptor is mobile in the cytoplasm or nucleus

19. __A__ Lipid

20. __A__ Regulates gene activity

21. __B__ Stored in secretory vesicles before release

22. __B__ One or more amino acids

23. __B__ Response time is usually several seconds to a few minutes

▶ *If you had difficulty with this section, review pages 547-556.*

II—PROSTAGLANDINS

Multiple Choice—select the best answer.

24. Prostaglandins are referred to as:
     a. growth hormones.
     b. tissue hormones.
     c. target cells.
     d. thyroxins.

25. Which of the following is *false*?
     a. Prostaglandins tend to integrate activities of neighboring cells.
     b. The first prostaglandin was discovered in semen.
     c. Aspirin produces some of its effects by increasing PGE synthesis.
     d. PGFs have been used to induce labor and accelerate delivery of a baby.

Fill in the blanks.

26. __paracrine__ hormones are hormones that regulate activity in nearby cells within the same tissue as their source.

27. __autocrine__ hormones regulate activity in the secreting cell itself.

28. The __seminal vesicles__ of the male reproductive system secretes prostaglandin in the semen.

29. Leukotrienes are regulators of __immunity__.

30. PGFs are required for normal __peristalsis__ to occur in the digestive tract.

▶ *If you had difficulty with this section, review pages 556-559.*

Labeling—using the terms provided, label the location and structure of the target cell concept.

capillary
hormone
target cells
receptors
nontarget cells

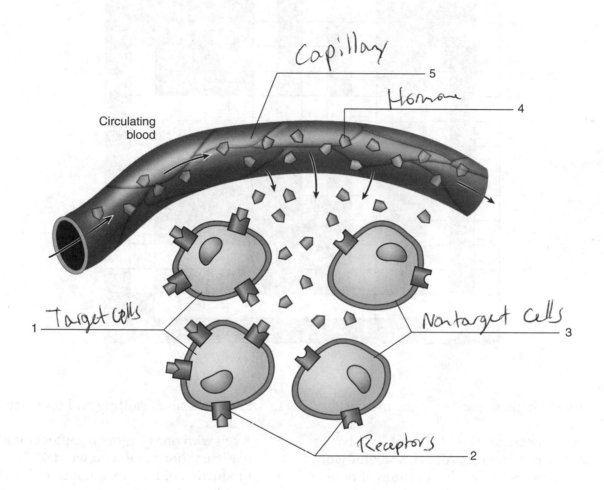

CROSSWORD PUZZLE

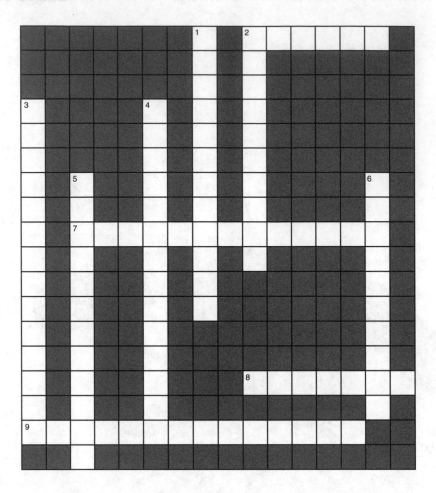

Across

2. Endocrine gland located in the mediastinum
7. Tissue hormone
8. Insulin, parathyroid, ACTH, and glucagon are examples of this classification of nonsteroid hormone
9. Cells that secrete chemical messengers that diffuse into the bloodstream rather than across a synapse

Down

1. Promotes blood clotting and constriction of blood vessels
2. A cell with one or more receptors for a particular hormone (two words)
3. Production of too much hormone by a diseased gland
4. Occurs when a small amount of one hormone allows a second hormone to have its full effect on a target cell
5. Releasing or inhibiting hormones are secreted by this gland
6. Hormones synthesized primarily from amino acids

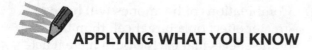

APPLYING WHAT YOU KNOW

31. India was pregnant and was 2 weeks past her due date. Her doctor suggested that she enter the hospital and he would induce labor. What local hormone might he give India to encourage labor?

32. Susie suffered a severe sprain while playing volleyball one day. She noticed her leg was swollen, red, warm to the touch, and very painful. X-rays indicated that there was no fracture but nonetheless, she was extremely uncomfortable. After reviewing the x-rays and lab reports, the doctor sent her home with instructions and suggested that she simply take aspirin for pain. Why did he make this recommendation for pain?

DID YOU KNOW

- People with dwarfism almost always have normal-sized children, even if both parents have dwarfism.

- The pituitary weighs little more than a small paper clip.

ONE LAST QUICK CHECK

Fill in the blanks.

33. Responses that result from the operation of feedback loops within the endocrine system are called ___Endocrine___ ___Reflexes___.

34. Unused hormones circulating in the blood are excreted by the ___Kidneys___.

35. In ___Antagonism___, one hormone produces the opposite effect of another hormone.

36. In second messenger systems, the hormone-receptor complexes may be taken into the cell by means of ___Endocytosis___.

37. The ___amount___ of steroid hormone present determines the magnitude of a target cell's response.

Circle the correct answer.

38. Endocrine target cells must have the appropriate receptor to be influenced by the signaling chemical—a process called (<u>signal transduction</u> or signal induction).

39. If too little hormone is produced, the condition is called (hypersecretion or <u>hyposecretion</u>).

40. Many nonsteroid hormones seem to use cAMP as the (first messenger or <u>second messenger</u>).

41. Some hormones produce their effects by triggering the opening of (<u>calcium</u> or potassium) channels.

42. The (<u>pituitary</u> or parathyroids) regulate(s) the thyroid by producing thyroid-stimulating hormone (TSH).

Matching—select the best choice for the following and insert the correct letter in the blanks.

a. tissue hormone
b. prostaglandins
c. ibuprofen
d. thromboxane
e. leukotrienes

43. ___D___ blood regulator important in blood clotting

44. ___E___ immunity regulator

45. ___A___ local hormone

46. ___B___ lipid molecules

47. ___C___ inhibits PGE synthesis

Multiple Choice—select the best answer.

48. If norepinephrine diffuses into the blood and then binds to an adrenergic receptor in a distant target cell, it is known as a:
    a. hormone.
    b. neurotransmitter.
    c. second messenger.
    d. none of the above.

49. All steroid hormones are derived from which common molecule?
    a. amino acid
    b. peptide
    c. cholesterol
    d. protein

50. Which of the following is *not* a peptide?
    a. antidiuretic hormone (ADH)
    b. oxytocin (OT)
    c. melanocyte-stimulating hormone (MSH)
    d. testosterone

51. Combinations of hormones will have a greater effect on a target cell than the sum of the effects that each would have if acting alone. This phenomenon is called:
    a. permissiveness.
    b. synergism.
    c. antagonism.
    d. transduction.

52. The target cell concept is an example of the _____ model of chemical reactions.
    a. lock-and-key
    b. signal transduction
    c. mobile-receptor
    d. nuclear-receptor

CHAPTER 19

Endocrine Glands

The endocrine system has often been compared to a fine concert symphony. When all instruments are playing properly, the sound is melodious. If one instrument plays too loud or too soft, however, it affects the overall quality and enjoyment of the entire performance.

The endocrine system is a ductless system that releases hormones into the bloodstream to help regulate body functions. The pituitary gland may be considered the conductor of the orchestra, because it stimulates many of the endocrine glands to secrete their powerful hormones. As mentioned in the previous chapter, all hormones, whether stimulated in this manner or by other control mechanisms, are interdependent. A change in the level of one hormone may affect the level of many other hormones. This fact makes the treatment of diseases or disorders of this system often very challenging. A hypersecretion of one gland may influence the secretion of another gland. It is therefore not uncommon for someone to have multiple disorders of the endocrine system.

This chapter reviews the individual glands and structures of the endocrine system and the effect that each has on the body individually and collectively. Your study of the "system of hormones" will result in a real appreciation for the critical role that the endocrine system plays in homeostasis and survival.

I—PITUITARY GLAND

Multiple Choice—select the best answer.

1. The pituitary is attached to the hypothalamus by a stalk called the:
   a. physis.
   b. infundibulum.
   c. pars intermedia.
   d. none of the above.

2. The vascular link between the hypothalamus and the adenohypophysis is called the:
   a. hypophyseal portal system.
   b. hepatic portal system.
   c. releasing hormone portal system.
   d. both a and c.

3. Which of the following links the nervous system with the endocrine system?
   a. pituitary
   b. pineal gland
   c. thalamus
   d. hypothalamus

4. Hypersecretion of prolactin can cause:
   a. insufficient milk production in nursing women.
   b. atrophy of breast tissue in non-nursing women.
   c. impotence in men.
   d. both a and b.

5. Psychosomatic and somatopsychic relationships between human body systems and the brain:
   a. are not believed to exist.
   b. are a real phenomenon.
   c. have a minimal effect on human physiology.
   d. none of the above.

Matching—identify each hormone with its corresponding function or description.

a. adrenocorticotropic hormone (ACTH)
b. antidiuretic hormone (ADH)
c. follicle-stimulating hormone (FSH)
d. growth hormone (GH)
e. luteinizing hormone (LH)
f. tropic hormone
g. oxytocin (OT)
h. prolactin (PRL)
i. thyroid-stimulating hormone (TSH)

6. _____ promotes development and secretion in the adrenal cortex

7. _____ promotes growth by stimulating protein anabolism and fat mobilization

8. _____ promotes development of ovarian follicles in females and sperm in males

9. _____ triggers ovulation in females and production of testosterone in males

10. _____ promotes milk secretion

11. _____ stimulates uterine contractions and milk ejection into mammary ducts

12. _____ stimulates the synthesis and secretion of target hormones

13. _____ stimulates development and secretion in the thyroid gland

14. _____ promotes water retention in kidney tubules

Labeling— using the terms provided, label the location and structure of the pituitary gland on the following illustration. Some terms may be used more than once.

pineal gland
adenohypophysis
nasal cavity
infundibulum
pituitary (hypophysis)
hypothalamus
third ventricle
thalamus

pars anterior
optic chiasma
neurohypophysis
pars intermedia
sella turcica (of sphenoid bone)
brainstem
mammillary body
pituitary diaphragm

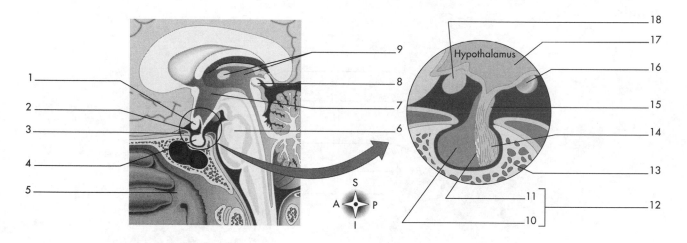

▶ *If you had difficulty with this section, review pages 563-571.*

II—PINEAL, THYROID, AND PARATHYROID GLANDS

Multiple Choice—select the best answer.

15. Which thyroid hormone is released in greatest quantity?
    a. T_3
    b. T_4
    c. triiodothyronine
    d. calcitonin

16. The principal thyroid hormone is:
    a. thyroxine.
    b. triiodothyronine.
    c. T_4.
    d. both a and c.

17. The two lobes of the thyroid are connected by the:
    a. infundibulum.
    b. isthmus.
    c. peninsula.
    d. islet.

18. High blood calcium levels can cause all of the following *except*:
    a. constipation.
    b. muscle spasms.
    c. lethargy.
    d. coma.

19. PTH increases calcium absorption in the intestines by activating:
    a. vitamin A.
    b. vitamin C.
    c. vitamin D.
    d. iron.

True or false

20. _____ Calcitonin in humans does not seem to have a great effect.

21. _____ The parathyroid glands are located on the anterior surface of the thyroid gland.

22. _____ Hypersecretion of thyroid hormone can cause Graves disease.

23. _____ The pineal gland functions to support the body's biological clock.

24. _____ The structural units of thyroid tissue are called *colloids*.

Labeling—label the following illustration showing the structure of the thyroid and parathyroid glands.

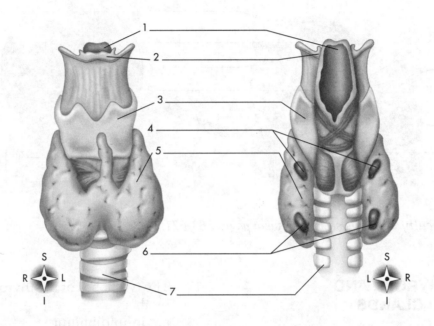

▶ *If you had difficulty with this section, review pages 571-577.*

III—ADRENAL GLANDS

Multiple Choice—select the best answer.

25. Which of the following hormones is *not* secreted by the adrenal cortex?
    a. aldosterone
    b. epinephrine
    c. adrenal androgens
    d. adrenal estrogens

26. Which of the following hormones is *not* secreted by the adrenal medulla?
    a. epinephrine
    b. norepinephrine
    c. adrenaline
    d. all of the above are secreted by adrenal medulla

27. The most physiologically important mineralocorticoid is:
    a. aldosterone.
    b. angiotensin II.
    c. renin.
    d. angiotensin I.

True or false

28. _____ The outer portion of the adrenal gland is called the *adrenal cortex.*

29. _____ Hypersecretion of cortisol from the adrenal cortex produces a collection of symptoms called *Addison disease.*

30. _____ The renin-angiotensin-aldosterone mechanism is a negative feedback mechanism that helps maintain homeostasis of blood pressure.

▶ *If you had difficulty with this section, review pages 577-580.*

IV—PANCREATIC ISLETS

Multiple Choice—select the best answer.

31. Glucagon functions to:
    a. promote the entry of glucose into cells.
    b. convert glucose into glycogen.
    c. increase blood glucose concentration.
    d. decrease blood glucose concentration.

32. Insulin functions to:
    a. decrease blood concentration of glucose, amino acids, and fatty acids.
    b. increase blood concentration of glucose, amino acids, and fatty acids.
    c. inhibit the secretion of growth hormone.
    d. both a and c.

True or false

33. _____ Somatostatin has the primary role of inhibiting the secretion of pancreatic hormones.

34. _____ Pancreatic polypeptide is the dominant pancreatic hormone in the regulation of blood glucose homeostasis.

Matching—identify each pancreatic islet cell type with its appropriate hormone secretion.

a. alpha cells
b. beta cells
c. delta cells
d. pancreatic polypeptide cells

35. _____ insulin
36. _____ somatostatin
37. _____ glucagon
38. _____ pancreatic polypeptide

▶ *If you had difficulty with this section, review pages 580-586.*

V—OTHER ENDOCRINE GLANDS AND TISSUES

Multiple Choice—select the best answer.

39. The major hormone produced by the corpus luteum is:
    a. progesterone.
    b. estrogen.
    c. human chorionic gonadotropin (hCG).
    d. none of the above.

40. Testosterone is produced by:
    a. seminiferous tubules.
    b. interstitial cells.
    c. LH.
    d. the scrotum.

41. The hormone that can be detected during the early part of a woman's pregnancy with an over-the-counter kit is:
    a. LH.
    b. estrogen.
    c. hCG.
    d. atrial natriuretic hormone (ANH).

True or false

42. _____ Thymosin is a major digestive hormone.

43. _____ ANH aids in the homeostasis of blood volume and blood pressure.

44. _____ Secretin plays a major regulatory role in the digestive process.

▶ *If you had difficulty with this section, review pages 586-587.*

VI—MECHANISMS OF DISEASE

Matching—identify the disease with its appropriate description.

a. hypersecretion of ACTH
b. lack of iodine
c. hypersecretion of thyroid hormone
d. hypersecretion of melatonin
e. hypersecretion of GH (adults)
f. extreme hyposecretion of thyroid (adult)
g. hyposecretion of estrogen in postmenopausal women
h. hyposecretion of adrenal cortex

45. _____ acromegaly
46. _____ Addison disease
47. _____ Cushing syndrome
48. _____ Graves disease
49. _____ myxedema
50. _____ osteoporosis
51. _____ simple goiter
52. _____ winter depression

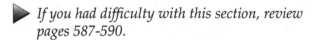 *If you had difficulty with this section, review pages 587-590.*

Crossword Puzzle

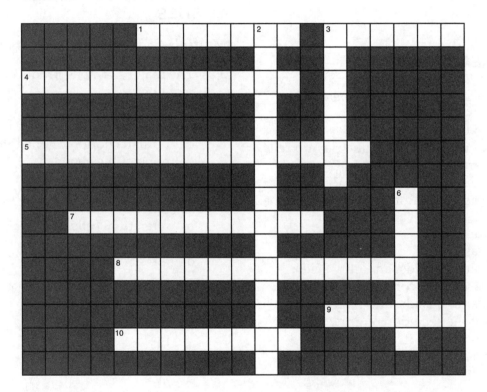

Across
1. Secreted by endocrine system
3. Located in the mediastinum beneath the sternum
4. Directly regulates the secretion of the "master gland"
5. Anterior pituitary
7. Secretes parathormone
8. Has a stimulating effect on other endocrine glands (two words)
9. Primary sex organs
10. Causes milk ejection from breasts of lactating women

Down
2. Posterior pituitary gland
3. Secretes thyroxin
6. Secretes aldosterone

APPLYING WHAT YOU KNOW

53. After a visit with the doctor, Amanda and Bill were elated to learn of the high levels of hCG in Amanda's urine. Why would this couple be so delighted? Which organ produced this hormone in her body and what is its function?

54. Dania has been experiencing excessive thirst, hunger, and copious urination. Which endocrine system syndrome may she be experiencing? What are the actual physiologic mechanisms that are causing her symptoms? How is she most likely to be treated?

DID YOU KNOW

- The total daily output of the pituitary gland is less than 1/1,000,000 of a gram, yet this small amount is responsible for stimulating the majority of all endocrine functions.

- The endocrine system is one of the primary means by which the body translates emotions into physical responses, such as love.

ONE LAST QUICK CHECK

Multiple Choice—select the best answer.

55. What does the outer zone of the adrenal cortex secrete?
    a. mineralocorticoids
    b. sex hormones
    c. glucocorticoids
    d. epinephrine

56. From what condition does diabetes insipidus result?
    a. low insulin levels
    b. high glucagon levels
    c. low antidiuretic hormone levels
    d. high steroid levels

57. Which of the following statements is true regarding a young child whose growth is stunted, metabolism is low, sexual development is delayed, and mental development is retarded?
    a. The child may suffer from cretinism.
    b. The child may have an underactive thyroid.
    c. Profound manifestations of the described condition may result in deformed dwarfism.
    d. All of the above.

58. What can result when too much growth hormone is produced by the pituitary gland?
    a. hyperglycemia
    b. a pituitary giant
    c. both a and b
    d. none of the above

59. Which of the following glands is/are *not* regulated by the pituitary?
    a. thyroid
    b. ovaries
    c. adrenals
    d. thymus

60. Which of the following statements about the antidiuretic hormone is true?
    a. It is released by the posterior lobe of the pituitary.
    b. It causes diabetes insipidus when produced in insufficient amounts.
    c. It decreases urine volume.
    d. All of the above.

61. What controls the development of the body's immune system?
    a. pituitary
    b. thymus
    c. pineal body
    d. thyroid

62. Administration of which of the following would best treat a person suffering from rheumatoid arthritis?
    a. gonadocorticoids
    b. glucagon
    c. mineralocorticoids
    d. glucocorticoids

63. Which endocrine gland is composed of cell clusters called the *islets of Langerhans*?
    a. adrenals
    b. thyroid
    c. pituitary
    d. pancreas

64. The normal adrenal cortex secretes small amounts of _____.
    a. epinephrine
    b. androgens
    c. ADH
    d. hCG

Matching—select the most correct answer for each item (only one answer is correct).

a. glucocorticoid hormones
b. antidiuretic hormone
c. mineralocorticoid
d. oxytocin
e. growth hormone
f. placenta
g. luteinizing hormone
h. insulin
i. prolactin
j. thyroid hormones

65. _____ goiter

66. _____ ovulation

67. _____ diabetes mellitus

68. _____ lactation

69. _____ diabetes insipidus

70. _____ human chorionic gonadotropin

71. _____ Cushing syndrome

72. _____ labor

73. _____ acromegaly

74. _____ aldosterone

CHAPTER 20

Blood

Blood, the river of life, is the body's primary means of transportation. Although it is the respiratory system that provides oxygen for the body, the digestive system that provides nutrients, and the urinary system that eliminates wastes, none of these functions could be provided for the individual cells without the blood. In less than 1 minute, a drop of blood will complete a trip through the entire body, distributing nutrients and collecting the wastes of metabolism.

Blood is divided into plasma (the liquid portion of blood) and the formed elements (the blood cells). There are three types of blood cells: red blood cells, white blood cells, and platelets. Together these cells and plasma provide a means of transportation that delivers the body's daily necessities.

Although all of us have red blood cells that are similar in shape, we have different blood types. Blood types are identified by the presence of certain antigens in the red blood cells. Every person's blood belongs to one of four main blood groups: Type A, B, AB, or O. Any one of the four groups or "types" may or may not have the Rh factor present in the red blood cells. If an individual has a specific antigen called the *Rh factor* present in his or her blood, the blood is Rh positive. If this factor is missing, the blood is Rh negative. Approximately 85% of the population have the Rh factor (Rh positive) while 15% do not have the Rh factor (Rh negative).

Your understanding of this chapter is necessary to prepare a proper foundation for the study of the circulatory system.

I—COMPOSITION OF BLOOD AND RED BLOOD CELLS

Multiple Choice—select the best answer.

1. The composition of blood is:
   a. 55% plasma, 45% formed elements.
   b. 45% plasma, 55% formed elements.
   c. 50% plasma, 50% formed elements.
   d. none of the above.

2. A hematocrit of 45% means that in every
    100 mL of whole blood:
    a. there are 45 mL of red blood cells and
        55 mL of plasma.
    b. there are 45 mL of plasma and 55 mL
        of red blood cells.
    c. 45% of the formed elements are red
        blood cells.
    d. plasma is 45% of the circulating whole
        blood.

3. Reduced red blood cell numbers cause:
    a. polycythemia.
    b. buffy coat.
    c. anemia.
    d. both a and c.

4. Which of the following formed elements
    carry oxygen?
    a. leukocytes
    b. erythrocytes
    c. thrombocytes
    d. monocytes

5. All formed elements arise from which
    stem cell?
    a. proerythroblast
    b. megakaryoblast
    c. lymphoblast
    d. hemocytoblast

True or false

6. _____ *Hematocrit* and *packed cell volume
    (PCV)* are synonymous terms.

7. _____ A reticulocyte count can indicate
    to a physician the rate of leuko-
    cyte formation.

8. _____ Oxygen deficiency increases RBC
    numbers by increasing the secre-
    tion of erythropoietin by the kid-
    neys.

9. _____ The life span of circulating RBCs
    is about 10 to 12 days.

10. _____ Heme is broken down into iron
    and amino acids for use in the
    synthesis of new RBCs.

▶ *If you had difficulty with this section, review
pages 597-605.*

II—WHITE BLOOD CELLS AND PLATELETS

*Matching—identify each term with its corre-
sponding description.*

a. agranulocytes
b. basophils
c. eosinophils
d. granulocytes
e. leukocytes
f. lymphocytes
g. megakaryocytes
h. monocytes
i. neutrophils
j. platelets

11. _____ classification of leukocytes that
    contain cytoplasmic granules

12. _____ most numerous leukocytes

13. _____ granulocytes that release heparin
    and histamine

14. _____ granulocytes that protect against
    infections from parasitic worms
    and allergic reactions

15. _____ agranulocytes that produce anti-
    bodies

16. _____ agranulocytes that enter tissue
    spaces as macrophages

17. _____ cell fragments that function in
    blood clotting and hemostasis

18. _____ cells from which platelets are
    formed

19. _____ classification of leukocytes with-
    out cytoplasmic granules

20. _____ classification of formed elements
    that are nucleated cells lacking
    hemoglobin

▶ *If you had difficulty with this section, review
pages 605-609.*

Human Blood Cells

Fill in the missing areas of the table.

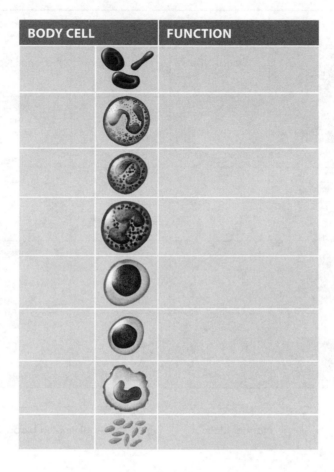

BODY CELL	FUNCTION

III—BLOOD TYPES

Multiple Choice—select the best answer.

21. A person with antibody A in his or her plasma would have which blood type?
    a. type A
    b. type B
    c. type AB
    d. type O

22. People with type O blood are considered to be universal donors because their blood contains:
    a. neither A nor B antigens on their RBCs.
    b. both A and B antigens in their blood plasma.
    c. the Rh antigen on their RBCs.
    d. none of the above.

23. A blood type and crossmatch is performed prior to transfusion. If this procedure is *not* completed:
    a. the blood may agglutinate.
    b. blood lysis may occur.
    c. a transfusion reaction may occur.
    d. all of the above.

True or false

24. _____ Type AB blood is considered to be the universal recipient.

25. _____ Type AB blood contains both the A and B antibodies in its plasma.

26. _____ Most blood contains the anti-Rh antibodies.

▶ *If you had difficulty with this section, review pages 609-613.*

Blood typing—Using the key below, draw the appropriate reaction with the donor's blood in the circles.

Recipient's blood		Reactions with donor's blood			
RBC antigens	Plasma antibodies	Donor type O	Donor type A	Donor type B	Donor type AB
None (Type O)	Anti-A Anti-B	◯	◯	◯	◯
A (Type A)	Anti-B	◯	◯	◯	◯
B (Type B)	Anti-A	◯	◯	◯	◯
AB (Type AB)	(none)	◯	◯	◯	◯

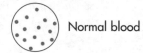 Normal blood   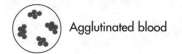 Agglutinated blood

IV—BLOOD PLASMA

True or false

27. _____ Plasma is a pale yellow fluid that accounts for more than half of the blood volume.

28. _____ Serum is whole blood minus the clotting elements.

29. _____ Synthesis of plasma proteins occurs in the spleen.

▶ *If you had difficulty with this section, review pages 613-614.*

V—BLOOD CLOTTING

Multiple Choice—select the best answer.

30. Which of the following is *not* a critical component of coagulation?
    a. thrombin
    b. fibrinolysis
    c. fibrinogen
    d. fibrin

31. For prothrombin to be synthesized by the liver, an adequate amount of which vitamin is required?
    a. vitamin A
    b. vitamin C
    c. vitamin D
    d. vitamin K

32. Which of the following does *not* hasten clotting?
    a. rough spot in the endothelium
    b. abnormally slow blood flow
    c. heparin
    d. all of the above hasten clotting

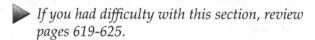 *If you had difficulty with this section, review pages 614-619.*

VI—MECHANISMS OF DISEASE

Fill in the blanks.

33. _____ is an excess of RBCs.

34. _____ _____ often results from the destruction of bone marrow by drugs, toxic chemicals, or radiation.

35. An anemia resulting from a dietary deficiency of vitamin B_{12} is _____ _____.

36. An example of a hemolytic anemia is _____ _____ _____.

37. _____ refers to an abnormally low WBC count.

38. A(n) _____ is a stationary clot.

39. A circulating clot is a(n) _____.

40. _____ is a type of X-linked inherited disorder that results from a failure to form blood-clotting factor VIII, IX, or XI.

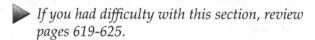 *If you had difficulty with this section, review pages 619-625.*

Crossword Puzzle

Across
2. Liquid portion of blood
4. WBC
7. Thrombocyte
8. Blood cells (two words)
10. Least numerous of the WBCs
12. RBC formation
13. Oxygen-carrying mechanism of blood
14. Largest of the leukocytes

Down
1. Movement of formed elements through a vessel wall
3. Agglutinogen
5. RBC
6. 65% of WBCs
9. 2-5% of circulating WBCs
11. Agglutinin

APPLYING WHAT YOU KNOW

41. Pepper is an elite competitive cyclist who wanted to gain a physiologic advantage over his competitors. He decided to have his own blood drawn and stored so that it could be infused into him prior to competition. What is the theory behind this practice? How effective is this procedure?

42. Mrs. Shearer's blood type is O positive. Her husband's type is O negative. Her newborn baby's blood type is O negative. Is there any need for concern with this combination?

43. After Mrs. Wiedeke's baby was born, the doctor applied a gauze dressing for a short time on the umbilical cord. He also gave the baby a dose of vitamin K. Why did the doctor perform these two procedures?

DID YOU KNOW

• In the second it takes to turn the page of a book, you will lose about 3 million red blood cells. During that same second, your bone marrow will have produced the same number of new ones.

• There is enough iron in a human to make a small nail.

✓ ONE LAST QUICK CHECK

Multiple Choice—select the best answer.

44. Which of the following statements is *false*?
    a. Sickle cell anemia is caused by a genetic defect.
    b. Leukemia is characterized by a low number of WBCs.
    c. Polycythemia is characterized by an abnormally high number of erythrocytes.
    d. Pernicious anemia is caused by a lack of vitamin B_{12}.

45. Deficiency in the number or function of erythrocytes is called:
    a. leukemia.
    b. anemia.
    c. polycythemia.
    d. leukopenia.

46. Which of the following statements does *not* describe a characteristic of leukocytes?
    a. They are disc-shaped cells that do not contain a nucleus.
    b. They have the ability to fight infection.
    c. They provide defense against certain parasites.
    d. They provide immune defense.

47. Which of the following substances is *not* found in serum?
    a. clotting factors
    b. water
    c. hormones
    d. all of the above are found in serum

48. Which of the following substances is *not* found in blood plasma?
    a. water
    b. oxygen
    c. hormones
    d. all of the above are found in blood plasma

49. An allergic reaction may increase the number of:
    a. eosinophils.
    b. neutrophils.
    c. lymphocytes.
    d. monocytes.

50. What is a blood clot that is moving through the body called?
    a. embolism
    b. fibrosis
    c. heparin
    d. thrombosis

51. When could difficulty with the Rh blood factor arise?
    a. Rh-negative man and woman produce a child.
    b. Rh-positive man and woman produce a child.
    c. Rh-positive woman and an Rh-negative man produce a child.
    d. Rh-negative woman and an Rh-positive man produce a child.

52. What is the primary function of hemoglobin?
    a. fight infection
    b. produce blood clots
    c. carry oxygen
    d. transport hormones

53. Are any of the following steps *not* involved in blood clot formation?
    a. A blood vessel is injured and platelet factors are formed.
    b. Thrombin is converted into prothrombin.
    c. Fibrinogen is converted into fibrin.
    d. All of the above are involved in blood clot formation.

Matching—select the most correct answer for each item.

a. heparin
b. contains anti-A and anti-B antibodies
c. clotting
d. immunity
e. erythroblastosis fetalis
f. anemia
g. cancer
h. contains A and B antigens
i. thin, white layer of leukocytes and platelets
j. phagocytosis
k. volume percent of RBCs in whole blood
l. decrease in WBCs

54. _____ lymphocytes

55. _____ erythrocyte disorder

56. _____ type AB

57. _____ basophils

58. _____ leukemia

59. _____ platelets

60. _____ type O

61. _____ Rh factor

62. _____ buffy coat

63. _____ neutrophils

64. _____ leukopenia

65. _____ hematocrit

CHAPTER 21

Anatomy of the Cardiovascular System

The heart is actually two pumps—one moves blood to the lungs, the other pushes it out into the body. These two functions seem rather elementary in comparison to the complex and numerous functions performed by most of the other body organs, and yet if this pump stops, within a few short minutes, life ceases.

The heart is divided into two upper compartments called *atria*, or receiving chambers, and two lower compartments, or discharging chambers, called *ventricles*. By age 45, approximately 300,000 tons of blood will have passed through these chambers to be circulated to the blood vessels. This closed system of circulation provides distribution of blood to the entire body (systemic circulation) and to specific regions, such as the pulmonary circulation or coronary circulation.

One hundred thousand miles of blood vessels make up the elaborate transportation system that circulates materials for energy, growth, and repair, and eliminates wastes from your body. These vessels are called *arteries, veins,* and *capillaries* (which are exchange vessels, or connecting links, between the arteries and veins). The pumping action of the heart keeps blood moving through the closed system of vessels. This closed system of circulation provides distribution of blood to the entire body and to specific regions such as the pulmonary circulation or hepatic portal circulation. Your review of the anatomy of this system will provide you with an understanding of the complex transportation mechanism necessary to provide oxygen and nutrients to our tissues.

I—HEART

Multiple Choice—select the best answer.

1. The visceral pericardium is found:
   a. inside the fibrous pericardium.
   b. adhering to the surface of the heart.
   c. lining the inside of the chambers of the heart.
   d. comprising the bulk of the heart tissue.

2. The correct layers of the heart, from superficial to deep, are:
   a. myocardium, pericardium, endocardium.
   b. epicardium, myocardium, pericardium.
   c. epicardium, myocardium, endocardium.
   d. endocardium, myocardium, epicardium.

3. The atrioventricular valves are also called:
    a. cuspid valves.
    b. semilunar valves.
    c. aortic valves.
    d. pulmonary valves.

4. Respectively, the right and left atrioventricular valves are also referred to as:
    a. tricuspid, mitral.
    b. bicuspid, tricuspid.
    c. mitral, bicuspid.
    d. bicuspid, mitral.

5. Semilunar valves prevent backflow of blood into the:
    a. atria.
    b. lungs.
    c. vena cava.
    d. ventricles.

6. The most abundant blood supply goes to the:
    a. right atrium.
    b. right ventricle.
    c. left atrium.
    d. left ventricle.

7. Branching of an artery as it progresses from proximal to distal is called:
    a. ischemia.
    b. infarction.
    c. anastomosis.
    d. both a and c.

8. The cavity of the heart that normally has the thickest wall is the:
    a. right atrium.
    b. right ventricle.
    c. left atrium.
    d. left ventricle.

9. Which of the following is a semilunar valve?
    a. aortic
    b. pulmonary
    c. mitral
    d. both a and b

10. The pacemaker of the heart is/are the:
    a. AV bundle.
    b. SA node.
    c. bundle of His.
    d. Purkinje fibers.

Labeling

11. Trace the blood flow through the heart by numbering the following structures in the correct sequence. Start with number 1 for the vena cava and proceed until you have numbered all the structures.

_____ right atrioventricular (tricuspid) valve

_____ pulmonary veins

_____ pulmonary arteries

_____ pulmonary semilunar valve

_____ left atrioventricular (mitral) valve

_____ left ventricle

_____ vena cava

_____ right atrium

_____ right ventricle

_____ left atrium

_____ aorta

_____ aortic semilunar valve

Labeling—using the terms provided, label the following illustration of the heart. Some terms may be used more than once.

openings to coronary arteries	interventricular septum
aorta	aortic (SL) valve
right atrium	chordae tendineae
pulmonary veins	papillary muscle
right AV (tricuspid) valve	pulmonary trunk
left AV (mitral) valve	superior vena cava
left ventricle	left atrium
right ventricle	

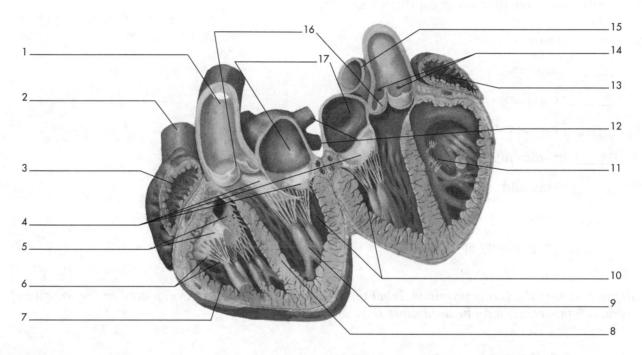

▶ *If you had difficulty with this section, review pages 629-642.*

Fill in the blanks.

12. A noninvasive technique for evaluating the internal structures and motions of the heart and great vessels is known as

_____ .

13. Increased serum levels in the blood are often indicative of a recent myocardial infarction. These levels are monitored by blood tests known as _____

_____ _____ .

14. Vagus fibers to the heart serve as

_____ or _____ nerves.

15. Rhythmic compressions of the heart combined with effective artificial respiration in cases of cardiac arrest are known as

_____

_____ .

▶ *If you had difficulty with this section, review pages 629-642.*

II—BLOOD VESSELS

Matching—identify the term with the proper selection.

a. smooth muscle cells that guard the entrance to capillaries
b. carry blood to the heart
c. carry blood into the venules
d. carry blood away from the heart
e. outermost layers of arteries and veins
f. capillary that has a large lumen and more tortuous course than other capillary vessels
g. endothelium

16. _____ arteries

17. _____ capillaries

18. _____ tunica externa

19. _____ tunica intima

20. _____ sinusoid

21. _____ veins

22. _____ precapillary sphincters

True or false

23. _____ Veins are the only blood vessels to contain semilunar valves.

24. _____ The walls of veins are much thicker than arteries.

25. _____ Arteries become progressively smaller as blood flows away from the heart and into branches feeding other areas of the body.

26. _____ Arteries are often referred to as *capacitance vessels*.

Labeling—using the terms provided, label the structure of blood vessels depicted in the following diagram. Some terms may be used more than once.

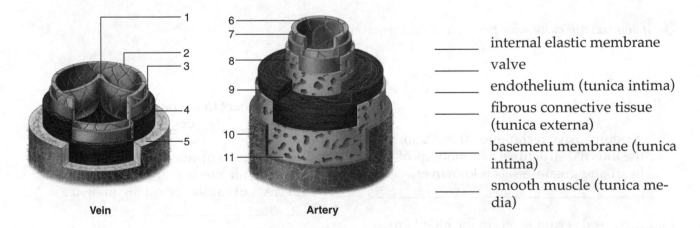

Vein   Artery

_____ internal elastic membrane

_____ valve

_____ endothelium (tunica intima)

_____ fibrous connective tissue (tunica externa)

_____ basement membrane (tunica intima)

_____ smooth muscle (tunica media)

▶ *If you had difficulty with this section, review pages 642-647.*

III—MAJOR BLOOD VESSELS

Multiple Choice—select the best answer.

27. The aorta carries blood out of the:
    a. right atrium.
    b. right ventricle.
    c. left atrium.
    d. left ventricle.

28. The superior vena cava returns blood to the:
    a. left atrium.
    b. left ventricle.
    c. right atrium.
    d. right ventricle.

29. Blood returns from the lungs during pulmonary circulation via the:
    a. pulmonary artery.
    b. pulmonary veins.
    c. aorta.
    d. inferior vena cava.

30. The hepatic portal circulation serves the body by:
    a. removing excess glucose and storing it in the liver as glycogen.
    b. detoxifying blood.
    c. assisting the body to maintain proper blood glucose.
    d. all of the above.

31. The structure used to bypass the liver in the fetal circulation is the:
    a. foramen ovale.
    b. ductus venosus.
    c. ductus arteriosus.
    d. umbilical vein.

32. The foramen ovale serves the fetal circulation by:
    a. connecting the aorta and the pulmonary artery.
    b. shunting blood from the right atrium directly into the left atrium.
    c. bypassing the liver.
    d. bypassing the lungs.

33. The structure used to connect the aorta and pulmonary artery in the fetal circulation is the:
    a. ductus arteriosus.
    b. ductus venosus.
    c. aorta.
    d. foramen ovale.

34. Which of the following is *not* an artery?
    a. femoral
    b. popliteal
    c. coronary
    d. inferior vena cava

Fill in the blanks.

35. Blood flow from the heart to all parts of the body and back again is known as _____ _____.

36. Small vessels join the anterior and posterior arteries to form an arterial circle at the base of the brain known as the _____ _____ _____.

37. _____ are the ultimate extensions of capillaries.

38. When blood is in the capillaries of abdominal digestive organs, it must flow through the _____ _____ _____.

39. If either hepatic portal circulation or venous return from the liver is interfered with, a condition known as _____ may occur.

40. Two _____ _____ carry circulation to the placenta and one _____ _____ returns blood from the placenta.

41. Many arteries have corresponding _____ with the same name.

Labeling—match each term with its corresponding number on the following illustration of the principal veins of the body. Some terms may be used more than once.

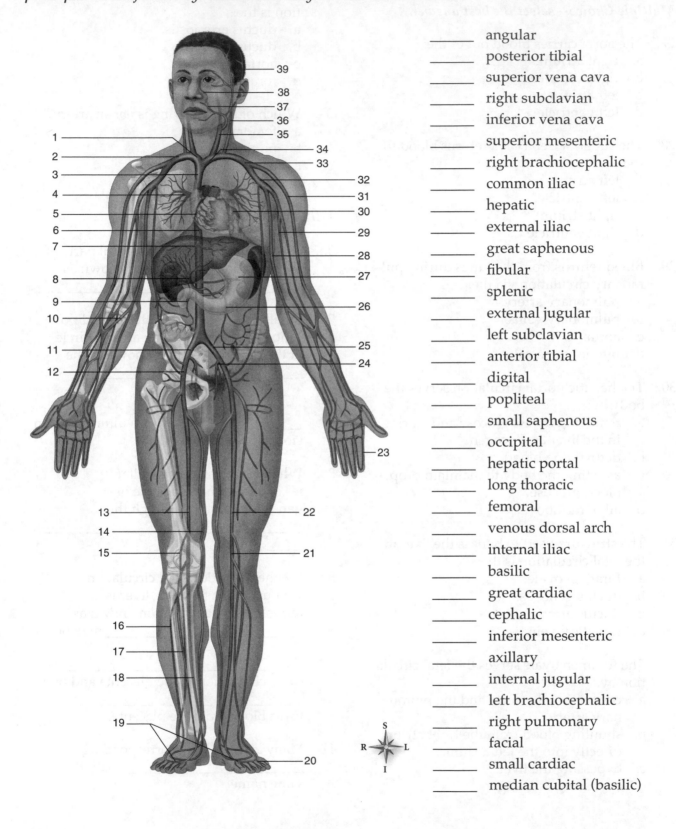

_____ angular
_____ posterior tibial
_____ superior vena cava
_____ right subclavian
_____ inferior vena cava
_____ superior mesenteric
_____ right brachiocephalic
_____ common iliac
_____ hepatic
_____ external iliac
_____ great saphenous
_____ fibular
_____ splenic
_____ external jugular
_____ left subclavian
_____ anterior tibial
_____ digital
_____ popliteal
_____ small saphenous
_____ occipital
_____ hepatic portal
_____ long thoracic
_____ femoral
_____ venous dorsal arch
_____ internal iliac
_____ basilic
_____ great cardiac
_____ cephalic
_____ inferior mesenteric
_____ axillary
_____ internal jugular
_____ left brachiocephalic
_____ right pulmonary
_____ facial
_____ small cardiac
_____ median cubital (basilic)

Labeling—match each term with its corresponding number on the following illustration of the principal arteries of the body. Some terms may be used more than once.

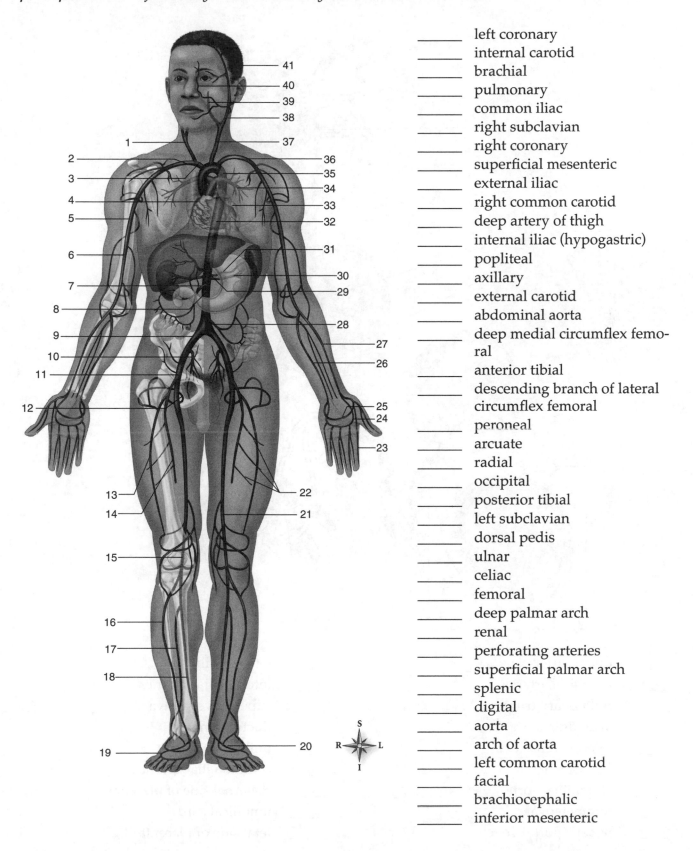

_____ left coronary
_____ internal carotid
_____ brachial
_____ pulmonary
_____ common iliac
_____ right subclavian
_____ right coronary
_____ superficial mesenteric
_____ external iliac
_____ right common carotid
_____ deep artery of thigh
_____ internal iliac (hypogastric)
_____ popliteal
_____ axillary
_____ external carotid
_____ abdominal aorta
_____ deep medial circumflex femoral
_____ anterior tibial
_____ descending branch of lateral circumflex femoral
_____ peroneal
_____ arcuate
_____ radial
_____ occipital
_____ posterior tibial
_____ left subclavian
_____ dorsal pedis
_____ ulnar
_____ celiac
_____ femoral
_____ deep palmar arch
_____ renal
_____ perforating arteries
_____ superficial palmar arch
_____ splenic
_____ digital
_____ aorta
_____ arch of aorta
_____ left common carotid
_____ facial
_____ brachiocephalic
_____ inferior mesenteric

Labeling—match each term with its corresponding number on the following depiction of fetal circulation.

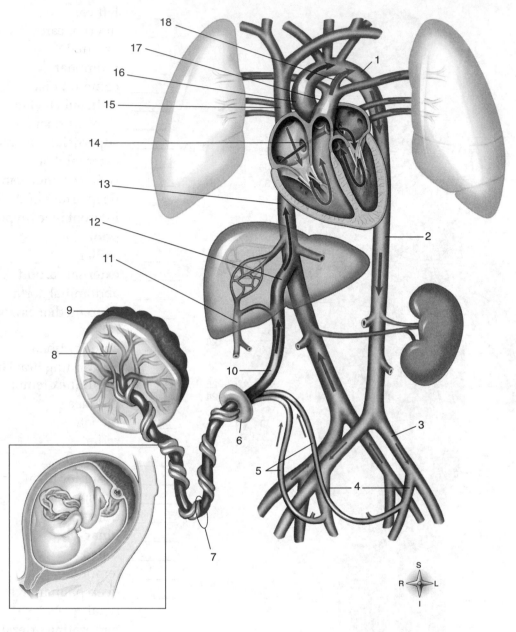

_____ ductus arteriosus

_____ umbilical arteries

_____ pulmonary trunk

_____ ascending aorta

_____ inferior vena cava

_____ aortic arch

_____ abdominal aorta

_____ foramen ovale

_____ hepatic portal vein

_____ fetal umbilicus

_____ internal iliac arteries

_____ superior vena cava

_____ ductus venosus

_____ umbilical vein

_____ common iliac arteries

_____ maternal side of placenta

_____ umbilical cord

_____ fetal side of placenta

Labeling—match each term with its corresponding number on this diagram of the hepatic portal circulation.

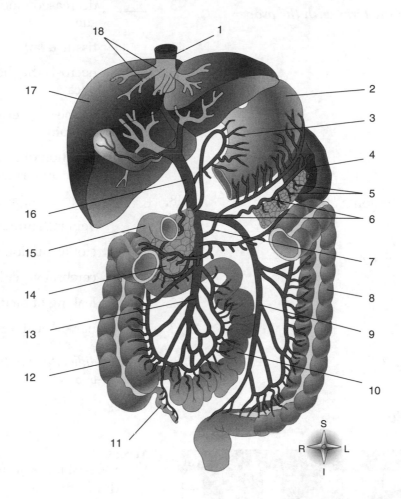

_____	liver	
_____	gastric vein	
_____	appendix	
_____	pancreas	
_____	hepatic veins	
_____	inferior vena cava	
_____	stomach	
_____	spleen	
_____	hepatic portal vein	

_____ superior mesenteric vein
_____ duodenum
_____ pancreatic vein
_____ splenic vein
_____ gastroepiploic vein
_____ descending colon
_____ inferior mesenteric vein
_____ small intestine
_____ ascending colon

▶ *If you had difficulty with this section, review pages 647-669.*

IV—MECHANISMS OF DISEASE

Matching—identify the term with the proper selection.

a. atherosclerosis
b. ischemia
c. aneurysm
d. necrosis
e. gangrene
f. hemorrhoids
g. phlebitis
h. stroke
i. myocardial infarction
j. thrombus
k. stenosed valves
l. mitral valve prolapse

42. _____ heart attack
43. _____ decreased blood supply to a tissue
44. _____ tissue death
45. _____ necrosis that has progressed to decay
46. _____ a type of arteriosclerosis caused by lipids
47. _____ a section of an artery that has become abnormally widened
48. _____ varicose veins in the rectum
49. _____ vein inflammation
50. _____ clot formation
51. _____ cerebral vascular accident
52. _____ leaking of bicuspid valve
53. _____ narrower-than-normal valve

▶ *If you had difficulty with this section, review pages 669-676.*

Crossword Puzzle

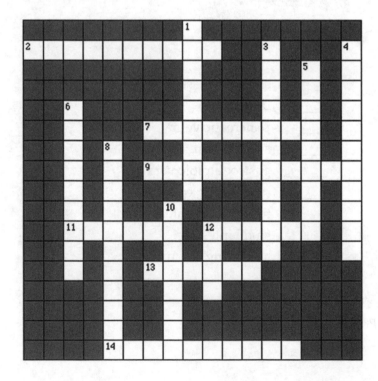

Across
2. Visceral layer of the serous pericardium
7. "Pumping chamber" of the heart
9. Membrane that surrounds the heart
11. Carries blood away from the heart
12. Small vein
13. "Receiving chamber" of the heart
14. Muscle of the heart

Down
1. _____ circulation (blood flow to lungs and back)
3. Delicate interior layer of the heart
4. Provides collateral circulation to a part
5. Small artery
6. Connects arterioles to venules
8. Cells that line the circulatory system
10. _____ circulation (blood flow throughout the system)
12. Vessel that returns blood to the heart

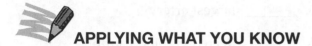

APPLYING WHAT YOU KNOW

54. Mr. Shearer was admitted to the emergency department with severe swelling in his extremities, difficulty breathing, and elevated blood pressure. His doctor advised him that he had "left-sided heart failure." What is the other name for this condition and could you elaborate on the possible serious outcome of this diagnosis if Mr. Shearer does not respond to this treatment?

55. Else was experiencing angina pectoris. Her doctor suggested a surgical procedure that would require the removal of a vein from another region of her body. What is the name of this surgical procedure?

56. Mr. Wertz called his doctor and informed him that during the night he had experienced some "heartburn" and "night sweats." His wife had insisted that he call the doctor even though he felt better. Mr. Wertz's doctor ordered bloodwork to be done and was not surprised when the serum levels of CPK, AST, and LDH came back elevated. How would you explain this elevation in blood serum levels?

DID YOU KNOW

* Your heart pumps more than 5 quarts of blood every minute… That's 2000 gallons a day!

* Capillaries are so small that it takes 10 of them to equal the thickness of a human hair.

* In one day, the blood travels a total of 12,000 miles… That's four times the distance across the U.S. from coast to coast!

ONE LAST QUICK CHECK

Multiple Choice—select the best answer.

57. The superior vena cava carries blood to the:
    a. left ventricle.
    b. coronary arteries.
    c. right atrium.
    d. pulmonary veins.

58. Which of the following statements is *false* regarding pericarditis?
    a. It may be caused by infection or trauma.
    b. It often causes severe chest pain.
    c. It may result in impairment of the pumping action of the heart.
    d. All of the above statements are true.

59. The outside covering that surrounds and protects the heart is called the:
    a. endocardium.
    b. myocardium.
    c. pericardium.
    d. ectocardium.

60. A valve that permits blood to flow from the right ventricle into the pulmonary artery is called the:
    a. tricuspid.
    b. mitral.
    c. aortic semilunar.
    d. pulmonary semilunar.

61. Hemorrhoids can best be described as:
    a. varicose veins.
    b. varicose veins in the rectum.
    c. thrombophlebitis of the rectum.
    d. clot formation in the rectum.

62. A common type of vascular disease that occludes arteries by lipids and other substances is:
    a. an aneurysm.
    b. atherosclerosis.
    c. varicose veins.
    d. thrombophlebitis.

Matching—select the most appropriate answer for each item (there is only one correct answer for each item).

a. ischemia
b. phlebitis
c. foramen ovale
d. aneurysm
e. vena cava
f. angioplasty
g. aorta
h. pulmonary
i. great saphenous vein
j. heart attack

63. _____ largest artery

64. _____ decreased blood supply

65. _____ leg vein

66. _____ fetal circulation

67. _____ arterial procedure

68. _____ vein inflammation

69. _____ lung circulation

70. _____ weakened artery

71. _____ large vein that returns venous blood to the heart

72. _____ myocardial infarction

CHAPTER 22

Physiology of the Cardiovascular System

The beating of the heart must be coordinated in a rhythmic manner if the heart is to pump effectively. That is achieved by electrical impulses that are stimulated by specialized structures embedded in the walls of the heart. The sinoatrial (SA) node, atrioventricular (AV) node, bundle of His, and Purkinje fibers combine efforts to produce the tiny electrical currents necessary to contract the heart. A healthy heart is necessary to pump blood throughout the body to nourish and oxygenate cells continuously. Any interruption or failure of this system may result in serious pathology.

Blood pressure is the force of blood in the vessels. This force is highest in the arteries and lowest in the veins. Normal blood pressure varies among individuals and depends upon the volume of blood in the arteries. The larger the volume of blood in the arteries, the more pressure is exerted on the walls of the arteries and the higher the arterial pressure. Conversely, the less blood in the arteries, the lower the blood pressure.

A functional cardiovascular system is vital for survival because without circulation, tissues would lack a supply of oxygen and nutrients. Waste products would begin to accumulate and could become toxic. Your review of this system will provide you with an understanding of the complex transportation mechanism of the body necessary for survival.

I—HEMODYNAMICS AND THE HEART AS A PUMP

1. Under resting conditions, the SA node fires at an intrinsic rhythmic rate of:
   a. 65 to 70 beats per minute.
   b. 70 to 75 beats per minute.
   c. 75 to 80 beats per minute.
   d. 80 to 85 beats per minute.

2. The normal pattern of impulse conduction through the heart is:
   a. AV node, SA node, AV bundle, Purkinje fibers.
   b. SA node, AV node, AV bundle, Purkinje fibers.
   c. AV bundle, AV node, SA node, Purkinje fibers.
   d. AV node, SA node, Purkinje fibers, AV bundle.

3. An ECG P wave represents:
    a. depolarization of the atria.
    b. repolarization of the atria.
    c. depolarization of the ventricles.
    d. repolarization of the ventricles.

4. Repolarization of the atria is:
    a. clearly depicted by the QRS complex.
    b. masked by the massive ventricular de-
        polarization.
    c. masked by the massive ventricular re-
        polarization.
    d. none of the above.

5. Contraction of the ventricles produces:
    a. the first heart sound (lub).
    b. the second heart sound (dupp).
    c. both of these.
    d. none of these.

True or false

6. _____ The contraction phase of the car-
    diac cycle is referred to as *systole*.

7. _____ Pacemakers other than the SA
    node are abnormal and are usu-
    ally *apical pacemakers*.

8. _____ The QRS complex represents re-
    polarization of the ventricles.

9. _____ *Rapid ejection* is characterized by
    a marked increase in ventricular
    and aortic pressure and in aortic
    blood flow.

10. _____ Isovolumetric ventricular con-
    traction occurs between the start
    of ventricular systole and the
    opening of the semilunar valves.

Labeling—label the following ECG deflection waves.

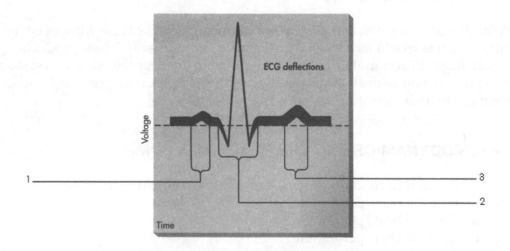

If you had difficulty with this section, review pages 681-690.

II—CIRCULATION AND BLOOD PRESSURE

Multiple Choice—select the best answer.

11. Blood pressure at the venae cavae and right atrium is:
    a. 120 mm Hg.
    b. 100 mm Hg.
    c. 80 mm Hg.
    d. 0 mm Hg.

12. Starling's law of the heart states that:
    a. blood flows from areas of high pressure to areas of low pressure.
    b. the volume of blood ejected from the ventricle is constant.
    c. the more stretched the heart fibers are at the beginning of a contraction, the stronger is their contraction.
    d. average heart rate is 72 beats per minute.

13. Parasympathetic control of the heart involves the:
    a. glossopharyngeal nerve (cranial nerve IX).
    b. vagus nerve (cranial nerve X).
    c. carotid sinus.
    d. aortic sinus.

14. The vagus nerve is said to act as a(n) _____ on the heart.
    a. temperature monitor
    b. positive feedback loop
    c. ejection mechanism
    d. brake

15. Under normal conditions, blood viscosity changes:
    a. frequently.
    b. during hemorrhage only.
    c. under stress.
    d. very little.

16. A dominance of sympathetic impulses increases heart rate and stroke volume and constricts reservoir vessels in response to:
    a. decreased O_2, increased CO_2, and/or decreased pH.
    b. increased O_2, increased CO_2, and/or decreased pH.
    c. decreased O_2, decreased CO_2, and/or decreased pH.
    d. decreased O_2, increased CO_2, and/or increased pH.

17. The difference between systolic and diastolic pressure is called:
    a. bruit pressure.
    b. pulse pressure.
    c. laminar pressure.
    d. none of the above.

18. The popliteal pulse point is found:
    a. at the bend of the elbow.
    b. on the dorsum of the foot.
    c. behind the knee.
    d. behind the medial malleolus.

19. Peripheral resistance is primarily affected by:
    a. the length of myocardial fibers.
    b. blood viscosity and the diameter of arterioles.
    c. the capacity of the blood reservoirs.
    d. the elasticity of the heart.

20. At rest, most of the body's blood supply resides in the:
    a. pulmonary loop.
    b. systemic arteries and arterioles.
    c. capillaries.
    d. systemic veins and venules.

True or false

21. _____ Stroke volume is determined by multiplying cardiac output and heart rate.

22. _____ A slow and weakly beating heart tends to have a decreased cardiac output.

23. _____ Starling's law operates in humans as a major regulator of stroke volume under ordinary conditions.

24. _____ Cardiac output can increase from 5 to 6 L/min during strenuous exercise.

25. _____ Skeletal muscle is of minor consequence in venous blood return to the heart.

26. _____ The fluid that leaves the capillaries at the arterial end is eventually recovered by the venous end of the capillary.

27. _____ Systolic blood pressure is the force with which the blood is pushing against the artery wall when the ventricles are contracting.

28. _____ Velocity of blood decreases as blood flows from the aorta toward the capillaries.

29. _____ The axillary artery is one of the six arteries identified to stop arterial bleeding.

30. _____ Hypercapnia acts as a major stimulant to chemoreceptors.

▶ *If you had difficulty with this section, review pages 690-712.*

Pulse Points

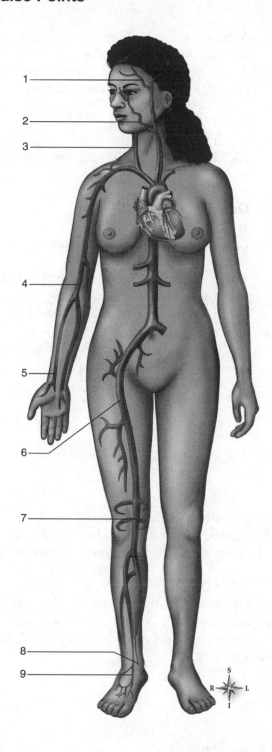

1 _____

2 _____

3 _____

4 _____

5 _____

6 _____

7 _____

8 _____

9 _____

III—MECHANISMS OF DISEASE

Fill in the blanks.

31. Complications of septicemia may result in
_____ _____.

32. _____ _____
results from any type of heart failure.

33. An acute type of allergic reaction called
_____ results in _____
_____.

34. _____ _____ re-
sults from widespread dilation of blood
vessels caused by an imbalance in autonomic stimulation of smooth muscles in
vessel walls.

35. *Hypovolemia* means_____
_____ _____.

36. A type of septic shock that results
from staphylococcal infections that
begin in the vagina of menstruat-
ing women and spread to the blood is

_____

_____ _____.

▶ *If you had difficulty with this section, review
pages 712-717.*

Crossword Puzzle

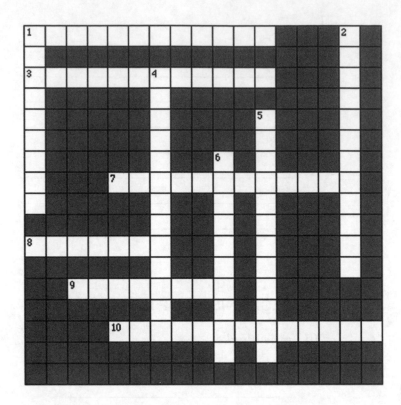

Across

1. Sensitive to pressure
3. Complete heartbeat (two words)
7. Volume pumped per heartbeat (two words)
8. Heart contracting
9. Heart at rest
10. Determined by stroke volume and heart rate (two words)

Down

1. SA node
2. Amount of blood returned to the heart by veins
4. Reflex that functions in hypoxia or hypercapnia emergencies
5. Increase in diameter of blood vessel
6. Resistance that helps determine arterial blood pressure

 APPLYING WHAT YOU KNOW

37. Kim received a gunshot wound to her leg during a robbery attempt. She experienced severe hemorrhaging that significantly decreased her blood volume. Which kind of shock is she at risk for? Name the physiologic mechanisms that her body has initiated to attempt to maintain circulatory homeostasis.

38. Upon examination with electrocardiogram, Brian was diagnosed with a cardiac dysrhythmia that displayed very slow ventricular contractions and large intervals between the P wave and the R peak of the QRS complex. What is the physiologic explanation for his symptoms? What can physicians do to restore his heart's conduction system?

 DID YOU KNOW

• Every pound of excess fat contains 200 miles of additional capillaries.

• If laid out in a straight line, the average adult's circulatory system would be nearly 60,000 miles long—enough to circle the earth 2.5 times.

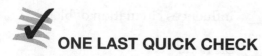

ONE LAST QUICK CHECK

Multiple Choice—select the best answer.

39. The medical term for high blood pressure is:
    a. arteriosclerosis.
    b. cyanosis.
    c. hypertension.
    d. central venous pressure.

40. Septic shock is caused by:
    a. complications of toxins in the blood.
    b. a nerve condition.
    c. a drop in blood pressure.
    d. blood vessel dilation.

41. Hypovolemic shock is caused by:
    a. heart failure.
    b. dilated blood vessels.
    c. a drop in blood pressure.
    d. a severe allergic reaction.

42. Which vessels collect blood from the capillaries and return it to the heart?
    a. arteries
    b. sinuses
    c. veins
    d. arterioles

43. Which of the following events, if any, would *not* cause the blood pressure to increase?
    a. hemorrhaging
    b. increasing viscosity of the blood
    c. increasing the strength of the heartbeat
    d. all of the above

44. The shift of the blood reservoir to the veins in the legs when standing is called the:
    a. orthostatic effect.
    b. total peripheral resistance effect.
    c. vasomotor mechanism.
    d. medullary ischemic reflex.

Fill in the blanks.

45. The four structures that make up the core of the electrical conduction system of the heart are the (a)_____, (b)_____, (c)_____, and (d)_____.

46. A graphic record of the heart's electrical activity is an _____ (when written) or _____ (when spoken).

47. A complete heartbeat may be referred to as a _____ _____.

48. The quantity of blood that remains in the ventricles at the end of the ejection period is called the _____ _____.

49. _____ _____ is the amount of blood that flows out of a ventricle of the heart per unit of time.

50. _____ _____ is the hormone most noted as a cardiac accelerator.

51. A principle stating whether fluids will move into or out of the plasma in the capillaries at a particular point is the _____ _____ _____ _____ _____.

Matching—identify the most appropriate answer for each item.

a.   P wave
b.   abnormal heart rate
c.   below 50 beats per minute
d.   baroreflexes
e.   hemodynamics
f.   inadequate blood supply
g.   diastole
h.   excess carbon dioxide
i.   residual volume
j.   occur in carotid arteries
k.   pacemaker
l.   dorsalis pedis

52. _____ influences circulation of blood

53. _____ SA node

54. _____ depolarization of atria

55. _____ dysrhythmia

56. _____ bradycardia

57. _____ heart at rest or relaxed

58. _____ blood remaining in ventricles

59. _____ pressoreflexes

60. _____ hypercapnia

61. _____ ischemia

62. _____ bruits

63. _____ pulse point

CHAPTER 23

Lymphatic System

The lymphatic system is similar to the circulatory system. Lymph, like blood, flows through an elaborate route of vessels. In addition to lymphatic vessels, the lymphatic system consists of lymph nodes, lymph, and the spleen. Unlike the circulatory system, the lymphatic vessels do not form a closed circuit. Lymph flows only once through the vessels before draining into the general blood circulation. This system is a filtering mechanism for microorganisms and serves as a protective device against foreign invaders, such as cancer.

As your text suggests, this system can also be likened to the wastewater system of our communities. Lymph circulates to bring contaminants to the system that are harmful to the body. Toxins are filtered and the fluid is returned cleansed, just as our wastewater systems remove harmful substances from the water and return it cleansed for our eventual use. Your knowledge of this system is necessary to understand the function of the lymphatic system in maintaining fluid balance in the tissues and the role that plays in the body's immune system.

I—LYMPHATIC VESSELS, LYMPH, AND CIRCULATION OF LYMPH

Multiple Choice—select the best answer.

1. The most important function(s) of the lymphatic system is/are:
   a. fluid balance of the internal environment.
   b. immunity.
   c. both a and b.
   d. none of the above.

2. Lymphatic capillaries that operate in the villi of the small intestine are called:
   a. lymphatics.
   b. lacteals.
   c. Peyer patches.
   d. lymph nodes.

3. Lymph from the entire body drains into the thoracic duct, *except* lymph from the:
   a. upper right quadrant.
   b. upper left quadrant.
   c. lower limbs.
   d. entire head and neck.

4. Which of the following is *not* a difference between lymphatics and veins?
   a. Lymphatics have thinner walls.
   b. Lymphatics contain more valves.
   c. Lymphatics contain lymph nodes.
   d. Lymphatics endure greater pressure.

5. If lymphatic return is blocked, which of the following will *not* occur?
   a. Blood protein concentration will fall.
   b. Blood osmotic pressure will fall.
   c. CO_2 levels in the blood will rise.
   d. Fluid imbalance will occur.

6. Lymphatic circulation is maintained by all of the following *except*:
   a. breathing movements.
   b. heart.
   c. skeletal muscle contractions.
   d. valves.

7. Lymphatic circulation begins with lymphatic:
   a. capillaries.
   b. veins.
   c. venules.
   d. arterioles.

True or false

8. _____ The lymphatic system could be referred to as a specialized component of the circulatory system.

9. _____ Lymphatic vessels, like vessels in the blood vascular system, form a closed loop of circulation.

10. _____ Both lymph and interstitial fluid closely resemble blood plasma in composition.

11. _____ Lymphatics have one-way valves much like veins.

12. _____ The milky lymph found in lacteals after digestion is called *chyle.*

13. _____ A dilated structure on the thoracic duct that serves as a storage area for lymph moving toward its point of entry into the venous system is the cisterna chyli.

14. _____ Activities that result in central movement, or flow, of lymph are called *lymphokinetic actions.*

▶ *If you had difficulty with this section, review pages 722-728.*

II—LYMPH NODES

Multiple Choice—select the best answer.

15. The small depression of a lymph node from which the efferent lymph vessel arises is termed the:
    a. sinus.
    b. hilum.
    c. capsule.
    d. nodule.

16. The lymph nodes located in front of the ear are called the:
    a. submaxillary groups.
    b. inguinal lymph nodes.
    c. cervical lymph nodes.
    d. none of the above.

17. An infection of a lymph node is called:
    a. adenitis.
    b. noditis.
    c. lymphitis.
    d. lysis.

18. The lymphatic tissue of lymph nodes serves as the final maturation site for:
    a. monocytes.
    b. lymphocytes.
    c. both a and b.
    d. none of the above.

True or false

19. _____ Even though some lymph nodes occur in clusters, most occur as single nodes.

20. _____ Cortical nodules are composed of packed lymphocytes that surround an area called the *germinal center.*

Labeling—identify the principal organs of the lymphatic system by matching each term with its corresponding number on the following illustration.

_____ spleen

_____ tonsils

_____ right lymphatic duct

_____ aggregated lymphoid nodules (Peyer patches) in intestinal wall

_____ entrance of thoracic duct into subclavian vein

_____ superficial cubital (supratrochlear) lymph nodes

_____ axillary lymph node

_____ red bone marrow

_____ cisterna chyli

_____ cervical lymph node

_____ thoracic duct

_____ inguinal lymph node

_____ thymus gland

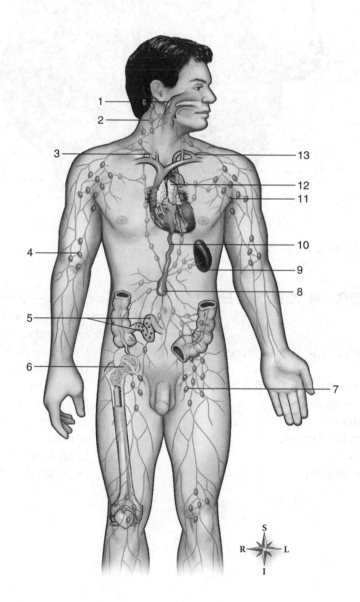

Labeling—using the terms provided, label the structure of a lymph node on the following diagram.

efferent lymph vessel   hilum
medullary cords   cortical nodules
afferent lymph vessel   sinuses
germinal center   capsule

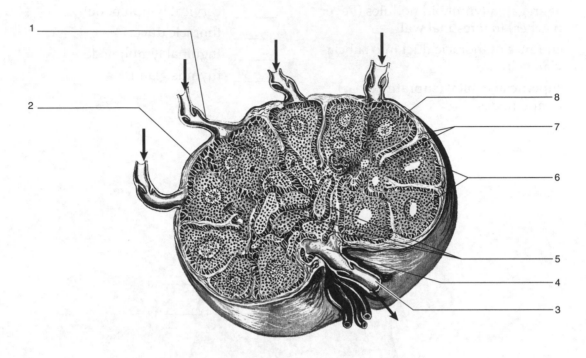

▶ *If you had difficulty with this section, review pages 728-732.*

III—LYMPHATIC DRAINAGE OF THE BREAST

Multiple Choice—select the best answer.

21. Over 85% of the lymph from the breast enters lymph nodes of the:
    a. axillary region.
    b. supraclavicular region.
    c. brachial region.
    d. subscapular region.

22. The breast—mammary gland and surrounding tissue—is drained by:
    a. lymphatics that originate in and drain the skin over the breast, with exception of the areola and nipple.
    b. lymphatics that originate in and drain the substance of the breast itself, including the skin of the areola and nipple.
    c. both a and b.
    d. none of the above.

Labeling—label the lymphatic drainage of the breast on the following illustration.

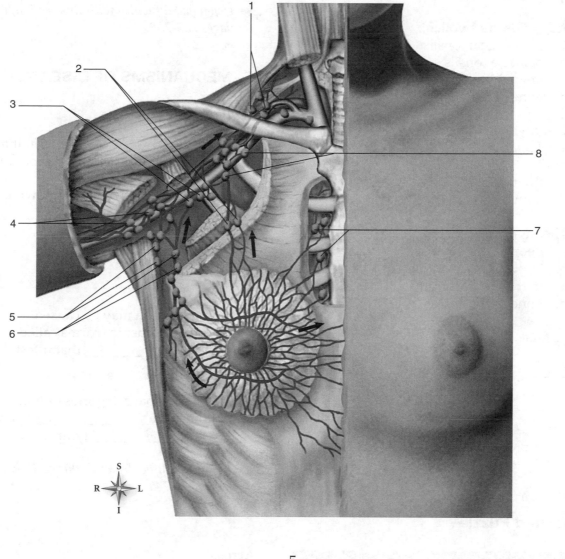

1 _____   5 _____

2 _____   6 _____

3 _____   7 _____

4 _____   8 _____

▶ *If you had difficulty with this section, review pages 732-733.*

IV—TONSILS, THYMUS, AND SPLEEN

Multiple Choice—select the best answer.

23. Adenoids are swollen:
    a. pharyngeal tonsils.
    b. palatine tonsils.
    c. lingual tonsils.
    d. none of the above.

24. The thymus secretes:
    a. T_3.
    b. T_4.
    c. thymosin.
    d. both a and c.

25. The thymus is located:
    a. deep to the thyroid.
    b. in the axillary region.
    c. in the mediastinum.
    d. none of the above.

True or false

26. _____ As a person ages, the thymus increases in size; this process is called *involution.*

27. _____ The spleen functions solely in defense from foreign microorganisms.

Crossword Puzzle

28. _____ The spleen removes imperfect platelets from the blood.

▶ *If you had difficulty with this section, review pages 733-738.*

V—MECHANISMS OF DISEASE

Fill in the blanks.

29. _____ is a term that refers to a tumor of the cells of lymphoid tissue.

30. A middle ear infection is known as
    _____ _____
    _____.

31. Septicemia is also known as
    _____ _____.

32. Lymphedema may be caused by small parasitic worms called _____ that infest the lymph nodes.

33. Two principal categories of lymphomas are _____ and _____ lymphoma.

▶ *If you had difficulty with this section, review pages 738-741.*

Across
4. Vessels that originate as lacteals in villi
5. Found in lacteals after digestion
6. Functions in defense and hematopoiesis (two words)
7. Palatine are an example
9. Active in production of T cells

Down
1. Activities that result in lymph flow
2. Destroys red blood cells
3. Located in villi
8. Fluid found in lymphatic vessels

APPLYING WHAT YOU KNOW

34. Ms. Langston was diagnosed with hemolytic anemia. Is a splenectomy a viable option? If so, why? Can she live without her spleen?

35. Baby Wilson was born without a thymus gland. Immediate plans were made for a transplant to be performed. In the meantime, baby Wilson was placed in strict isolation. For what reason was he placed in isolation?

DID YOU KNOW

• According to the Centers for Disease Control and Prevention, 18 million courses of antibiotics are prescribed for the common cold in the United States per year. Research shows that colds are caused by viruses. Fifty million unnecessary antibiotics are prescribed for viral respiratory infections every year.

ONE LAST QUICK CHECK

Matching—select the best response.

a. thymus
b. tonsils
c. spleen

36. _____ palatine, pharyngeal, tubal, and lingual are examples

37. _____ hematopoiesis

38. _____ destroys worn-out red blood cells

39. _____ located in the mediastinum

40. _____ serves as a reservoir for blood

41. _____ T-lymphocytes

42. _____ largest at puberty

True or false

43. _____ The cisterna chyli is a dilated structure on the thoracic duct that serves as a storage area for lymph moving into the venous system.

44. _____ Healthy capillaries "leak" proteins.

45. _____ Thoracic duct lymph is "pumped" into the venous system during inspiration.

46. _____ Lymph nodes have several afferent and efferent vessels.

47. _____ Lymphedema is swelling due to an accumulation of lymph.

48. _____ An anastomosis is the removal of a part.

49. _____ The spleen is located below the diaphragm, above the right kidney and descending colon.

50. _____ Splenomegaly is removal of the spleen.

CHAPTER 24

Immune System

The immune system is the armed forces division of the body. Ready to attack at a moment's notice, the immune system defends us against the major enemies of the body: microorganisms, foreign transplanted tissue cells, and our own cells that have turned malignant.

The most numerous cells of the immune system are the lymphocytes. These cells circulate in the body's fluids seeking invading organisms and destroying them with powerful lymphotoxins, lymphokines, or antibodies.

Phagocytes, another large group of immune system cells, assist with the destruction of foreign invaders by a process known as *phagocytosis.* Neutrophils and macrophages ingest and digest the invaders, rendering them harmless to the body.

Another weapon that the immune system possesses is complement. Normally a group of inactive enzymes present in the blood, complement can be activated to kill invading cells by drilling holes in their cytoplasmic membranes, which allows fluid to enter the cell until it bursts. Your review of this chapter will give you an understanding of how the body defends itself from the daily invasion of destructive substances.

I—INNATE IMMUNITY

Multiple Choice—select the best answer.

1. Which of the following cells is *not* involved with innate immunity?
   a. natural killer cells
   b. neutrophils
   c. macrophages
   d. all of the above are involved with innate immunity

2. The "first line of defense" in innate immunity is:
   a. inflammation.
   b. phagocytosis.
   c. mechanical and chemical barriers.
   d. complement.

3.   About 15% of the total number of lympho-
cyte cells are:
a.   natural killer (NK) cells.
b.   macrophages.
c.   neutrophils.
d.   interferon.

4.   The most numerous type of phagocyte is
the:
a.   neutrophil.
b.   macrophage.
c.   histocyte.
d.   Kupffer cell.

5.   Which of the following is a phagocytic
monocyte that migrates out of the bloodstream?
a.   neutrophil
b.   macrophage
c.   phagosome
d.   none of the above

True or false

6.   _____   The immune mechanism that
provides a general defense by acting against anything recognized
as nonself is termed *adaptive immunity.*

7.   _____   Species resistance is the genetic
characteristics of the human spe-
cies that protect the body from
certain pathogens.

8.   _____   Interferon has been proven effective as a treatment against most
cancers.

9.   _____   The complement cascade causes
phagocytosis of the foreign cell
that triggered it.

10.   _____   Natural killer cells are a group of
lymphocytes that kill many types
of tumor cells and cells infected
by different kinds of viruses.

▶ *If you had difficulty with this section, review
pages 745-756.*

II—ADAPTIVE IMMUNITY

Multiple Choice—select the best answer.

11.   B cells and T cells are examples of:
a.   monocytes.
b.   lymphocytes.
c.   neutrophils.
d.   macrophages.

12.   Cell-mediated immunity involves:
a.   B cells.
b.   T cells.
c.   both a and b.
d.   neither a nor b.

13.   The T cell subsets that are clinically important in diagnosing AIDS are:
a.   CD4.
b.   CD8.
c.   neither a nor b.
d.   both a and b.

14.   An antibody consists of:
a.   two heavy and two light polypeptide
chains.
b.   two heavy and one light polypeptide
chains.
c.   one heavy and two light polypeptide
chains.
d.   one heavy and one light polypeptide
chain.

15.   The amount of antibodies in a person's
blood in response to exposure to a pathogen is called:
a.   toxoid.
b.   titer.
c.   both a and b.
d.   none of the above.

16.   The most abundant circulating antibody
is:
a.   IgM.
b.   IgG.
c.   IgA.
d.   IgE.

17. The specific cells that secrete antibodies are:
    a. B cells.
    b. T cells.
    c. plasma cells.
    d. none of the above.

18. T cells are sensitized by:
    a. direct exposure to an antigen.
    b. presentation of an antigen by an antigen-presenting cell.
    c. antibodies produced by B cells.
    d. lymphokines.

19. *Complement* can best be described as:
    a. an antibody.
    b. an enzyme in the blood plasma.
    c. a hormone.
    d. a lymphokine.

20. The chemical messengers that T cells release into inflamed tissues are called:
    a. pathogens.
    b. cytokines
    c. lymphotoxins.
    d. suppressor cells.

Fill in the blanks.

21. Antibodies are proteins of the family called _____.

22. _____ is the predominant class of antibody produced after initial contact with an antigen.

23. The first vaccination was against the _____ _____.

24. Some vaccines use _____ (weakened) pathogens.

25. _____ _____ generally lasts longer than passive immunity.

26. Abnormal antigens or _____ _____ are present in the plasma membranes of some cancer cells in addition to self-antigens.

27. _____ is elevated in both benign and malignant prostate disease.

28. Helper T cells and suppressor T cells help regulate _____ _____ function by regulating B cell and T cell function.

29. A fetus receives protection from the mother through _____ _____ immunity.

30. A vaccination provides _____ _____ immunity.

▶ *If you had difficulty with this section, review pages 756-772.*

T Cell Development

Labeling—label the T cell as it progresses from the thymus through activation.

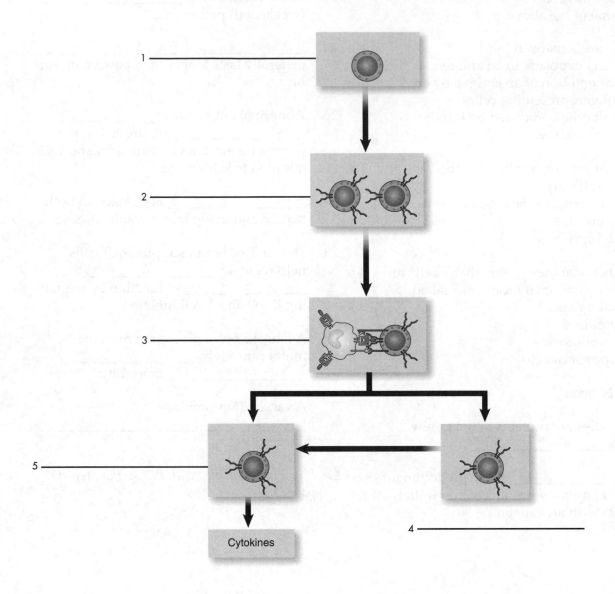

Cytokines

III—MECHANISMS OF DISEASE

Matching—match the term with the proper selection.

a. HIV
b. AZT
c. SCID
d. HLAs
e. SLE

31. _____ Stem cells are missing or unable to grow properly

32. _____ Retrovirus

33. _____ Inhibits symptoms of AIDS

34. _____ Chronic autoimmune inflammatory disease of the joints, blood vessels, skin, kidney, and nervous system

35. _____ Involved in transplant rejection

▶ *If you had difficulty with this section, review pages 772-777.*

Crossword Puzzle

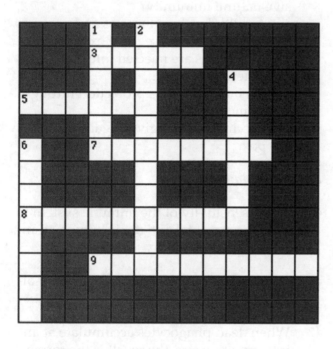

Across
3. Family of cells descended from one cell
5. Cell-mediated immunity (two words)
7. Immunity that recognizes specific threatening agents and responds to these only
8. Inhibits spread of a viral infection
9. Enlarged monocytes that are giant phagocytic cells

Down
1. Produce antibodies (two words)
2. Immunity that resists various threatening agents (general defense)
4. Foreign protein
6. Plasma protein (immunoglobulin)

APPLYING WHAT YOU KNOW

36. Trent, a newborn, received immune protection from his mother through the placenta and breast milk. Which specific type of immunity is this? His older sister, Carrie, also recently received immune protection from a host of illnesses; however, hers was achieved deliberately via immunization by her pediatrician. What specific types of immunity is she experiencing? How do her types of immunity differ from her brother's?

37. Marcia is an intravenous drug user. She has developed a type of skin cancer known as Kaposi sarcoma. What, most likely, is Marcia's primary diagnosis? What are some of the medications that might be used to inhibit symptoms for a while?

DID YOU KNOW

- The swine flu vaccine in 1976 caused more deaths and illness than the disease that it was intended to prevent.

- In the United States, the HIV infection rate is increasing four times faster in women than in men. Women tend to underestimate their risk.

ONE LAST QUICK CHECK

Multiple Choice—select the best answer.

38. T cells do which of the following?
    a. develop in the thymus
    b. form memory cells
    c. form plasma cells
    d. all of the above

39. Acquired immune deficiency syndrome is characterized by which of the following?
    a. caused by a retrovirus
    b. causes inadequate T cell formation
    c. can result in death from cancer
    d. all of the above

40. Interferon is:
    a. produced by B cells.
    b. a protein compound that protects other cells by interfering with the ability of a virus to reproduce.
    c. a group of inactive enzyme proteins normally present in blood.
    d. all of the above.

41. B cells do which of the following?
    a. develop into plasma cells and memory cells
    b. secrete antibodies
    c. develop from primitive cells in bone marrow called *stem cells* and then into naïve B cells
    d. all of the above

42. Which of the following functions to kill invading cells by drilling a hole in their plasma membrane?
    a. interferon
    b. complement
    c. antibody
    d. memory cell

43. What is a rapidly growing population of identical cells that produce large quantities of specific antibodies called?
    a. complementary
    b. lymphotoxic
    c. chemotactic
    d. monoclonal

44. Which of the following is a form of passive natural immunity?
    a. A child develops measles and acquires immunity to subsequent exposure.
    b. Antibodies are injected into an infected individual.
    c. An infant receives protection through its mother's milk.
    d. Vaccinations are given against smallpox.

Fill in the blanks.

45. Hypersensitivity of the immune system to an environmental antigen is known as an _____.

46. Drugs used to relieve the symptoms of allergies are called _____.

47. When dead phagocytes accumulate at an inflammation site, the result is the formation of _____.

48. _____ is a powerful poison that acts directly and quickly to kill any cell it attacks.

49. Adaptive immunity is also known as _____ _____.

50. The _____ _____ is the second line of defense for the body.

True or false

51. _____ The human immunodeficiency virus has a profound impact on a person's number of CD12 subset of T cells.

52. _____ Once inside a cell, HIV uses its viral RNA to produce DNA; this process is called *reverse transcription.*

53. _____ A common autoimmune disease is SLE or "lupus."

54. _____ SCID is an immunosuppressive drug.

55. _____ Glomerulonephritis is an autoimmune disease of the neuromuscular junction.

CHAPTER 25

Stress

Life without any stress would be very dull and boring. Often it is stress that stimulates us to achieve our dreams and experience success and happiness. However, too much stress becomes unpleasant and tiring and can seriously interfere with our ability to function effectively. The challenge is to keep stress at a level that is healthy and enjoyable.

Although we react differently and in various degrees to stressors, we must acknowledge that in most individuals, stress leads to a physiologic stress response. These responses may be as simple as an increase in heart rate or perspiration or as complex as a disease syndrome. And although we may not be aware of it on a day-to-day basis, stress can be cumulative and manifest itself long after apparent stressors have been resolved. Your study of this unit will alert you to the impact of stress on your body and the significant role it plays in homeostasis.

I—SELYE'S CONCEPT OF STRESS

Multiple Choice—select the best answer.

1. The stages of general adaptation syndrome in the correct order are:
   a. alarm reaction, stage of exhaustion, stage of resistance.
   b. alarm reaction, stage of resistance, stage of exhaustion.
   c. stage of exhaustion, alarm reaction, stage of resistance.
   d. stage of exhaustion, stage of resistance, stage of alarm.

2. The "stress triad" refers to:
   a. alarm, exhaustion, resistance.
   b. hypertrophied adrenals, atrophied thymus and lymph nodes, and bleeding ulcers.
   c. stressor, stress, and response.
   d. health, stress, and disease.

3. Which of the following is *not* an alarm reaction response resulting from hypertrophy of the adrenal cortex?
   a. hyperglycemia
   b. hypertrophy of thymus
   c. decreased immunity
   d. decreased allergic responses

4.   All of the following are true statements *except:*
     a.   stressors are extreme stimuli.
     b.   stressors are always unpleasant, injurious, or painful.
     c.   the emotions of fear, anxiety, and grief can act as stressors.
     d.   stressors differ in individuals.

5.   What determines which stimuli are stressors for each individual?
     a.   past experience
     b.   diet
     c.   heredity
     d.   all of the above

True or false

6.   _____   Selye's stage of exhaustion is reached in each exposure to stressors.

7.   _____   High-stress, hard-driving, competitive individuals who may be at greater risk of coronary heart disease are classified as "Type B."

8.   _____   The *stage of resistance* can also be described as *adaptation*.

9.   _____   Stressors are "bad" stimuli that should always be avoided.

10. _____   The stress response commonly referred to as "fight or flight" is evoked by increased sympathetic activity.

Matching—identify the best answer from the choices given and insert the letter in the answer blank.

a.   FAS
b.   resistance stage
c.   general adaptation syndrome
d.   alarm stage
e.   exhaustion state
f.   stressor

11. _____   group of changes that make the presence of stress in the body known

12. _____   occurs when stress is extremely severe or continues over long periods

13. _____   increased activity of the sympathetic nervous system

14. _____   agent that produces stress

15. _____   *fight or flight* reaction disappears

16. _____   can occur as the result of stress in a developing fetus

▶ *If you had difficulty with this section, review pages 782-788.*

II—SOME CURRENT CONCEPTS ABOUT STRESS

Multiple Choice—select the best answer.

17. Corticotropin-releasing hormone (CRH) stimulates the anterior pituitary gland to secrete increased amounts of:
     a.   glucocorticoids.
     b.   aldosterone.
     c.   ACTH.
     d.   ADH.

18. All of the following are effects of cortisol *except:*
     a.   increased protein catabolism.
     b.   decreased immune responses.
     c.   decreased allergic responses.
     d.   "fight or flight" responses.

19. The dominant subjective reaction that occurs with psychological stress is:
     a.   guilt.
     b.   anxiety.
     c.   depression.
     d.   fear.

True or false

20. _____   The current definition of *stress* is "any stimulus that directly or indirectly stimulates neurons of the hypothalamus to release corticotropin-releasing hormone (CRH)."

21. _____ It is accepted among physiologists that a higher-than-normal blood level of corticoids results in a greater ability to resist stress.

22. _____ Physiologic stress and psychological stress are clearly different phenomena.

23. _____ Hypervolemia and antidiuresis are common responses to stress.

24. _____ Stress is an issue only among adolescents and adults.

25. _____ The brain's limbic system is often called the "emotional brain."

▶ *If you had difficulty with this section, review pages 788-794.*

Crossword Puzzle

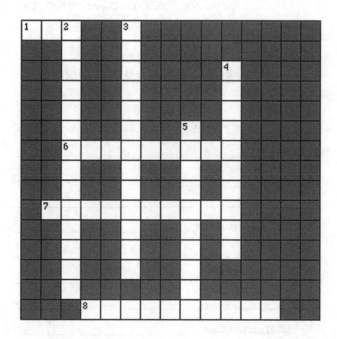

Across
1. General adaptation syndrome (abbrev.)
6. Agents that produce stress
7. Coping successfully with stress
8. General adaptation syndrome stage that develops only when stress is severe

Down
2. Also known as the *stress response* (two words)
3. Stage of general adaptation syndrome (two words)
4. General adaptation syndrome stage where sympathetic activity returns to normal
5. Hormones that increase during stress

 APPLYING WHAT YOU KNOW

26. Merrilee has an adolescent crush on John. Whenever she is near him, she feels anxious, her pupils dilate, heart rate elevates, systolic blood pressure rises, blood glucose levels are above normal, and blood and urine levels of epinephrine and norepinephrine are elevated. What is the physiologic term used to describe this syndrome? Beginning in the hypothalamus, trace the mechanisms that are causing this response. If this physiologic scenario were extended and intense, what illnesses might Merrilee be at risk for?

27. Bill is going to his boss for his annual evaluation. He is planning to ask for a raise and hopes the evaluation will be good. Which subdivision of the autonomic nervous system will be active during this stressful conference? Should he have a large meal before his appointment? Support your answer with facts.

DID YOU KNOW

- Laughing lowers levels of stress hormones and strengthens the immune system. Six-year-olds laugh an average of 300 times a day. Adults only laugh 15–100 times a day.

- A survey conducted at Iowa State College in 1969 suggests that a parent's stress at the time of conception plays a major role in determining a baby's sex. The child tends to be of the same sex as the parent who is under less stress.

ONE LAST QUICK CHECK

Fill in the blanks.

28. _____ _____ _____ is the term for the group of changes that make the presence of stress in the body known.

29. The stage of _____ develops only when stress is extremely severe or continues over a long period.

30. The hypothalamus releases _____ _____ _____, which acts as a trigger that initiates many diverse changes in the body.

31. The term that describes the stress responses that occur as a result of stimulation of the sympathetic centers is known as the _____ _____ _____ _____.

32. _____ investigates physiologic responses made by individuals to psychological stressors.

True or False

33. _____ Type B personalities are at greater risk of coronary disease than Type A personalities.

34. _____ Stress causes disruption in homeostasis.

35. _____ Smoking increases plasma adrenocorticoids by as much as 77%.

36. _____ Identical psychological stressors induce identical physiologic responses in different individuals.

37. _____ Hans Selye identified a group of changes classic to stress and called them the *stress triad*.

38. _____ Prolonged stress is thought to produce the hormone neuropeptide Y.

Fill in the blanks—provide an example of a disease or condition for each of the target organs or systems.

39. Cardiovascular system _____

_____

40. Muscles _____

_____

41. Connective tissue _____

_____

42. Pulmonary system _____

_____

43. Immune system _____

_____

44. Gastrointestinal system _____

_____

45. Genitourinary system _____

_____

46. Skin _____

_____

47. Endocrine system _____

_____

48. Central nervous system _____

_____

CHAPTER 26

Anatomy of the Respiratory System

A s you sit reviewing this system, your body needs 16 quarts of air per minute. Walking requires 24 quarts of air and running requires 50 quarts per minute. The respiratory system provides the air necessary for you to perform your daily activities and eliminates the waste gases from the air that you breathe. Take a deep breath and think of the air as it enters some 250 million tiny air sacs similar in appearance to clusters of grapes. These microscopic air sacs expand to let air in and contract to force it out. These tiny sacs, or *alveoli*, are the functioning units of the respiratory system. They provide the necessary volume of oxygen and eliminate carbon dioxide 24 hours a day.

Air enters either through the mouth or the nasal cavity. Next it passes through the pharynx and past the epiglottis, through the glottis and the rest of the larynx. It then continues down the trachea, into the bronchi to the bronchioles, and finally through the alveoli. The reverse occurs for expelled air. Your review of this system is necessary to provide you with an understanding of this essential homeostatic mechanism—the breath of life.

I—UPPER RESPIRATORY TRACT

Multiple Choice—select the best answer.

1. Which of the following structures is *not* part of the upper respiratory tract?
    a. trachea
    b. larynx
    c. oropharynx
    d. nose

2. Which part of the respiratory system does *not* function as an air distributor?
    a. trachea
    b. bronchioles
    c. alveoli
    d. bronchi

3. Which sequence is the correct pathway for air movement through the nose and into the pharynx?
   a. anterior nares, posterior nares, vestibule, nasal cavity meatuses
   b. anterior nares, vestibule, posterior nares, nasal cavity meatuses
   c. nasal cavity meatuses, anterior nares, vestibule, posterior nares
   d. anterior nares, vestibule, nasal cavity meatuses, posterior nares

4. Which of the following is *not* a paranasal sinus?
   a. frontal
   b. maxillary
   c. mandibular
   d. sphenoid

5. The true vocal cords and the rima glottidis are called the:
   a. glottis.
   b. epiglottis.
   c. vestibular fold.
   d. both a and b.

True or false

6. _____ Failure of the palatine bones to unite is called *cribriform palate.*

7. _____ The pharynx is a tubelike structure that opens only into the mouth and larynx.

8. _____ Enlarged pharyngeal tonsils are called *adenoids.*

9. _____ The more common name for the thyroid cartilage is the *voicebox.*

10. _____ The epiglottis moves up and down during swallowing to prevent food or liquids from entering the trachea.

Labeling—match each term with its corresponding number on the following illustration of the respiratory system.

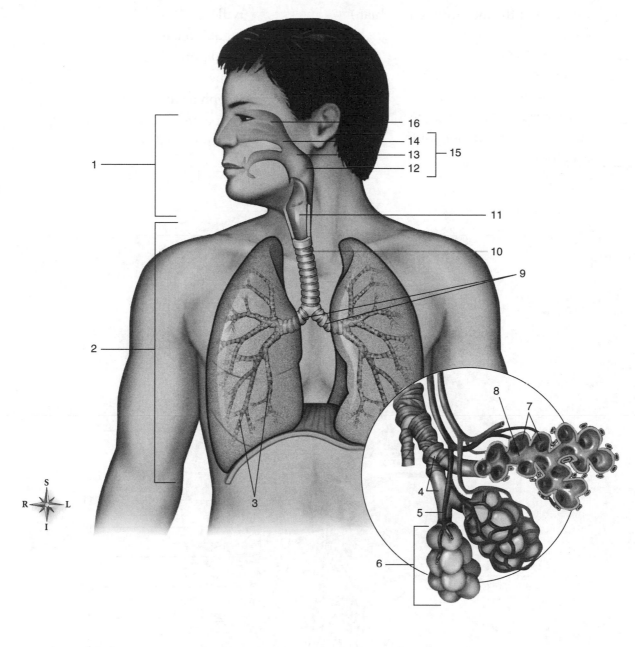

_____ bronchioles	_____ pharynx
_____ nasal cavity	_____ left and right primary bronchi
_____ bronchioles	_____ laryngopharynx
_____ upper respiratory tract	_____ capillary
_____ alveoli	_____ trachea
_____ lower respiratory tract	_____ larynx
_____ alveolar duct	_____ alveolar sac
_____ nasopharynx	_____ oropharynx

Labeling—using the terms provided, label the three divisions of the pharynx and nearby structures on the following illustration.

_____ opening of the auditory (eustachian) tube

_____ laryngopharynx

_____ esophagus

_____ oropharynx

_____ vocal cords

_____ pharyngeal tonsil (adenoids)

_____ epiglottis

_____ uvula

_____ lingual tonsil

_____ hyoid bone

_____ trachea

_____ nasopharynx

_____ soft palate

_____ palatine tonsil

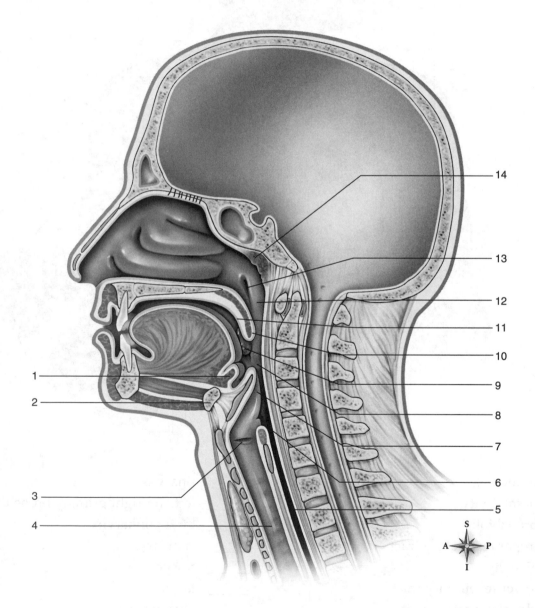

Labeling—label the structures related to the paranasal sinuses on the following illustration. Some terms may be used more than once.

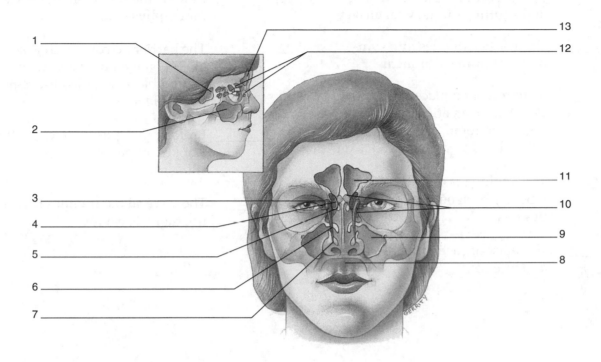

▶ *If you had difficulty with this section, review pages 797-807.*

II—LOWER RESPIRATORY TRACT

Multiple Choice—select the best answer.

11. Aspirated objects tend to lodge in the:
    a. right bronchus.
    b. left bronchus.
    c. either right or left bronchus.
    d. none of the above.

12. The fluid coating the alveoli that reduces surface tension is called:
    a. bronchus.
    b. surfactant.
    c. alveolus.
    d. none of the above.

13. Which of the following is *not* an area of the lungs?
    a. oblique fissure
    b. horizontal fissure
    c. superior fissure
    d. hilum

14. Which of the following is *false*?
    a. When the diaphragm relaxes, it returns to a domelike shape.
    b. When the diaphragm contracts, it pulls the floor of the thoracic cavity downward.
    c. Changes in thorax size bring about inspiration and expiration.
    d. Raising the ribs decreases the depth and width of the thorax.

True or false

15. _____ The rings of cartilage that form the trachea are complete rings that prevent it from collapsing and shutting off the vital airway.

16. _____ The trachea divides into symmetrical primary bronchi.

17. _____ A tube is often placed in the trachea before a patient leaves the operating room, especially if he or she has had a muscle relaxant.

18. _____ The left lung is divided into three lobes by horizontal and oblique fissures.

19. _____ The apex of each lung is lateral and inferior.

20. _____ The exchange of gases between air and blood occurs in the alveoli.

21. _____ LVRS is the treatment of choice for emphysema.

22. _____ The barrier across which gases are exchanged between alveolar air and blood is called the *respiratory membrane*.

23. _____ Prolonged exposure to cigarette smoke can paralyze respiratory cilia.

24. _____ The visceral pleura lines the entire thoracic cavity.

Labeling—identify the lobes and fissures of the lungs by matching each term with its corresponding number on the following illustration (anterior view).

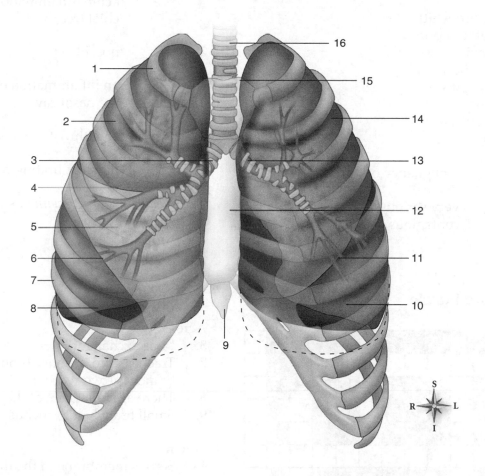

_____ right primary bronchus	_____ right inferior lobe
_____ oblique fissure	_____ right middle lobe
_____ trachea	_____ oblique fissure
_____ right superior lobe	_____ sternum (xiphoid process)
_____ sternum (manubrium)	_____ body of sternum
_____ horizontal fissure	_____ first rib
_____ seventh rib	_____ left superior lobe
_____ left primary bronchus	_____ left inferior lobe

▶ *If you had difficulty with this section, review pages 807-816.*

III—MECHANISMS OF DISEASE

Matching—identify each disorder with its corresponding description.

a. acute bronchitis
b. deviated septum
c. epistaxis
d. lung cancer
e. pharyngitis
f. rhinitis
g. tuberculosis
h. croup

25. _____ malignancy of pulmonary tissue

26. _____ very serious, chronic, and highly contagious infection

27. _____ displacement of the nasal septum

28. _____ a common infection of the lower respiratory tract characterized by acute inflammation of the bronchial tree

29. _____ nosebleed

30. _____ an inflammation of the mucosa of the nasal cavity

31. _____ sore throat

32. _____ harsh, vibrating cough

▶ *If you had difficulty with this section, review pages 816-820.*

Crossword Puzzle

Across
3. "Gas exchanger"
7. Trachea, two primary bronchi, and their branches (two words)
8. There are four pairs of these sinuses
9. Small branch of bronchus

Down
1. Serous membrane in the thoracic cavity
2. "Windpipe"
4. "Voice box"
5. "Throat"
6. Conchae

APPLYING WHAT YOU KNOW

33. Mrs. Metheny's 6-year-old child had trouble swallowing. She had a high fever, appeared very anxious, and was drooling from her mouth. Mrs. Metheny called the EMS personnel who assessed the child, inserted an airway, and transported her immediately to the emergency department. What is a possible explanation for why the child is experiencing these symptoms? What is the causative agent for these symptoms? Is this a serious threat to the child?

34. Dr. Harry is a pediatrician who recently examined a 2-year-old boy who awakened in the middle of the night frightened and with the following symptoms: labored inspiration, harsh and vibrating cough, and a normal body temperature. What diagnosis might Dr. Harry give his patient? Is this life-threatening?

35. Mr. Gorski is a heavy smoker. Recently, he has noticed that when he gets up in the morning, he has a bothersome cough that brings up a large accumulation of mucus. This cough persists for several minutes and then leaves until the next morning. What is a possible explanation for this problem?

 DID YOU KNOW

- If the roof of your mouth is narrow, you are more likely to snore because you are not getting enough oxygen through your nose.

- Only about 10% of the air in the lungs is actually changed with each cycle of inhaling and exhaling when an at-rest person is breathing, but up to 80% can be exchanged during deep breathing or strenuous exercise.

 ONE LAST QUICK CHECK

Matching—choose the correct response.

a. nose
b. pharynx
c. larynx

36. _____ warms and humidifies air

37. _____ air and food pass through here

38. _____ sinuses

39. _____ conchae

40. _____ septum

41. _____ tonsils

42. _____ middle ear infections

43. _____ epiglottis

44. _____ rhinitis

45. _____ sore throat

46. _____ epistaxis

Fill in the blanks.

The organs of the respiratory system are designed to perform two basic functions. They serve as an (47) _____ _____ and as a (48) _____ _____. In addition to the above, the respiratory system (49) _____, (50) _____, and (51) _____ the air we breathe. Respiratory organs include the (52) _____, (53) _____, (54) _____, (55) _____ (56) _____, and the (57) _____. The respiratory system ends in millions of tiny, thin-walled sacs called (58) _____. (59) _____ of gases takes place in these sacs. Two aspects of the structure of these sacs assist them in the exchange of gases. First, an extremely thin membrane, the (60) _____ _____, allows for easy exchange and second, the large number of air sacs makes an enormous (61) _____ area.

CHAPTER 27

Physiology of the Respiratory System

The respiratory system functions to diffuse gases into and out of the blood so that the organs of our body receive blood that is rich in oxygen and low in carbon dioxide. The exchange of gases that occurs within the body is a complex operation and each component of the pulmonary system contributes to successful ventilation. Air must enter the lungs (inspiration) from the external environment, an exchange must occur between the blood and the cells, and then air high in CO_2 is returned to the environment (expiration).

Numerous anatomic and physiologic mechanisms influence the successful exchange of gases throughout the process. The rate, depth, and pressure of pulmonary ventilation are dependent upon these structures to successfully perform their respiratory function. Your review of this system is necessary to provide you with an understanding of this essential homeostatic mechanism necessary for survival.

I—PULMONARY VENTILATION

Multiple Choice—select the best answer.

1. Boyle's law states that:
   a. fluids move from areas of high pressure to low.
   b. the volume of a gas is inversely proportional to its pressure.
   c. the atmosphere exerts a pressure of 760 mm Hg.
   d. volume is directly proportional to temperature.

2. When the diaphragm contracts, the volume of the thorax increases, thoracic pressure:
   a. increases, and air is forced from the lungs.
   b. decreases, and air is forced from the lungs.
   c. decreases, and air rushes into the lungs.
   d. increases, and air rushes into the lungs.

3. Quiet inspiration is the function of:
   a. the diaphragm and internal intercostal.
   b. the diaphragm and external intercostal.
   c. the internal intercostal and external intercostal.
   d. none of the above.

4. During normal, quiet respiration, the amount of air exchanged between the lungs and atmosphere is called _____ and has a volume of _____ mL.
    a. tidal volume; 1200
    b. vital capacity; 4500
    c. tidal volume; 500
    d. residual volume; 1200

5. Functional residual capacity (FRC) equals:
    a. TV + IRV.
    b. TV + IRV + ERV + RV.
    c. TV + IRV + ERV.
    d. ERV + RV.

6. *Eupnea* is a term used to describe:
    a. rapid, deep respiration.
    b. cessation of respiration.
    c. slow, shallow respiration.
    d. normal breathing.

7. Under normal conditions, air in the atmosphere exerts a pressure of:
    a. 500 mm Hg.
    b. 560 mm Hg.
    c. 660 mm Hg.
    d. 760 mm Hg.

8. Areas where gas exchange cannot take place are:
    a. anatomical dead spaces.
    b. nose, pharynx, larynx.
    c. trachea and bronchi.
    d. all of the above.

9. All of the following are regulated processes associated with the functioning of the respiratory system *except*:
    a. control of cell reproduction.
    b. gas exchange in lungs and tissue.
    c. pulmonary ventilation.
    d. transport of gases.

10. Dalton's law is also known as:
    a. Henry's law.
    b. Boyle's law.
    c. Charles' law.
    d. the law of partial pressures.

True or false

11. _____ Temperature is the measurement of the motion of molecules.

12. _____ The largest amount of air that can enter and leave the lungs during respiration is termed *total lung capacity (TLC)*.

13. _____ Residual volume (RV) is the volume remaining in the respiratory tract after maximum expiration.

14. _____ The temporary cessation of breathing is termed *apnea*.

15. _____ It is not possible to exhale all of the air from your lungs.

Labeling—label the following diagram with the correct terminology for the lung volumes displayed.

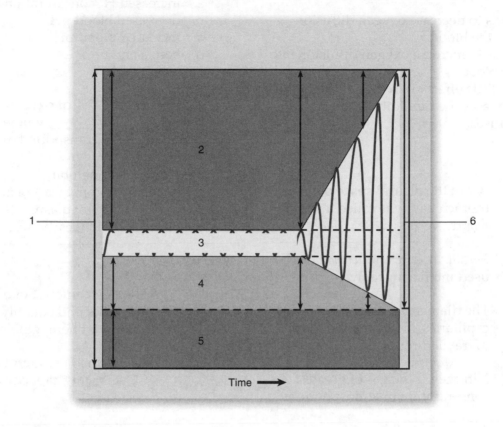

Time ⟶

1 _____   4 _____

2 _____   5 _____

3 _____   6 _____

▶ *If you had difficulty with this section, review pages 823-838.*

II—PULMONARY GAS EXCHANGE

Multiple Choice—select the best answer.

16. If oxygen is 21% of the atmosphere, it will contribute _____ of the total atmospheric pressure.
    a. 21%
    b. 79%
    c. 0.21%
    d. .79%

17. The amount of oxygen that diffuses into blood each minute depends on the:
    a. total functional surface area of the respiratory membrane.
    b. respiratory minute volume.
    c. alveolar ventilation.
    d. all of the above.

18. P_{O_2} at standard atmospheric pressure is approximately:
    a. 21 mm Hg.
    b. 0.2 mm Hg.
    c. 160 mm Hg.
    d. 760 mm Hg.

19. Anything that decreases the total functional surface area of the respiratory membrane:
    a. tends to decrease oxygen diffusion into the blood.
    b. tends to increase oxygen diffusion into the blood.
    c. has little effect on oxygen diffusion.
    d. increases the humidity of oxygen as it diffuses.

True or false

20. _____ Air in the pleural space of the thoracic cavity is called a *pneumothorax*.

21. _____ *Partial pressure* and *tension* can be used interchangeably.

22. _____ The diameter of the pulmonary capillaries allows red blood cells to travel through at 10 abreast.

23. _____ Nitrogen is the gas of greatest concentration in atmospheric air.

▶ *If you had difficulty with this section, review pages 838-841.*

III—BLOOD TRANSPORTATION OF GASES AND SYSTEMIC GAS EXCHANGE

Multiple Choice—select the best answer.

24. Oxygen is carried in blood:
    a. as oxyhemoglobin.
    b. dissolved in plasma.
    c. molecularly as HbO_2.
    d. all of the above.

25. Which of the following is *not* a manner in which CO_2 is transported in the blood?
    a. dissolved in plasma
    b. bound to the heme group of the hemoglobin molecule
    c. as bicarbonate ions
    d. bound to the polypeptide chains of hemoglobin

26. Increasing the carbon dioxide content of blood results in:
    a. increased H^+ concentration of plasma.
    b. decreased blood pH.
    c. increased blood pH.
    d. both a and b.
    e. both a and c.

27. Approximately 97% of oxygen is transported as _____, whereas the remaining 3% is transported dissolved in _____.
    a. plasma; hemoglobin
    b. oxyhemoglobin; bicarbonate ion
    c. oxyhemoglobin; plasma
    d. bicarbonate ion; carbonic acid

True or false

28. _____ The exact amount of oxygen in blood depends mainly upon the amount of hemoglobin present.

29. _____ As plasma P_{CO_2} increases, the CO_2 carrying capacity of blood decreases.

30. _____ Interstitial fluid P_{O_2} and intracellular fluid P_{O_2} are essentially the same.

31. _____ A right shift of the oxygen-hemoglobin dissociation curve due to increased P_{CO_2} is known as the *Bohr effect*.

▶ *If you had difficulty with this section, review pages 841-848.*

IV—REGULATION OF BREATHING

Multiple Choice—select the best answer.

32. The basic rhythm of the respiratory cycle seems to be influenced by:
    a. the medullary rhythmicity area.
    b. the pneumotaxic center.
    c. the apneustic center.
    d. all of the above.

33. The diving reflex:
    a. explains why some people can hold their breath for extended periods while under water.
    b. is responsible for the astonishing recovery of near-drowning victims in cold water.
    c. forces a submerged individual to exhale prior to surfacing.
    d. both a and c.

True or false

34. _____ Input from the apneustic center in the pons inhibits the inspiratory center, causing a decrease in the length and depth of inspiration.

35. _____ Irritation of the phrenic nerve can cause extended periods of hiccups.

Labeling—identify the respiratory centers of the brain stem by matching each term to its corresponding number on the following illustration.

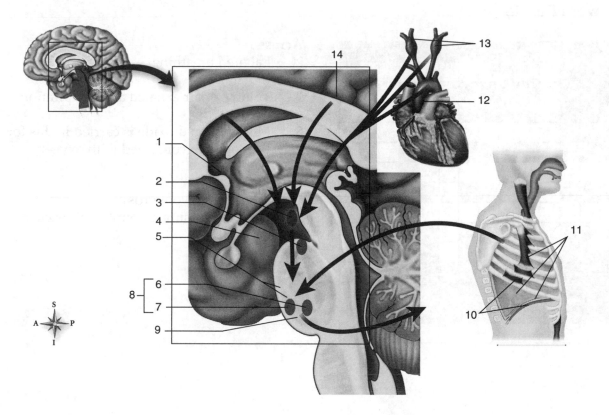

_____ carotid chemoreceptors and baroreceptors

_____ respiratory muscles

_____ apneustic center

_____ DRG

_____ limbic system (emotional responses)

_____ aortic chemoreceptors and baroreceptors

_____ PRG

_____ pons

_____ VRG

_____ medulla

_____ stretch receptors in lungs and thorax

_____ cortex (voluntary control)

_____ medullary rhythmicity area

_____ central chemoreceptors

▶ *If you had difficulty with this section, review pages 848-854.*

V—MECHANISMS OF DISEASE

Fill in the blanks.

36. _____ or _____
_____ _____
_____ is a broad term used to
describe conditions of progressive, irre-
versible obstruction of expiratory air flow.

37. _____ results from exces-
sive tracheobronchial secretions that obstruct air flow.

38. _____ may result from
the progression of chronic bronchitis or
other conditions as air becomes trapped
within alveoli causing them to enlarge
and eventually rupture.

39. _____ is an obstruc-
tive disorder characterized by recurring
spasms of the smooth muscle in the walls
of the bronchial air passages.

▶ *If you had difficulty with this section, review
pages 854-857.*

Crossword Puzzle

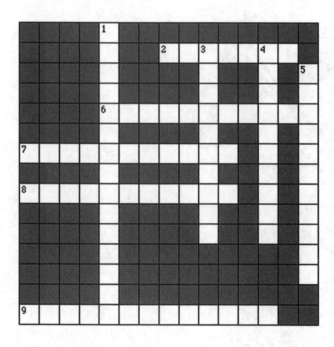

Across
2. Labored breathing
6. Inhaling
7. Volume of air exhaled after inspiration
(two words)
8. Most carbon dioxide is carried in this form
9. Hemoglobin combined with oxygen

Down
1. "Tension" (two words)
3. Used to measure amount of air exchanged
in breathing
4. Exhaling
5. Breathing

APPLYING WHAT YOU KNOW

40. Mr. Gaines has smoked a considerable number of cigars and cigarettes during the last two de-
cades. He is beginning to have difficulty breathing—especially upon exhalation. Which broad
category of diseases may he be exhibiting symptoms of? What other diseases is he at risk for?
What are the physiologic mechanisms of these diseases?

41. While sledding on a frozen creek, Heather, a 12-year-old girl, fell through the ice. Her situation wasn't discovered for about half an hour. Upon rescue, she displayed fixed, dilated pupils;
cyanosis; and no pulse. Miraculously, she recovered. Identify and explain the physiologic phenomena that resulted in this astonishing recovery.

DID YOU KNOW

- Sinusitis affects 37 million Americans causing difficulty in breathing and chronic headaches.

- A person's nose and ears continue to grow throughout his or her life.

ONE LAST QUICK CHECK

Multiple Choice—select the best answer.

42. The term that means the same thing as *breathing* is:
    a. gas exchange.
    b. respiration.
    c. inspiration.
    d. pulmonary ventilation.

43. Carbaminohemoglobin is formed when _____ bind(s) to hemoglobin.
    a. oxygen
    b. amino acids
    c. carbon dioxide
    d. nitrogen

44. Most of the oxygen transported by the blood is:
    a. dissolved to white blood cells.
    b. bound to white blood cells.
    c. bound to hemoglobin.
    d. bound to carbaminohemoglobin.

45. Which of the following does *not* occur during inspiration?
    a. elevation of the ribs
    b. the diaphragm relaxes
    c. alveolar pressure decreases
    d. chest cavity becomes longer from top to bottom

46. A young adult male would have a vital capacity of about _____ mL.
    a. 500
    b. 1200
    c. 3300
    d. 4800

47. The amount of air that can be forcibly exhaled after expiring the tidal volume is known as the:
    a. total lung capacity.
    b. vital capacity.
    c. inspiratory reserve volume.
    d. expiratory reserve volume.

48. Which one of the following is correct?
    a. VC = TV – IRV + ERV
    b. VC = TV + IRV – ERV
    c. VC = TV + IRV x ERV
    d. VC = TV + IRV + ERV

Matching—identify the term with the proper selection.

a. collapsed lung
b. quaternary protein
c. approximately 3300 mL
d. P_{O_2}
e. normal exhalation volume
f. increased in emphysema
g. helps control respirations
h. respiratory stimulant
i. cessation of breathing
j. sensitive to changes in arterial CO_2 and pH

49. _____ tidal volume

50. _____ inspiratory reserve volume

51. _____ pneumothorax

52. _____ physiologic dead space

53. _____ oxygen tension

54. _____ hemoglobin

55. _____ apneusis

56. _____ chemoreceptors

57. _____ Hering-Breuer reflexes

58. _____ CO_2

CHAPTER 28

Anatomy of the Digestive System

Think of the last meal you ate. The different shapes, sizes, tastes, and textures that you so recently enjoyed. Think of those items circulating in your bloodstream in those same original shapes and sizes. Impossible? Of course. Because of this impossibility you can begin to understand and marvel at the close relationship of the digestive system to the circulatory system. It is the digestive system that changes our food, both mechanically and chemically, into a form that is acceptable to the blood and the body.

This change begins the moment you take the very first bite. Digestion starts in the mouth, where food is chewed and mixed with saliva. It then moves down the pharynx and esophagus by peristalsis and enters the stomach. In the stomach it is churned and mixed with gastric juices to continue the digestive process. As the food continues into the small intestine, it is further broken down chemically by intestinal fluids, bile, and pancreatic juice. These secretions prepare the food for absorption all along the course of the small intestine (duodenum, jejunum, and ileum). Products that are not absorbed pass on and enter the cecum of the large intestine and continue through the ascending colon, transverse colon, descending colon, sigmoid colon, into the rectum, and out the anus.

Products that are used in the cells undergo absorption. Absorption allows newly processed nutrients to pass through the walls of the digestive tract and into the bloodstream to be distributed to the cells. Your review of this system will help you understand the anatomy that provides the mechanical and chemical processes necessary to convert food into energy sources and compounds necessary for survival.

I—OVERVIEW OF THE DIGESTIVE SYSTEM

Multiple Choice—select the best answer.

1. Starting from the deepest layer and moving toward the most superficial, the layers of the wall of the GI tract are:
   a. mucosa, submucosa, serosa, muscularis.
   b. submucosa, mucosa, muscularis, serosa.
   c. mucosa, submucosa, muscularis, serosa.
   d. submucosa, serosa, muscularis, mucosa.

2. The serosa is actually:
   a. parietal peritoneum.
   b. visceral peritoneum.
   c. mesentery.
   d. none of the above.

True or false

3. _____ *Gastrointestinal tract* and *alimentary canal* are often used synonymously.

4. _____ The tissue layers of the GI tract are constant, with no variation in the different organs.

Matching—identify each digestive organ with its correct classification.

a. GI tract segment   b. accessory organ

5. _____ mouth

6. _____ jejunum

7. _____ cecum

8. _____ pancreas

9. _____ teeth

10. _____ liver

11. _____ salivary glands

12. _____ vermiform appendix

13. _____ oropharynx

14. _____ sigmoid colon

Labeling—identify the principal organs of the digestive system by matching each term with its corresponding number on the following illustration.

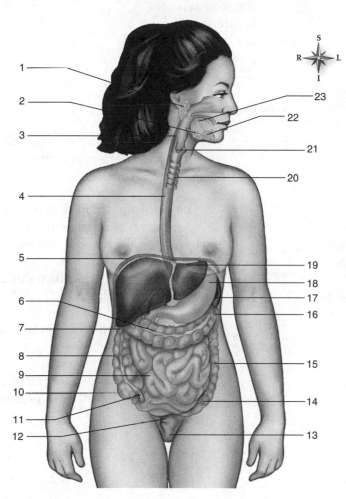

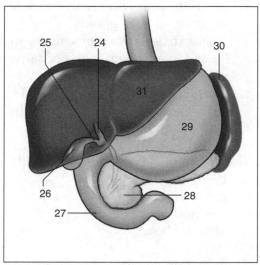

_____ submandibular salivary gland
_____ ascending colon
_____ liver
_____ esophagus
_____ transverse colon
_____ parotid gland
_____ spleen
_____ cystic duct
_____ ileum
_____ gallbladder
_____ vermiform appendix
_____ splenic flexure of colon
_____ cecum
_____ diaphragm
_____ duodenum
_____ common hepatic duct
_____ rectum

_____ descending colon
_____ anal canal
_____ spleen
_____ pancreas
_____ liver
_____ hepatic flexure of colon
_____ sigmoid colon
_____ tongue
_____ stomach
_____ trachea
_____ larynx
_____ sublingual salivary gland
_____ stomach
_____ pharynx

▶ *If you had difficulty with this section, review pages 861-864.*

II—MOUTH AND PHARYNX

Multiple Choice—select the best answer.

15. The hard palate consists of portions of:
    a. three bones: two maxillae and one palatine.
    b. two bones: one maxillae and one palatine.
    c. three bones: one maxillae and two palatine.
    d. four bones: two maxillae and two palatine.

16. Which of the following is an accurate description of salivary glands?
    a. There are four pairs of salivary glands.
    b. They secrete about 1 liter of saliva per day.
    c. They are associated with buccal glands that secrete about 50% of the saliva.
    d. Both b and c are true.

17. The crown of a tooth is covered with:
    a. dentin.
    b. cementum.
    c. enamel.
    d. alveolar bone.

18. Teeth that do *not* appear as deciduous teeth are:
    a. incisors.
    b. canines.
    c. second molars.
    d. premolars.

19. The act of swallowing moves a mass of food called a _____ from the mouth to the stomach.
    a. dentin
    b. bolus
    c. fauces
    d. philtrum

True or false

20. _____ A typical tooth can be divided into three main parts: crown, neck, and root.

21. _____ The *philtrum* is a fold of mucous membrane that helps anchor the tongue to the floor of the mouth.

22. _____ There are 20 deciduous teeth and 30 permanent teeth.

23. _____ The act of swallowing is termed *deglutition*.

24. _____ The soft palate forms a partition between the mouth and oropharynx.

Labeling—label the structures of the tooth on the following illustration.

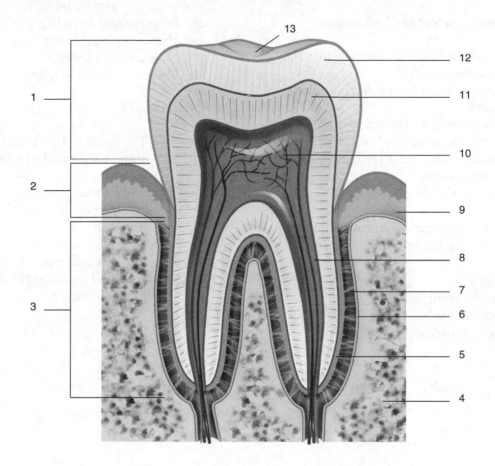

1 _____	8 _____
2 _____	9 _____
3 _____	10 _____
4 _____	11 _____
5 _____	12 _____
6 _____	13 _____
7 _____	

▶ *If you had difficulty with this section, review pages 864-870.*

III—ESOPHAGUS AND STOMACH

Multiple Choice—select the best answer.

25. Which of the following statements is *not* true of the esophagus?
    a. It extends from the pharynx to the stomach.
    b. It lies anterior to the trachea and posterior to the heart.
    c. It resides in both the thoracic and abdominal cavities.
    d. It pierces the diaphragm.

26. Which of the following controls the opening of the stomach into the small intestine?
    a. pylorus
    b. cardiac sphincter
    c. duodenal bulb
    d. pyloric sphincter

27. Which of the layers of the muscularis is present only in the stomach?
    a. longitudinal muscle layer
    b. circular muscle layer
    c. oblique muscle layer
    d. horizontal muscle layer

True or false

28. _____ The folds in the lining of the stomach are called *rugae*.

29. _____ The cardiac sphincter controls the opening of the esophagus into the stomach.

30. _____ Parietal cells secrete hydrochloric acid and are thought to produce intrinsic factor.

Labeling—match each term with its corresponding number on the following illustration of the stomach.

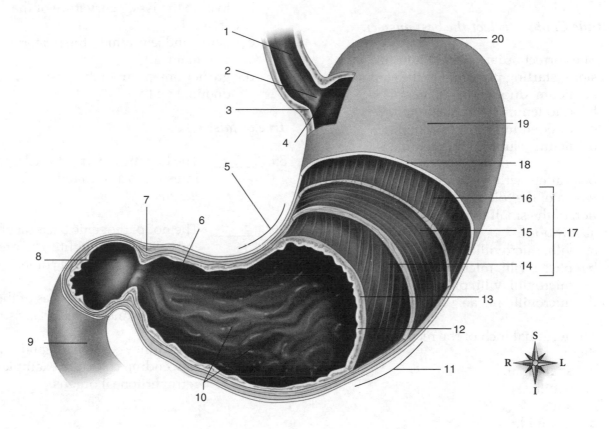

_____ rugae

_____ fundus

_____ mucosa

_____ lower esophageal sphincter (LES)

_____ cardia

_____ longitudinal muscle layer

_____ pylorus

_____ esophagus

_____ oblique muscle layer

_____ duodenum

_____ serosa

_____ duodenal bulb

_____ greater curvature

_____ submucosa

_____ lesser curvature

_____ circular muscle layer

_____ pyloric sphincter

_____ muscularis

_____ gastroesophageal opening

_____ body of stomach

▶ *If you had difficulty with this section, review pages 870-875.*

IV—SMALL INTESTINE, LARGE INTESTINE, APPENDIX, AND PERITONEUM

Multiple Choice—select the best answer.

31. The correct order of small intestine divisions, starting proximal to the stomach, is:
    a. ileum, duodenum, jejunum.
    b. duodenum, ileum, jejunum.
    c. duodenum, jejunum, ileum.
    d. ileum, jejunum, duodenum.

32. Beginning with the largest structures, which of the following is a correct description of the small intestine's adaptation for absorption?
    a. villi, microvilli, plicae
    b. plicae, villi, microvilli
    c. microvilli, villi, plicae
    d. microvilli, plicae, villi

33. The terminal inch of the rectum is called the:
    a. anal canal.
    b. fistula.
    c. anus.
    d. sigmoid.

34. The lesser omentum attaches the:
    a. transverse colon to the posterior abdominal wall.
    b. liver to the lesser curvature of the stomach.
    c. ileum and jejunum to the posterior abdominal wall.
    d. greater omentum to the posterior abdominal wall.

True or false

35. _____ The hepatic flexure of the large intestine is also called the *left colic flexure.*

36. _____ The nonpathogenic bacteria of the colon are thought to be produced in the sigmoid colon.

37. _____ The pouchlike structures of the large intestine are called *haustra.*

38. _____ The kidneys, adrenal glands, and descending colon are examples of retroperitoneal organs.

Labeling—using the terms provided, label the wall of the small intestine on the following illustration.

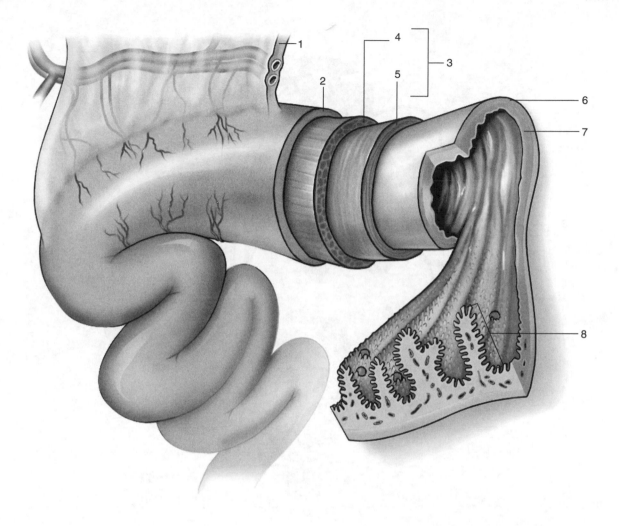

_____ circular muscle

_____ plica (fold)

_____ serosa

_____ longitudinal muscle

_____ mesentery

_____ muscularis

_____ submucosa

_____ mucosa

Labeling—using the terms provided, label the divisions of the large intestine on the following illustration.

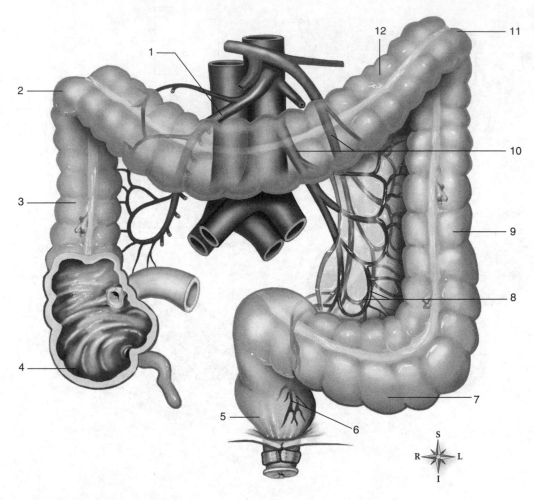

_____ hepatic (right colic) flexure		_____ cecum	
_____ splenic (left colic) flexure		_____ sigmoid colon	
_____ superior rectal artery and vein		_____ transverse colon	
_____ inferior mesenteric artery and vein		_____ sigmoid artery and vein	
_____ ascending colon		_____ rectum	
_____ superior mesenteric artery		_____ descending colon	

▶ *If you had difficulty with this section, review pages 875-882.*

V—LIVER, GALLBLADDER, AND PANCREAS

Multiple Choice—select the best answer.

39. The anatomic units of the liver are called:
    a. lobes.
    b. lobules.
    c. sinusoids.
    d. none of the above.

40. Blood flows to hepatic lobules via branches of the:
    a. hepatic artery.
    b. hepatic portal vein.
    c. hepatic vein.
    d. both a and b.

41. A merger of the hepatic duct and cystic duct form the:
    a. common hepatic duct.
    b. common bile duct.
    c. right hepatic duct.
    d. left hepatic duct.

42. Bile salts aid in the absorption of:
    a. fat.
    b. carbohydrates.
    c. proteins.
    d. waste products.

True or false

43. _____ The liver consists of two lobes separated by the falciform ligament.

44. _____ Bile is manufactured by the Kupffer cells of the liver.

45. _____ The pancreas is both an endocrine and exocrine gland.

46. _____ Surgical removal of the gallbladder is called *cholecystectomy*.

Labeling—match each term with its corresponding number on the following illustration of the liver.

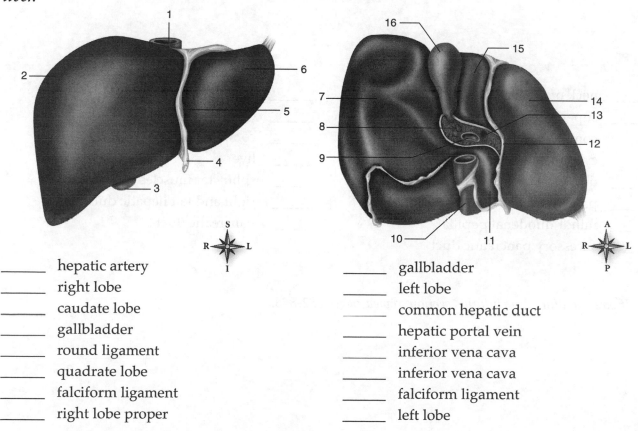

_____ hepatic artery	_____ gallbladder
_____ right lobe	_____ left lobe
_____ caudate lobe	_____ common hepatic duct
_____ gallbladder	_____ hepatic portal vein
_____ round ligament	_____ inferior vena cava
_____ quadrate lobe	_____ inferior vena cava
_____ falciform ligament	_____ falciform ligament
_____ right lobe proper	_____ left lobe

Labeling—match each term with its corresponding number on the following illustration of the common bile duct and its tributaries.

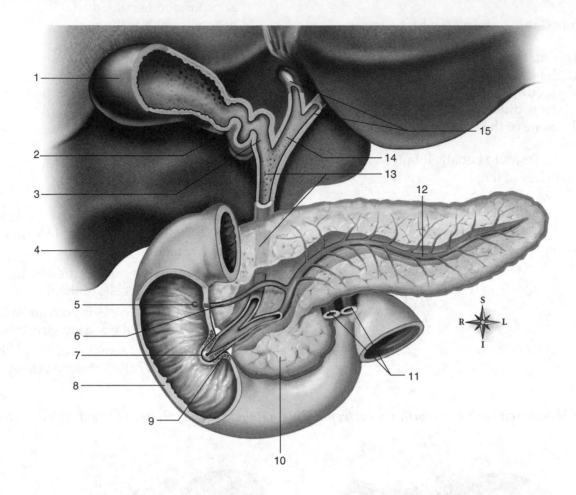

_____	neck of gallbladder	_____	major duodenal papilla
_____	superior mesenteric artery and vein	_____	corpus (body) of gallbladder
_____	common bile duct	_____	common hepatic duct
_____	cystic duct	_____	liver
_____	duodenum	_____	sphincter muscles
_____	pancreas	_____	right and left hepatic ducts
_____	minor duodenal papilla	_____	pancreatic duct
_____	accessory pancreatic duct		

▶ *If you had difficulty with this section, review pages 882-888.*

VI—MECHANISMS OF DISEASE

Matching—identify the term with the appropriate description.

a. corrects malocclusion
b. swelling of parotid glands
c. inflammation of rectal mucosa
d. dilated veins
e. autoimmune disease that targets salivary and tear glands
f. obstructive narrowing
g. low incidence in older adults
h. minor laceration
i. causes most gastric and duodenal ulcers
j. gastric reflux
k. infection of gums

47. _____ hemorrhoids
48. _____ appendicitis
49. _____ pyloric stenosis
50. _____ Sjögren's syndrome
51. _____ *Helicobacter pylori*
52. _____ orthodontics
53. _____ anal fissures
54. _____ mumps
55. _____ proctitis
56. _____ gingivitis
57. _____ heartburn

▶ *If you had difficulty with this section, review pages 888-897.*

Crossword Puzzle

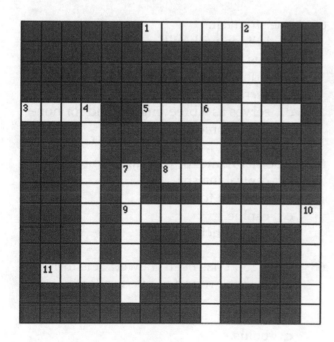

Across

1. Alimentary canal (abbrev., two words)
3. Stored in gallbladder
5. Division of small intestine
8. Small projection in small intestine
9. Large sheet of serous membrane
11. Chewing

Down

2. Large intestine
4. First segment of digestive tube
6. Swallowing
7. Refers to liver
10. Innermost layer of GI tract

APPLYING WHAT YOU KNOW

58. Brian is experiencing difficulty digesting fatty foods and is displaying a yellow discoloration of his skin. What may be causing his condition? What is the clinical term used to describe the yellow appearance of his skin and what is the physiology? How could doctors treat his condition and what are the names of the procedures?

59. Baby Billy has been regurgitating his bottle-feeding at every meal. The milk is curdled, but does not appear to be digested. He has become dehydrated, so his mother, Amanda, is taking him to the pediatrician. What is a possible diagnosis from your textbook reading?

DID YOU KNOW

- The human stomach lining replaces itself every 3 days.

- If one were to unravel the entire human alimentary canal (esophagus, stomach, small and large intestines), it would reach the height of a three-story building.

ONE LAST QUICK CHECK

Multiple Choice—select the best answer.

60. The first baby tooth, on an average, appears at age:
    a. 2 months.
    b. 1 year.
    c. 1 month.
    d. 6 months.

61. The dentin of the tooth contains the _____, which consists of connective tissue, blood and lymphatic vessels, and nerves.
    a. pulp cavity
    b. neck
    c. root
    d. crown

62. Which of the following teeth is missing from the deciduous arch?
    a. central incisor
    b. canine
    c. second premolar
    d. first molar

63. The permanent central incisor erupts between the ages of _____.
    a. 9 and 13
    b. 5 and 6
    c. 7 and 10
    d. 8 and 9

64. A general term for infection of the gums is:
    a. dental caries.
    b. leukoplakia.
    c. Vincent's angina.
    d. gingivitis.

65. The ducts of the _____ glands open into the floor of the mouth.
    a. sublingual
    b. submandibular
    c. parotid
    d. carotid

66. The stomach:
    a. is lined with villi.
    b. lies in a vertical position of the left side of the abdomen.
    c. secretes intrinsic factor.
    d. serves as a breeding ground for non-pathogenic bacteria.

67. Another name for the third molar is:
    a. central incisor.
    b. wisdom tooth.
    c. canine.
    d. lateral incisor.

68. After food has been chewed, it is formed into a small rounded mass called a:
    a. moat.
    b. chyme.
    c. bolus.
    d. protease.

69. Which one is *not* part of the small intestine?
    a. jejunum
    b. ileum
    c. cecum
    d. duodenum

70. The union of the cystic duct and the _____ forms the common bile duct.
    a. hepatic duct
    b. major duodenal papilla
    c. minor duodenal papilla
    d. pancreatic duct

71. Each villus in the intestine contains a lymphatic vessel or _____ that serves to absorb lipid or fat materials from the chyme.
    a. plica
    b. lacteal
    c. villa
    d. microvilli

72. *Cholelithiasis* is the term used to describe:
    a. biliary colic.
    b. jaundice.
    c. portal hypertension.
    d. gallstones.

73. The largest gland in the body is the:
    a. pituitary.
    b. thyroid.
    c. liver.
    d. thymus.

True or false

74. _____ The splenic flexure is the bend between the ascending colon and the transverse colon.

75. _____ The splenic colon is the S-shaped segment that terminates in the rectum.

76. _____ Following mastication, deglutition occurs.

77. _____ The oral cavity is also known as the *buccal cavity*.

78. _____ The esophagus is voluntary in the upper third, mixed in the middle, and involuntary in the lower third.

79. _____ The upper lip is marked near the midline by a shallow vertical groove called the *philtrum*.

80. _____ The mesentery is a fan-shaped projection of the parietal peritoneum.

81. _____ The complete process of altering the physical and chemical composition of ingested food material so that it can be absorbed and used by the body is called *digestion*.

82. _____ The fundus, pylorus, and plicae are the three main divisions of the stomach.

CHAPTER 29

Physiology of the Digestive System

Digestion is the process of breaking down complex nutrients into simpler units suitable for absorption. It involves two major processes: mechanical and chemical. Mechanical digestion occurs during mastication and the churning and propelling mechanisms that take place along the alimentary canal. Chemical digestion occurs with the help of the many digestive enzymes and various substances that are added to the nutrients as they progress the length of the digestive tube. These substances include saliva and gastric, pancreatic, and intestinal enzymes. Delicate nervous and hormonal reflex mechanisms control the flow of these juices so that the proper amount is released at the appropriate time.

Absorption is the passage of substances (digested foods, water, salts, and vitamins) through the intestinal mucosa and into the blood or lymph. After the body has determined the nutrients necessary for absorption, it sends the residue of digestion to the final segment of the GI tract to be eliminated as feces.

Your review of this system will help you understand the mechanical and chemical processes necessary to convert food into energy sources and compounds necessary for survival.

I—DIGESTION

Multiple Choice—select the best answer.

1. Which of the following describes the pharyngeal stage of deglutition?
    a. mouth to oropharynx
    b. oropharynx to esophagus
    c. esophagus to stomach
    d. none of the above

2. Which step of deglutition is under voluntary control?
    a. oral
    b. pharyngeal
    c. esophageal
    d. all of the above

3. The final product of carbohydrate digestion is a:
    a. disaccharide.
    b. monosaccharide.
    c. polysaccharide.
    d. fatty acid.

4. Enzymes that catalyze the hydrolysis of proteins are:
    a. proteases.
    b. amylases.
    c. lactases.
    d. lipases.

5. A micelle is:
    a. a disaccharide attached to the brush border of the small intestine.
    b. a tiny sphere of lipid and water.
    c. a thick, milky material comprised of food and digestive enzymes.
    d. synonymous with *bolus*.

6. Which of the following is *not* true concerning the gastric emptying of water?
    a. Large volumes of water leave the stomach more rapidly than small volumes.
    b. Warm fluids empty more quickly than cool fluids.
    c. High-solute concentration fluids empty slower than dilute concentrations.
    d. All of the above are true.

7. The process of fat emulsification consists of:
    a. chemically breaking down fat molecules.
    b. absorption of fats.
    c. breaking down fats into small droplets.
    d. the secretion of digestive juices for fat digestion.

True or false

8. _____ Peristalsis can be described as a mixing movement.

9. _____ The volumes of the stomach and the duodenum are approximately equal.

10. _____ Enzymes are organic catalysts.

11. _____ Digestive enzymes catalyze chemical reactions with great efficiency within a wide range of pH.

12. _____ Cellulose resists digestion and is eliminated in feces.

13. _____ Water is readily absorbed in the stomach.

14. _____ Amino acids are the end product of protein digestion.

▶ *If you had difficulty with this section, review pages 901-914.*

II—SECRETION AND CONTROL OF DIGESTIVE GLAND SECRETION

Multiple Choice—select the best answer.

15. The principal enzyme of saliva is:
    a. protease.
    b. amylase.
    c. lipase.
    d. salivase.

16. Which of the following is true?
    a. Saliva contains large amounts of lipase.
    b. Pepsinogen is converted into pepsin by hydrochloric acid.
    c. Chief cells secrete pepsin.
    d. Zymogenic cells produce intrinsic factor.

17. Which of the following is present in bile?
    a. lecithin
    b. gastrin
    c. bile salts
    d. both a and c

18. The hormone that stimulates the gallbladder to release bile is:
    a. enterogastrone.
    b. insulin.
    c. gastrin.
    d. cholecystokinin.

True or false

19. _____ Pancreatic juice is secreted by exocrine acinar cells of the pancreas.

20. _____ Olfactory and visual stimuli are factors concerning the control of digestive gland secretion.

21. _____ The cephalic phase is initiated by the presence of food in the stomach.

22. _____ Chyme is liquefied food found in the stomach.

▶ *If you had difficulty with this section, review pages 914-921.*

CHEMICAL DIGESTION

Fill in the blank areas on the chart below.

Digestive Juices and Enzymes	Substance Digested (or Hydrolyzed)	Resulting Product
Saliva		
1. Amylase	1.	1. Maltose
Gastric Juice		
2. Protease (pepsin) plus hydrochloric acid	2. Proteins	2.
Pancreatic Juice		
3. Protease (trypsin)	3. Proteins (intact or partially digested)	3.
4. Lipase	4.	4. Fatty acids, monoglycerides, and glycerol
5. Amylase	5.	5. Maltose
Intestinal Juice		
6. Peptidases	6.	6. Amino acids
7.	7. Sucrose	7. Glucose and fructose
8. Lactase	8.	8. Glucose and galactose (simple sugars)
9. Maltase	9. Maltose	9.
10. Nucleotidases and phosphatases		10. Nucleosides

III—ABSORPTION AND ELIMINATION

Multiple Choice—select the best answer.

23. Fats are absorbed primarily into which of the following structures?
    a. blood in intestinal capillaries
    b. lymph in intestinal lacteals
    c. villi in large intestine
    d. none of the above

24. Movement of lower colon and rectum contents at a rate slower than normal can cause:
    a. defecation.
    b. constipation.
    c. diarrhea.
    d. both b and c.

25. Which blood vessel carries absorbed nutrients from the GI tract to the liver?
    a. hepatic artery
    b. hepatic vein
    c. portal vein
    d. inferior vena cava

True or false

26. _____ Both water and sodium are absorbed via simple diffusion.

27. _____ The majority of substances are absorbed in the small intestine.

28. _____ Cholera is an intestinal infection that kills more than 600,000 infants and children worldwide each year.

29. _____ Vitamins A, C, D, and E are known as "fat-soluble" vitamins.

30. _____ Impaired fat absorption produces large, greasy, foul-smelling stools known as *steatorrhea*.

Labeling—fill in the functions of each organ of digestion in the boxes provided below.

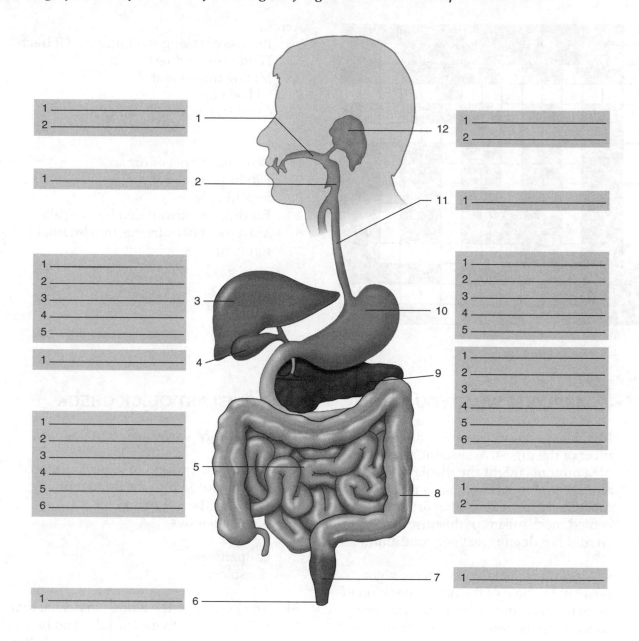

1 _____
2 _____

1 _____

1 _____
2 _____
3 _____
4 _____
5 _____

1 _____

1 _____
2 _____
3 _____
4 _____
5 _____
6 _____

1 _____

1 _____
2 _____

1 _____

1 _____
2 _____
3 _____
4 _____
5 _____

1 _____
2 _____
3 _____
4 _____
5 _____
6 _____

1 _____
2 _____

1 _____

▶ *If you had difficulty with this section, review pages 921-927.*

Crossword Puzzle

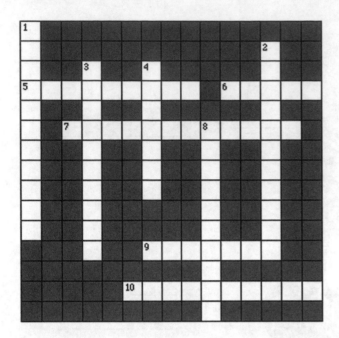

Across

5. Process of taking food into the GI tract
6. Food leaving the stomach
7. Mixing movement
9. GI hormones
10. Chemical process in digestion

Down

1. Wavelike ripple of organ
2. Fat droplet
3. Expelling feces
4. Fat droplet surrounded by bile salts
8. Movement of nutrients into internal environment

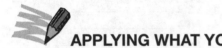

APPLYING WHAT YOU KNOW

31. Mrs. Haygood was diagnosed with an ulcer of the digestive system. What kind of symptoms might she display? Where along her alimentary canal is this lesion most likely to reside? What are the two accepted mechanisms of this disease? How should her doctor treat her condition?

32. Cliff and Pete like to play soccer vigorously in the heat of the day. What kind of recommendations should they observe concerning the replacement of fluids? Be sure to consider parameters such as fluid temperature, volume, and solute concentration.

DID YOU KNOW

* There are 35 million digestive glands in the stomach.

* Even if the stomach, the spleen, 75% of the liver, 80% of the intestines, one kidney, one lung, and virtually every organ from the pelvic and groin area are removed, the human body can still survive!

ONE LAST QUICK CHECK

Multiple Choice—select the best answer.

33. During the process of digestion, stored bile is poured into the duodenum by which of the following?
    a. gallbladder
    b. liver
    c. pancreas
    d. spleen

34. The portion of the alimentary canal that mixes food with gastric juice and breaks it down into a mixture called *chyme* is the:
    a. gallbladder.
    b. small intestine.
    c. stomach.
    d. large intestine.

35. What is the middle portion of the small intestine called?
    a. jejunum
    b. ileum
    c. duodenum
    d. cecum

36. Which of the following is *not* a stage of deglutition?
    a. oral
    b. pharyngeal
    c. esophageal
    d. gastric

37. Protein digestion begins in the:
    a. esophagus.
    b. small intestine.
    c. stomach.
    d. large intestine.

38. The enzyme pepsin is concerned primarily with the digestion of which of the following?
    a. sugars
    b. starches
    c. proteins
    d. fats

39. The enzyme amylase converts which of the following?
    a. starches to sugars
    b. sugars to starches
    c. proteins to amino acids
    d. fatty acids and glycerols to fats

40. Which of the following substances does *not* contain any enzymes?
    a. saliva
    b. bile
    c. gastric juice
    d. intestinal juice

41. Which of the following is a simple sugar?
    a. maltose
    b. sucrose
    c. lactose
    d. glucose

42. Fats are broken down into:
    a. amino acids.
    b. simple sugars.
    c. fatty acids.
    d. disaccharides.

43. Which hormone decreases peristalsis and slows the passage of food from the stomach to the duodenum?
    a. CCK
    b. GIP
    c. secretin
    d. gastrin

44. The union of the cystic duct and hepatic duct form the:
    a. common bile duct.
    b. major duodenal papilla.
    c. minor duodenal papilla.
    d. pancreatic duct.

45. The process of swallowing is known as:
    a. mastication.
    b. segmentation.
    c. peristalsis.
    d. deglutition.

46. Peristalsis begins in the:
    a. mouth.
    b. pharynx.
    c. esophagus.
    d. stomach.

True or false

47. _____ The mechanical process that occurs in the rectum is churning.

48. _____ Mechanical digestion begins in the mouth.

49. _____ The hormones secretin and CCK stimulate ejection of bile.

50. _____ Segmentation is a mixing movement.

51. _____ Bilirubin is the result of hemolysis by the liver.

52. _____ Most digestive enzymes are synthesized and secreted as inactive kinases.

CHAPTER 30

Nutrition and Metabolism

Most of us love to eat, but do the foods we enjoy provide us with the basic food types necessary for good nutrition? The body, a finely tuned machine, requires a balance of carbohydrates, fats, proteins, vitamins, and minerals to function properly. These nutrients must be digested, absorbed, and circulated to cells constantly to accommodate the numerous activities that occur throughout the body. The use the body makes of foods once these processes are completed is called *metabolism*.

Although the body relies on many organs to prepare nutrients, the liver plays a major role in the metabolism of food. It helps maintain a normal blood glucose level, removes toxins from the blood, processes blood immediately after it leaves the gastrointestinal tract, and initiates the first steps of protein and fat metabolism.

The study of metabolism is not complete without a discussion of the basal metabolic rate (BMR). The BMR is the rate at which food is catabolized under basal conditions. The total metabolic rate (TMR) is the amount of energy, expressed in calories, used by the body each day. This chapter also demonstrates the use of metabolic testing to measure thyroid functioning.

Finally, the hypothalamus appears to be a critical component in determining appetite and satiety. While many theories suggest various ways that the hypothalamus might perform these functions, it is imperative that we acknowledge its importance in nutrition and metabolism. Review of this chapter is necessary to provide you with an understanding of the *fuel*, or nutrition, necessary to maintain that complex homeostatic machine—the body.

I—OVERVIEW OF NUTRITION AND METABOLISM

Multiple Choice—select the best answer.

1. The universal biological currency is:
    a. ATP.
    b. ADP.
    c. carbohydrates.
    d. NADH.

2. *Nutrition* refers to the:
    a. complex set of chemical processes that make life possible.
    b. breaking down of food into small molecular compounds.
    c. release of energy in two main forms.
    d. food we eat and the nutrients they contain.

True or false

3. _____ Catabolism is a process that breaks down molecules into smaller molecular compounds.

4. _____ Metabolism is identical in all cells.

▶ *If you had difficulty with this section, review pages 931-934.*

II—CARBOHYDRATES

Multiple Choice—select the best answer.

5. Glucose, fructose, and galactose are important:
    a. monosaccharides.
    b. disaccharides.
    c. polysaccharides.
    d. starches.

6. The carbohydrate most useful to the human cell is:
    a. cellulose.
    b. glucose.
    c. fructose.
    d. galactose.

7. The process of glucose phosphorylation forms the molecule:
    a. ATP.
    b. ADP.
    c. glucose-6-phosphate.
    d. glycogen.

8. The breakdown of one glucose molecule into two pyruvic acid molecules is called:
    a. glycolysis.
    b. glycogenesis.
    c. glycogenolysis.
    d. glycogen.

9. The amount of heat necessary to raise the temperature of 1 g of water by 1° C is a:
    a. calorie.
    b. Celsius.
    c. kilocalorie.
    d. none of the above.

10. To enter the citric acid cycle, glucose must be transformed into:
    a. pyruvic acid.
    b. acetyl-CoA.
    c. ATP.
    d. NADH.

11. Which of the following defines *glycogenesis?*
    a. process of glycogen formation
    b. joining of glucose molecules
    c. catabolism of glycogen
    d. both a and b

12. Which of the following hormones helps glucose enter cells, and therefore decreases blood glucose?
    a. glucagon
    b. insulin
    c. epinephrine
    d. growth hormone

True or false

13. _____ Glycolysis is an anaerobic process.

14. _____ Glycolysis prepares glucose for the citric acid cycle.

15. _____ Glycolysis occurs in the mitochondria, whereas the citric acid cycle occurs in the cytoplasm.

16. _____ Erythrocytes rely upon aerobic respiration.

17. _____ The process of gluconeogenesis synthesizes new glucose molecules.

18. _____ Glycogenesis is a homeostatic mechanism that functions when blood glucose levels increase above normal.

19. _____ Hyperglycemia occurs when the blood glucose dips below the normal set point level.

20. _____ The conversion of proteins to glucose is an example of gluconeogenesis.

21. _____ Glucagon stimulates glycogenolysis in the liver.

22. _____ ACTH decreases blood glucose concentration.

23. _____ Disaccharides do *not* need to be chemically digested before they can be absorbed.

24. _____ The *citric acid cycle*, the *TCA cycle*, and the *Krebs cycle* are all synonymous.

25. _____ *Oxidative phosphorylation* refers to the joining of a phosphate group to ADP to form ATP.

26. _____ The breakdown of ATP molecules provides 50% of all of the energy needed for cellular work.

27. _____ Glycogenolysis is consistent in all cells.

▶ *If you had difficulty with this section, review pages 934-946.*

III—LIPIDS

Multiple Choice—select the best answer.

28. _____ contains fatty acid chains in which all available bonds of its hydrocarbon chain are filled with hydrogen atoms.
    a. Saturated fat
    b. Unsaturated fat
    c. Cholesterol
    d. Both a and b

29. The most common lipids in the diet are:
    a. phospholipids.
    b. cholesterol.
    c. triglycerides.
    d. prostaglandins.

30. A high risk for atherosclerosis is associated with a high blood concentration of:
    a. LDL.
    b. HDL.
    c. CVA.
    d. both a and b.

31. All of the following hormones control lipid metabolism *except*:
    a. ACTH.
    b. glucocorticoids.
    c. epinephrine.
    d. insulin.

32. Which of the following lab results would indicate high risk for atherosclerosis?
    a. 100 mg LDL/100 mL of blood
    b. 180 mg HDL/100 mL of blood
    c. 60 mg HDL/100 mL of blood
    d. 200 mg LDL/100 mL of blood

True or false

33. _____ A diet high in saturated fats and cholesterol tends to increase blood concentration of high-density lipoproteins.

34. _____ Lipid catabolism yields 9 kcal/g.

35. _____ Essential fatty acids are not synthesized by the body and must be obtained through the diet.

36. _____ Lipids are transported in the blood as chylomicrons, lipoproteins, and free fatty acids.

37. _____ The liver is the chief site of ketogenesis.

▶ *If you had difficulty with this section, review pages 946-948.*

IV—PROTEINS

Multiple Choice—select the best answer.

38. Which of the following is a nonessential amino acid?
    a. lysine
    b. alanine
    c. tryptophan
    d. valine

39. The process by which proteins are synthesized by the ribosomes in all cells is called:
    a. protein catabolism.
    b. protein anabolism.
    c. protein metabolism.
    d. both a and b.

40. Which of the following hormones tends to promote protein anabolism?
    a. testosterone
    b. growth hormone
    c. thyroid hormone
    d. all of the above

True or false

41. ＿＿＿＿＿ In protein metabolism, catabolism is primary and anabolism is secondary.

42. ＿＿＿＿＿ Foods from animal sources high in proteins contain the essential amino acids.

43. ＿＿＿＿＿ Glucocorticoids are protein catabolic hormones.

44. ＿＿＿＿＿ Growth and pregnancy usually result in a negative nitrogen balance.

45. ＿＿＿＿＿ The first step in protein catabolism takes place in the liver and is called *deamination*.

▶ *If you had difficulty with this section, review pages 948-952.*

V—VITAMINS AND MINERALS

Multiple Choice—select the best answer.

46. Which of the following plays an important role in detecting light in the sensory cells of the eye?
    a. vitamin D
    b. retinal
    c. biotin
    d. pantothenic acid

47. Which of the following vitamins is fat-soluble?
    a. vitamin A
    b. vitamin B
    c. vitamin C
    d. none of the above

48. Which of the following illnesses can result from an iodine deficiency?
    a. anemia
    b. bone degeneration
    c. goiter
    d. acid-base imbalance

True or false

49. ＿＿＿＿＿ Athletic performance can be enhanced by vitamin supplementation.

50. ＿＿＿＿＿ Vitamin E is thought to neutralize free radicals.

51. ＿＿＿＿＿ Vitamin C deficiency could result in scurvy.

52. ＿＿＿＿＿ Coenzymes are inorganic catalysts.

▶ *If you had difficulty with this section, review pages 952-955.*

VI—METABOLIC RATE AND MECHANISMS FOR REGULATING FOOD INTAKE

Multiple Choice—select the best answer.

53. Which of the following is *not* a condition required for the BMR?
    a. The individual is lying down and not moving.
    b. The individual is sleeping.
    c. It has been 12 to 18 hours since the individual's last meal.
    d. The individual is in a comfortable, warm environment.

54. Which of the following does *not* influence BMR?
    a. age
    b. gender
    c. ethnicity
    d. size

55. One pound of adipose tissue equals:
    a. 1000 kcal.
    b. 350 kcal.
    c. 3500 kcal.
    d. 10,000 kcal.

56. The appetite center is most likely located in the:
    a. cerebrum.
    b. hypothalamus.
    c. small intestine.
    d. stomach.

True or false

57. _____ Males have a BMR approximately 15–20% higher than females.

58. _____ Increases in blood temperature and glucose concentration may be linked to satiety.

59. _____ Body weight is linked to both energy input and energy output.

60. _____ When body temperature decreases, metabolism increases.

61. _____ Metabolic rate is the amount of energy released in the body in a given time by anabolism.

▶ *If you had difficulty with this section, review pages 955-961.*

VII—MECHANISMS OF DISEASE

Matching—choose the correct response.

a. phenylketonuria
b. anorexia nervosa
c. bulimia
d. obesity
e. protein-calorie malnutrition
f. marasmus
g. ascites

62. _____ characterized by a refusal to eat

63. _____ results from a deficiency of calories in general and protein in particular

64. _____ inborn error of metabolism

65. _____ advanced form of PCM

66. _____ not a disorder, but may be a symptom of abnormal behavior

67. _____ binge-purge syndrome

68. _____ abdominal bloating

▶ *If you had difficulty with this section, review pages 961-965.*

Crossword Puzzle

(crossword grid with numbered cells: 1, 2, 3, 4, 5, 6, 7, 8, 9)

Across

1. Decomposition process
4. Synthesis process
8. The food and nutrients we eat
9. Discovered citric acid cycle

Down

2. Does not require oxygen
3. Forms body fat from food
5. Requires oxygen
6. Chemical processes that make life possible
7. Organ molecule needed to assist enzyme functioning

APPLYING WHAT YOU KNOW

69. Dr. Reeder was concerned about Myrna. Her daily food intake provided fewer calories than her TMR. If this trend continues, what will be the result? If it continues over a long period of time, what eating disorder might Myrna develop?

70. Tom was experiencing fatigue and a blood test revealed that he was slightly anemic. What mineral(s) will his doctor most likely prescribe? What dietary sources might you suggest that he emphasize in his daily diet?

DID YOU KNOW

- The body's daily requirement of vitamins and minerals is less than a thimbleful.

- The average person consumes 2000 to 2500 calories a day but if you had the metabolism of a shrew you would need to consume approximately 200,000 calories a day! Smaller animals have higher metabolic rates because they have to work harder to keep their bodies warm.

ONE LAST QUICK CHECK

Multiple Choice—select the best answer.

71. What is the process by which pyruvic acid is broken down into carbon dioxide and high-energy electrons called?
    a. glycogenesis
    b. citric acid cycle
    c. glycolysis
    d. pyruvic acid cycle

72. The anabolism of glucose produces which of the following?
    a. glycogen
    b. amino acid
    c. rennin
    d. starch

73. Which of the following is a major hormone in the body that aids carbohydrate metabolism?
    a. oxytocin
    b. prolactin
    c. insulin
    d. ADH

74. The total metabolic rate is which of the following?
    a. the amount of fats we consume in a 24-hour period
    b. the same as the BMR
    c. the amount of energy expressed in calories used by the body per day
    d. cannot be calculated

75. When your consumption of calories equals your TMR, your weight will do which of the following?
    a. increase
    b. remain the same
    c. fluctuate
    d. decrease

76. What is the primary molecule the body usually breaks down as an energy source?
    a. amino acids
    b. pepsin
    c. maltose
    d. glucose

77. When glucose is *not* available, the body will next catabolize which of the following energy sources?
    a. fats
    b. hormones
    c. minerals
    d. vitamins

Circle the word or phrase that does **not** *belong.*

78. glycolysis   citric acid cycle

    ATP   bile

79. adipose   amino acids

    triglycerides   lipid

80. A   D

    M   K

81. iron   protein

    amino acids   essential

82. ACTH   insulin

    growth hormone   epinephrine

83. sodium   calcium

    zinc   folic acid

84. thiamine   niacin

    ascorbic acid   riboflavin

Matching—identify the term that best matches the definition.

a. carbohydrate
b. fat
c. protein
d. vitamins
e. minerals

85. _____ preferred energy food

86. _____ amino acids

87. _____ fat-soluble

88. _____ required for nerve conduction

89. _____ glycolysis

90. _____ inorganic elements found naturally in the earth

91. _____ pyruvic acid

92. _____ chylomicrons

93. _____ triglycerides

CHAPTER 31

Urinary System

Living produces wastes. Wherever people live or work or play, wastes accumulate. To keep these areas healthy, there must be a method of disposing of these wastes such as a sanitation department.

Wastes also accumulate in your body. The conversion of food and gases into substances and energy necessary for survival results in waste products. A large percentage of these wastes is removed by the urinary system.

Two vital organs, the kidneys, cleanse the blood of the many waste products that are continually produced as a result of the metabolism of food in the body cells. They eliminate these wastes in the form of urine.

Urine formation is the result of three processes: filtration, reabsorption, and secretion. These processes occur in successive portions of the microscopic units of the kidneys known as *nephrons*. The amount of urine produced by the nephrons is controlled primarily by the hormones antidiuretic hormone (ADH) and aldosterone. After the urine is produced, it is drained from the renal pelvis by the ureters to flow into the bladder. The bladder then stores the urine until it is voided through the urethra.

If waste products are allowed to accumulate in the body, they soon become poisonous, a condition called *uremia*. A knowledge of the urinary system is necessary to understand how the body rids itself of waste and avoids toxicity.

I—ANATOMY OF THE URINARY SYSTEM

Multiple Choice—select the best answer.

1. Which of the following is regulated by the kidneys?
   a. water content of the blood
   b. blood pH level
   c. blood ion concentration
   d. all of the above

2. The medial surface of each kidney has a notch called the:
   a. medulla.
   b. cortex.
   c. hilum.
   d. pelvis.

3. At the beginning of the "plumbing system" of the urinary system, urine leaving the renal papilla is collected in the cuplike structures called:
   a. renal columns.
   b. renal pyramids.
   c. calyces.
   d. ureters.

4. The functional unit of the kidney is the:
   a. renal corpuscle.
   b. nephron.
   c. juxtaglomerular apparatus.
   d. Bowman's capsule.

5. Which of the following is a component of the renal corpuscle?
   a. glomerulus
   b. Bowman's capsule
   c. afferent arteriole
   d. both a and b

6. Which of the following structures secretes renin when blood pressure in the afferent arteriole drops?
   a. renal tubule
   b. proximal convoluted tubule
   c. juxtaglomerular apparatus
   d. both a and b

7. Substances pass from the glomerulus and into the Bowman's capsule by:
   a. diffusion.
   b. active transport.
   c. filtration.
   d. osmosis.

8. The juxtaglomerular cells reside in the:
   a. afferent arteriole.
   b. efferent arteriole.
   c. proximal convoluted tubule.
   d. distal convoluted tubule.

True or false

9. _____ The left kidney is often slightly larger and positioned slightly lower than the right kidney.

10. _____ Blood is brought to the kidneys by the renal vein.

11. _____ *Micturition* and *urination* are synonymous terms.

12. _____ The glomerulus is one of the most important capillary networks for survival.

13. _____ Once urine enters the renal pelvis, it then travels to the renal calyces.

14. _____ As the basic functional unit of the kidney, the nephron's function is blood processing and urine formation.

15. _____ The kidneys are covered with visceral peritoneum.

Labeling—match each term with its corresponding number on the following illustration of the kidney.

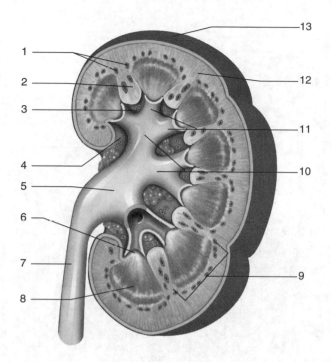

_____ renal pelvis	_____ renal sinus
_____ renal papilla of pyramid	_____ interlobular arteries
_____ minor calyces	_____ capsule (fibrous)
_____ renal column	_____ medulla
_____ cortex	_____ major calyces
_____ hilum	_____ medullary pyramid
_____ ureter	

Labeling—match each term with its corresponding number on the following illustration of the nephron.

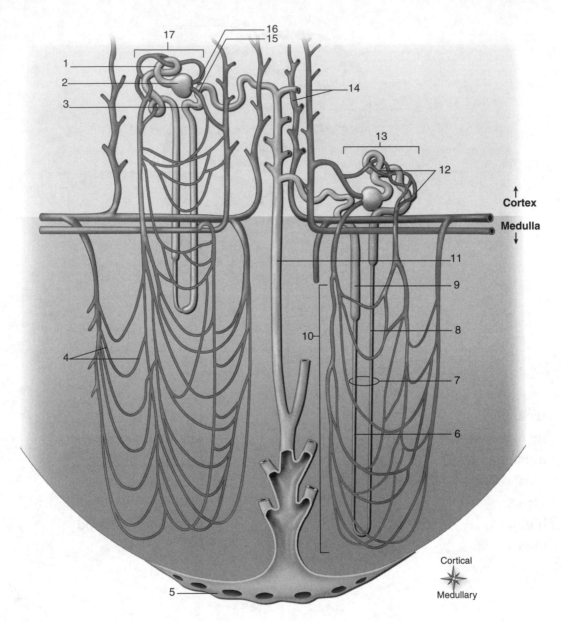

_____ renal corpuscle

_____ thick ascending limb of Henle loop (TAL)

_____ peritubular capillaries

_____ arcuate artery and vein

_____ proximal convoluted tubule (PCT)

_____ efferent arteriole

_____ thin ascending limb of Henle loop (tALH)

_____ cortical nephron

_____ Henle loop

_____ vasa recta

_____ papilla of renal pyramid

_____ afferent arteriole

_____ descending limb of Henle loop

_____ collecting duct (CD)

_____ juxtamedullary nephron

_____ distal convoluted tubule (DCT)

_____ interlobular artery and vein

Labeling—label the following structure of the male urinary bladder.

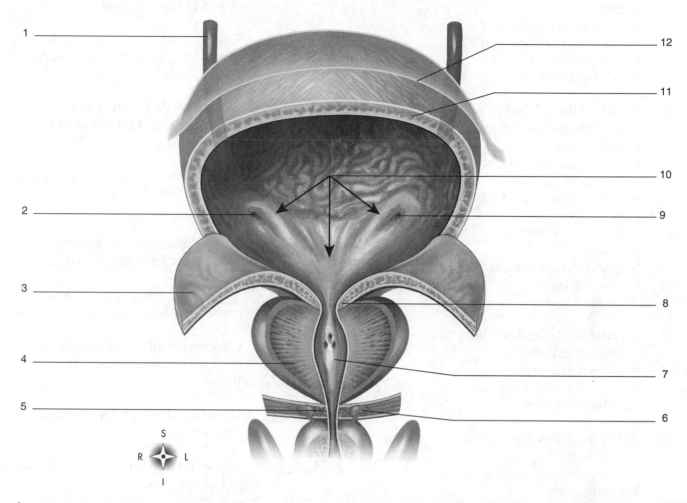

▶ *If you had difficulty with this section, review pages 970-982.*

II—PHYSIOLOGY OF THE URINARY SYSTEM

Multiple Choice—select the best answer.

16. Which of the following is *not* one of the processes of urine formation?
    a. filtration
    b. diffusion
    c. reabsorption
    d. secretion

17. The movement of water and solutes from the plasma in the glomerulus, across the glomerular-capsular membrane, and into the capsular space of the Bowman's capsule, is termed:
    a. filtration.
    b. diffusion.
    c. reabsorption.
    d. secretion.

18. The movement of molecules out of the peritubular blood and into the tubule for excretion is:
    a. filtration.
    b. diffusion.
    c. reabsorption.
    d. secretion.

19. Under normal conditions, most water, electrolytes, and nutrients are reabsorbed in the:
    a. proximal convoluted tubule.
    b. distal convoluted tubule.
    c. Henle loop.
    d. collecting duct.

20. Which of the following is considered a countercurrent structure?
    a. glomerulus
    b. proximal convoluted tubule
    c. Henle loop
    d. distal convoluted tubule

21. Water loss from the blood is reduced by:
    a. ADH.
    b. atrial natriuretic hormone (ANH).
    c. aldosterone.
    d. both a and c.

22. *Dysuria* is a term describing:
    a. blood in the urine.
    b. pus in the urine.
    c. painful urination.
    d. absence of urine.

23. All of the following are normal contents of urine *except*:
    a. nitrogenous wastes.
    b. hormones.
    c. pigments.
    d. plasma proteins.

24. Which of the following is *not* symptomatic of diabetes mellitus?
    a. copious urination
    b. glycosuria
    c. anuria
    d. diuresis

True or false

25. _____ Proximal convoluted tubules reabsorb nutrients from the tubule fluid, notably glucose and amino acids, into peritubular blood by a special type of active transport mechanism called *sodium cotransport*.

26. _____ Postexercise proteinuria is considered serious and often indicative of kidney disease.

27. _____ Fluid exiting the Henle loop becomes less concentrated with Na^+ and Cl^- ions.

28. _____ A hydrostatic pressure gradient drives the filtration out of the plasma and into the nephron.

29. _____ The efferent arteriole has a larger diameter than the afferent arteriole.

30. _____ Stress causes an increase in glomerular hydrostatic pressure.

31. _____ In the renal tubule, Na^+ is reabsorbed via active transport.

32. _____ Glomerular filtration separates only harmful substances from the blood.

33. _____ Urine consists of approximately 75% water.

34. _____ Urine has a pH of 4.6 to 8.0 and is generally alkaline.

35. _____ More than 99% of filtrates must be reabsorbed from the tubular segments of the nephron.

▶ *If you had difficulty with this section, review pages 982-994.*

III—MECHANISMS OF DISEASE

Matching—select the correct disorder from the choices provided.

a. pyelonephritis
b. renal colic
c. renal calculi
d. acute glomerulonephritis
e. proteinuria
f. uremia
g. neurogenic bladder
h. acute renal failure
i. hydronephrosis
j. chronic renal failure
k. cystitis
l. urethritis

36. _____ urine backs up into the kidneys causing swelling of the renal pelvis and calyces

37. _____ kidney stones

38. _____ final stage of chronic renal failure

39. _____ involuntary retention of urine with subsequent distention of the bladder

40. _____ inflammation of the bladder

41. _____ inflammation of the renal pelvis and connective tissues of the kidney

42. _____ an abrupt reduction in kidney function characterized by oliguria and a sharp rise in nitrogenous compounds in the blood

43. _____ progressive condition resulting from gradual loss of nephrons

44. _____ intense kidney pain caused by destruction of the ureters by large kidney stones

45. _____ most common form of kidney disease caused by a delayed immune response to streptococcal infection

46. _____ albumin in the urine

47. _____ inflammation of the urethra that commonly results from bacterial infection

▶ *If you had difficulty with this section, review pages 994-999.*

Crossword Puzzle

Across
1. Capillary network in renal corpuscles
4. Movement of molecules back into the blood
8. Tube from kidney to bladder
9. Mouth of nephron (two words)
10. Outer region of kidney (two words)

Down
2. Inner region of kidney (two words)
3. Opening from bladder to exterior
5. Osmotic concentration of a solution
6. Functional unit of kidney
7. Amount of substance removed from blood by kidneys per minute

APPLYING WHAT YOU KNOW

48.   Mr. Dietz, an accident victim, was admitted to the hospital several hours ago. His chart indicates that he had been hemorrhaging at the scene of the accident. Nurse Petersen has been closely monitoring his urinary output and has noted that it has dropped to 10 mL/hr (the normal urine output for a healthy adult is approximately 30 to 60 mL/hr). What might explain this drop in urine output?

49.   Madison developed chronic renal failure. Describe the progression of each of the three phases of chronic renal failure.

DID YOU KNOW

*   If the tubules in a kidney were stretched and untangled, there would be 70 miles of them.

*   While examining urine, German chemist Hennig Brand discovered phosphorus.

✔ ONE LAST QUICK CHECK

Multiple Choice—select the best answer.

50.   Which of the following processes is used by the artificial kidney to remove waste materials from the blood?
    a.   pinocytosis
    b.   dialysis
    c.   catheterization
    d.   active transport

51.   Failure of the kidneys to remove wastes from the blood will result in which of the following?
    a.   retention
    b.   anuria
    c.   incontinence
    d.   uremia

52.   Hydrogen ions are transferred from blood into the urine during which of the following processes?
    a.   secretion
    b.   filtration
    c.   reabsorption
    d.   all of the above

53.   Which of the following conditions would be considered normal in an infant younger than 2 years of age?
    a.   retention
    b.   cystitis
    c.   incontinence
    d.   anuria

54.   Which of the following steps involved in urine formation allows the blood to retain most body nutrients?
    a.   secretion
    b.   filtration
    c.   reabsorption
    d.   all of the above

55.   Voluntary control of micturition is achieved by the action of which of the following?
    a.   internal urethral sphincter
    b.   external urethral sphincter
    c.   trigone
    d.   bladder muscles

56.   What is the structure that carries urine from the kidney to the bladder called?
    a.   urethra
    b.   Bowman's capsule
    c.   ureter
    d.   renal pelvis

57. What are the capillary loops contained within Bowman's capsule called?
    a. convoluted tubules
    b. glomeruli
    c. limbs of Henle
    d. collecting ducts

58. The triangular divisions of the medulla of the kidney are known as:
    a. pyramids.
    b. papillae.
    c. calyces.
    d. nephrons.

59. The trigone is located in the:
    a. kidney.
    b. bladder.
    c. ureter.
    d. urethra.

Matching—select the best answer to describe the terms.

a. involuntary voiding
b. passes through prostate gland
c. absence of urine
d. urination
e. blood in the urine
f. inflammation of the kidney
g. large amount of protein in urine
h. large amount of urine
i. folds that line the bladder
j. scanty amount of urine
k. test for renal dysfunction

60. _____ hematuria

61. _____ anuria

62. _____ nephritis

63. _____ micturition

64. _____ oliguria

65. _____ polyuria

66. _____ incontinence

67. _____ proteinuria

68. _____ rugae

69. _____ urethra

70. _____ BUN

CHAPTER 32

Fluid and Electrolyte Balance

R eferring to the very first chapter in your text, you will recall that survival depends on the body's ability to maintain or restore homeostasis. Specifically, *homeostasis* means that the body fluids remain constant within very narrow limits. These fluids are classified as either intracellular fluid (ICF) or extracellular fluid (ECF). As their names imply, intracellular fluid lies within the cells and extracellular fluid is located outside the cells. A balance between these two fluids is maintained by several body mechanisms. Among them are: 1) the adjustment of fluid output to fluid intake under normal circumstances, 2) the concentration of electrolytes, 3) the capillary blood pressure, and 4) the concentration of proteins in the blood. Knowledge of how these mechanisms maintain and restore fluid balance is necessary for an understanding of the complexities of homeostasis and its relationship to the survival of the individual.

I—OVERVIEW OF FLUID AND ELECTROLYTE BALANCE

Multiple Choice—select the best answer.

1. The majority of total body water is found in the:
   a. plasma.
   b. interstitial fluid.
   c. ICF.
   d. ECF.

2. The most abundant intracellular cation is:
   a. Na^+.
   b. Cl^-.
   c. K^+.
   d. Mg^{++}.

3. The most abundant extracellular cation is:
   a. Na^+.
   b. Cl^-.
   c. K^+.
   d. Mg^{++}.

4. The most abundant anion in ECF is:
   a. Na^+.
   b. Cl^-.
   c. K^+.
   d. Mg^{++}.

5. Electrolyte reactivity is measured in:
   a. mg/100 L.
   b. milliequivalents.
   c. mEq/L.
   d. both b and c.

6. Which of the following mechanisms varies fluid output so that it equals input?
   a. antidiuretic device
   b. aldosterone mechanism
   c. renin-angiotensin-aldosterone mechanism
   d. both b and c

7. Which of the following is *not* one of the seven basic solutions used for parenteral therapy?
   a. ammonium chloride
   b. carbohydrate in water
   c. liquid protein
   d. Ringer's solution

True or false

8. _____ Obese people have a higher water content per kilogram of body weight than slender people.

9. _____ When compared chemically, plasma and interstitial fluid are nearly identical.

10. _____ Fluid intake usually equals fluid output.

11. _____ Electrolytes are substances that bind in water.

12. _____ Thirst is associated with any condition that decreases total volume of body water.

13. _____ Water exits the body only through the urinary and digestive systems.

14. _____ *Hypervolemia* refers to excess blood volume.

▶ *If you had difficulty with this section, review pages 1003-1010.*

II—MECHANISMS THAT MAINTAIN HOMEOSTASIS OF TOTAL FLUID VOLUME

Multiple Choice—select the best answer.

15. The two factors that determine urine volume are:
    a. the amount of antidiuretic hormone (ADH) and aldosterone secretion.
    b. the amount of adrenocorticotropic hormone (ACTH) and ADH secretion.
    c. fluid intake and ADH secretion.
    d. the glomerular filtration rate and the rate of water reabsorption by the renal tubules.

16. Which of the following is an example of obligatory fluid output?
    a. water vapor in expired air
    b. water diffusion through the skin
    c. both a and b
    d. none of the above

True or false

17. _____ If a person takes nothing by mouth for several days, fluid output decreases to zero to compensate and maintain homeostasis.

18. _____ Dehydration is often detected by loss of skin elasticity.

▶ *If you had difficulty with this section, review pages 1010-1012.*

III—REGULATION OF WATER AND ELECTROLYTE LEVELS IN PLASMA, INTERSTITIAL FLUID, AND INTRACELLULAR FLUID

Multiple Choice—select the best answer.

19. Blood hydrostatic pressure:
    a. tends to force fluid out of capillaries and into interstitial fluid.
    b. tends to force fluid out of interstitial fluid and into capillaries.
    c. allows for an equilibrium across the capillary membrane.
    d. none of the above.

20. Which of the following is *not* a correct statement regarding severe dehydration?
    a. Loss of skin turgor is a symptom of severe dehydration.
    b. The relative loss of water in sweat is greater than the loss of electrolytes.
    c. Sweating serves the body by increasing body heat.
    d. Treatment of dehydration requires appropriate electrolyte replacement therapy.

21. The formula representing Starling's law of the capillaries is:
    a. (BHP + BCOP) – (IFCOP + IFHP) = EFP.
    b. (BHP + IFHP) – (IFCOP + BCOP) = EFP.
    c. (BHP + IFCOP) – (IFHP + BCOP) = EFP.

22. Which large molecules are retained by the selectively permeable cell membrane?
    a. sodium ions
    b. potassium ions
    c. proteins
    d. water

True or false

23. _____ *Edema* can be defined as "the presence of abnormally large amounts of fluid in the intercellular spaces of the body."

24. _____ The most common cause of edema is glomerulonephritis.

25. _____ The most significant player regulating ICF composition is the plasma membrane.

26. _____ Osmotic pressure is influenced by large protein molecules in the intracellular fluid.

▶ *If you had difficulty with this section, review pages 1012-1017.*

IV—REGULATION OF SODIUM AND POTASSIUM LEVELS IN BODY FLUIDS

True or false

27. _____ The release of ADH causes an increase in the reabsorption of sodium and water by the renal tubules.

28. _____ Over 8 liters of various internal secretions are produced daily.

29. _____ Potassium deficit is termed *hypokalemia*.

30. _____ ECF depletion is said to be the "last line of defense" against dehydration.

31. _____ By volume, intestinal secretions are the largest sodium-containing internal secretions.

▶ *If you had difficulty with this section, review page 1013 and pages 1017-1019.*

V—MECHANISMS OF DISEASE

Matching—identify the best answer for the terms.

a. dehydration
b. excessive perspiration
c. excess fluid volume
d. increased serum potassium
e. decreased serum sodium

32. _____ hypovolemia

33. _____ hyperkalemia

34. _____ hyponatremia

35. _____ diaphoresis

36. _____ hypervolemia

True or false

37. _____ Skin turgor is an important indicator of fluid volume stability.

38. _____ Cushing syndrome can cause hypokalemia.

39. _____ Overuse of diuretics can result in hyponatremia.

40. _____ Hyperkalemia is *not* a serious threat to the body.

▶ *If you had difficulty with this section, review pages 1019-1021.*

Crossword Puzzle

Across
1. Detect decreased blood pressure when dehydration occurs
4. Fluid volume excess
8. Fluid located within cells
9. Excessive loss of fluid from the body
10. Low serum potassium
11. Water found outside the cells

Down
2. Swelling
3. MEq
5. Fluid that surrounds the cells
6. Chloride deficiency
7. Administration of fluids by injection

APPLYING WHAT YOU KNOW

41. Ms. Titus was asked to keep an accurate record of her fluid intake and output. She was concerned because the two did not balance, even though the physician assured her that she had no kidney pathology. What is a possible explanation for this?

42. Jack Sprat was 6′ 5″ and weighed 185 lbs. His wife was 5′ 6″ and weighed 185 lbs. Whose body contained more water?

DID YOU KNOW

• The best fluid replacement drink is to add 1/2 tsp of table salt to one quart of water.

• If all of the water were drained from the body of an average 160-lb. man, the body would weigh 64 lbs.

ONE LAST QUICK CHECK

Circle the correct answer.

43. The largest volume of water by far lies (inside or outside) cells.

44. Interstitial fluid is (intracellular or extracellular).

45. Plasma is (intracellular or extracellular).

46. Obese people have a (lower or higher) water content per pound of body weight than thin people.

47. Infants have (more or less) water in comparison to body weight than adults of either sex.

48. In general, as age increases, the amount of water per pound of body weight (increases or decreases).

Multiple Choice—select the best answer.

49. Which one of the following is *not* a positively charged ion?
    a. chloride
    b. calcium
    c. sodium
    d. potassium

50. Which one of the following is *not* a negatively charged ion?
    a. chloride
    b. bicarbonate
    c. phosphate
    d. sodium

51. The smallest amount of water comes from:
    a. water in foods that are eaten.
    b. ingested food.
    c. water formed from catabolism.
    d. none of the above.

52. The greatest amount of water lost from the body is from the:
    a. lungs.
    b. skin by diffusion.
    c. skin by sweat.
    d. feces.
    e. kidneys.

53. Excessive water loss and fluid imbalance can result from which of the following?
    a. diarrhea
    b. vomiting
    c. severe burns
    d. all of the above

54. Signals generated by osmoreceptors in the subfornical organ and hypothalamus stimulate the secretion of:
    a. aldosterone.
    b. insulin.
    c. ADH.
    d. ANH.

55. If blood sodium concentration decreases, what does blood volume do?
    a. increases
    b. decreases
    c. remains the same

56. Which of the following is true of body water?
    a. It is obtained from the liquids we drink.
    b. It is obtained from the foods we eat.
    c. It is formed by the catabolism of food.
    d. All of the above are true.

57. Edema may result from which of the following?
    a. retention of electrolytes
    b. decreased blood pressure
    c. increased concentration of blood plasma proteins
    d. all of the above

58. The most abundant and important positive plasma ion is which of the following?
    a. sodium
    b. chloride
    c. calcium
    d. oxygen

59. Which of the following is true when ECF volume decreases?
    a. Aldosterone secretion increases.
    b. Kidney tubule reabsorption of sodium increases.
    c. Urine volume decreases.
    d. All of the above are true.

True or false

60. _____ Interstitial fluid contains hardly any protein anions.

61. _____ No net transfer of water occurs between blood and interstitial fluid as long as effective filtration pressure (EFP) equals 0.

62. _____ Any change in the solute concentration of ECF will have a direct effect on water movement across the cell

CHAPTER 33

Acid-Base Balance

It has been established in previous chapters that an equilibrium between intracellular and extracellular fluid volume must exist for homeostasis. Equally important to homeostasis is the chemical acid-base balance of the body fluids. The degree of acidity or alkalinity of a body fluid is expressed as pH value. The neutral point, where a fluid would be neither acid nor alkaline, is pH 7. Increasing acidity is expressed as less than 7, and increasing alkalinity as greater than 7. Examples of body fluids that are acidic are gastric juice (pH 1.6) and urine (pH 6.0). Blood, on the other hand, is considered alkaline with a pH of 7.4.

Buffers are substances that prevent a sharp change in the pH of a fluid when an acid or base is added to it. They are one of several mechanisms that are constantly monitoring the pH of fluids in the body. If for any reason these mechanisms do not function properly, a pH imbalance occurs. These two kinds of imbalances are known as *alkalosis* and *acidosis*.

Maintaining the acid-base balance of body fluids is a matter of vital importance. If this balance varies even slightly, necessary chemical and cellular reactions cannot occur. Your review of this chapter is necessary to understand the delicate fluid balance necessary for survival.

I—MECHANISMS THAT CONTROL pH OF BODY FLUIDS

Multiple Choice—select the best answer.

1. As pH goes down, a:
   a. solution becomes more basic.
   b. solution's hydrogen ion concentration decreases.
   c. solution becomes more acidic.
   d. solution thickens.

2. The most acidic body substance of the following is:
   a. gastric juice.
   b. pancreatic juice.
   c. bile.
   d. urine.

3. Which of the following is an acid-forming food?
   a. grapefruit
   b. meat
   c. orange juice
   d. coffee

4. Which of the following is a base-forming food?
   a. fruit
   b. vegetable
   c. egg
   d. both a and b

5. Which of the following describes the narrow pH range of blood?
   a. 7.21 to 7.49
   b. 7.00 to 7.20
   c. 7.36 to 7.41
   d. 7.50 to 7.77

6. An acid-forming element is:
   a. sulfur.
   b. calcium.
   c. potassium.
   d. sodium.

7. Acidic ketone bodies are associated with cellular metabolism of:
   a. proteins.
   b. carbohydrates.
   c. fats.
   d. minerals.

True or false

8. _____ Blood is slightly alkaline.

9. _____ Citrus fruits, such as oranges and grapefruit, have a significant effect on acid-base balance.

10. _____ Chemical buffer systems are fast-acting.

11. _____ The carbon dioxide present in venous blood causes it to become slightly more basic than arterial blood.

12. _____ A vegetarian diet would tend to produce an alkaline state in body fluids.

13. _____ The respiratory and urinary systems can serve as physiologic buffer systems.

▶ *If you had difficulty with this section, review pages 1025-1028.*

II—BUFFER MECHANISMS FOR CONTROLLING pH OF BODY FLUIDS

Multiple Choice—select the best answer.

14. Potassium salts of hemoglobin inside the red blood cell primarily buffer:
    a. carbonic acid.
    b. lactic acid.
    c. phosphoric acid.
    d. sulfuric acid.

15. A serious complication of vomiting is:
    a. carbonic acid.
    b. bicarbonate deficit.
    c. metabolic alkalosis.
    d. metabolic acidosis.

True or false

16. _____ The process of exchanging a bicarbonate ion formed in the red blood cell with a chloride ion from the plasma is called *chloride shift*.

17. _____ Buffers control pH in a manner that requires no other mechanism of pH control to maintain homeostasis.

18. _____ The blood buffer system normally converts a strong acid to a weak acid.

19. _____ Bicarbonate loading by athletes has proven to be mildly successful in diminishing the muscle soreness and fatigue associated with strenuous exercise.

20. _____ Elevated CO_2 levels result in increased formation of carbonic acid in red blood cells.

▷ *If you had difficulty with this section, review pages 1028-1032.*

III—RESPIRATORY AND URINARY MECHANISMS OF pH CONTROL

Multiple Choice—select the best answer.

21. With each expiration, which substances leave the body?
    a. CO_2
    b. H_2O
    c. O_2
    d. both a and b

22. All of the following would increase the respiration rate *except*:
    a. decreased blood pH.
    b. decreased carbon dioxide.
    c. increased arterial blood CO_2.
    d. all increase respirations.

23. The kidney tubules secrete hydrogen ions in exchange of:
    a. K^+.
    b. Na^+.
    c. Ca^{++}.
    d. Cl^-.

24. Acidosis causes:
    a. hyperventilation.
    b. hypoventilation.
    c. an increase in blood pH.
    d. increase in potassium ion excretion.

25. A decrease in blood pH accelerates tubule excretion of:
    a. hydrogen.
    b. ammonia.
    c. both a and b.
    d. none of the above.

True or false

26. _____ Prolonged hyperventilation may increase blood pH enough to cause alkalosis.

27. _____ Respiratory mechanisms are much more effective in expelling hydrogen ions than are urinary mechanisms.

28. _____ The more hydrogen ions secreted by the renal tubule, the fewer potassium ions secreted.

29. _____ Intravenous administration of normal saline is used for metabolic acidosis.

30. _____ An increase in blood pH above normal (alkalosis) causes hypoventilation.

▷ *If you had difficulty with this section, review pages 1032-1036.*

IV—MECHANISMS OF DISEASE

Matching—write the letter of the correct term on the blank next to the appropriate definition.

a. metabolic acidosis
b. metabolic alkalosis
c. respiratory acidosis
d. respiratory alkalosis
e. treatment for metabolic and respiratory acidosis
f. uncompensated metabolic acidosis
g. hyperventilation

31. _____ result of untreated diabetes

32. _____ sodium lactate

33. _____ bicarbonate deficit

34. _____ bicarbonate excess

35. _____ rapid breathing

36. _____ carbonic acid excess

37. _____ carbonic acid deficit

▷ *If you had difficulty with this section, review pages 1036-1039.*

Crossword Puzzle

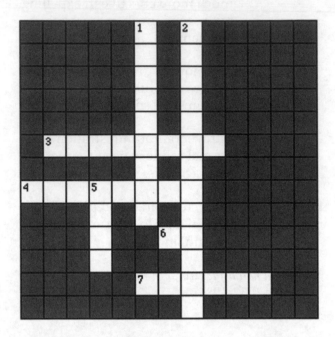

Across

3. May be caused by prolonged hypoventilation
4. pH greater than 7.0
6. Degree of acidity or alkalinity
7. Prevents swing in pH

Down

1. Complication of vomiting
2. Maintains electrical neutrality of red blood cells (two words)
5. pH less than 7.0

 APPLYING WHAT YOU KNOW

38. Desi was pregnant and was experiencing repeated vomiting episodes for several days. Her doctor became concerned, admitted her to the hospital, and began intravenous administrations of normal saline. How will this help Desi?

39. Ginny had a minor bladder infection. She had heard that this is often the result of the urine being less acidic than necessary and that she should drink cranberry juice to correct the acid problem. She had no cranberry juice, so she decided to substitute orange juice. What was wrong with this substitution?

 **DID YOU KNOW**

- English ships carried limes to protect the sailors from scurvy. American ships carried cranberries.

 ONE LAST QUICK CHECK

Multiple Choice—select the best answer.

40. What happens as blood flows through lung capillaries?
    a. Carbonic acid in blood decreases.
    b. Hydrogen ions in blood decrease.
    c. Blood pH increases from venous to arterial blood.
    d. All of the above are true.

41. Which of the following organs is considered the most effective regulator of blood carbonic acid levels?
    a. kidneys
    b. intestines
    c. lungs
    d. stomach

42. Which of the following organs is/are considered the most effective regulator(s) of blood pH?
    a. kidneys
    b. intestines
    c. lungs
    d. stomach

43. What is the pH of the blood?
    a. 7.0 to 8.0
    b. 7.6 to 7.8
    c. 6.2 to 7.4
    d. 7.3 to 7.4

44. If the ratio of sodium bicarbonate to carbonate ions is lowered (perhaps 10 to 1) and blood pH is also lowered, what is the condition called?
    a. uncompensated metabolic acidosis
    b. uncompensated metabolic alkalosis
    c. compensated metabolic acidosis
    d. compensated metabolic alkalosis

45. If a person hyperventilates for a sufficient time period, which of the following will probably develop?
    a. metabolic acidosis
    b. metabolic alkalosis
    c. respiratory acidosis
    d. respiratory alkalosis

46. Normal saline is a therapy option for severe vomiting because this solution provides _____ ions, which replace bicarbonate ions that are responsible for the metabolic imbalance.
    a. hydrogen
    b. sodium
    c. potassium
    d. chloride

47. In the presence of a strong acid, which of the following is true?
    a. Sodium bicarbonate will react to produce carbonic acid.
    b. Sodium bicarbonate will react to produce more sodium bicarbonate.
    c. Carbonic acid will react to produce sodium bicarbonate.
    d. Carbonic acid will react to form more carbonic acid.

Matching—select the best answer for each item.

a. untreated diabetes mellitus
b. excessive vomiting
c. alkaline solution
d. "fixed" acid
e. barbiturate overdose
f. fever
g. acidic solution
h. prevent sharp pH changes

48. _____ pH lower than 7.0

49. _____ pH higher than 7.0

50. _____ buffers

51. _____ decrease in respirations

52. _____ increase in respirations

53. _____ metabolic acidosis

54. _____ metabolic alkalosis

55. _____ lactic acid

CHAPTER 34

Male Reproductive System

The reproductive system consists of those organs that participate in propagating the species. It is a unique body system in that its organs differ between the two sexes, and yet the goal of creating a new being is the same. Of interest also is the fact that this system is the only one not necessary to the survival of the individual, and yet survival of the species depends on the proper functioning of the reproductive organs. The male reproductive system is divided into the external genitals, testes, duct system, and accessory glands. The testes, or gonads, are considered essential organs because they produce the sex cells—sperm—which join with the female sex cells—ova—to form a new human being. They also secrete testosterone, the male sex hormone, which is responsible for the physical transformation of a boy to a man.

Sperm are formed in the testes by the seminiferous tubules. From there they enter a long narrow duct, the epididymis. They continue onward through the vas deferens into the ejaculatory duct, down the urethra, and out of the body. Throughout this journey, various glands secrete substances that add motility to the sperm and create a chemical environment conducive to reproduction.

Knowledge of the male reproductive system is necessary to understand the role of the male and the phenomena necessary to produce an offspring.

I—MALE REPRODUCTIVE ORGANS

Multiple Choice—select the best answer.

1. The male gonads are known as the:
    a. testes.
    b. prostate.
    c. epididymis.
    d. perineum.

2. The region within a "triangle" created by the ischial tuberosities and the symphysis is the:
    a. anal triangle.
    b. urogenital triangle.
    c. perineal triangle.
    d. testicular triangle.

3. Which of the following is *not* a supporting structure?
   a. penis
   b. scrotum
   c. prostate
   d. spermatic cord

4. Each testicular lobule contains:
   a. seminiferous tubules.
   b. interstitial cells.
   c. Leydig cells.
   d. all of the above.

5. The blood-testis barrier is formed by tight junctions between which cells?
   a. Leydig cells
   b. interstitial cells
   c. sustentacular cells
   d. all of the above

6. Sperm production occurs in the:
   a. seminiferous tubules.
   b. interstitial cells.
   c. Sertoli cells.
   d. prostate.

7. Which hormone is responsible for the stimulation of sperm production?
   a. follicle-stimulating hormone (FSH)
   b. luteinizing hormone (LH)
   c. testosterone
   d. both b and c

8. Which of the following is *not* a specific region of a spermatozoon?
   a. head
   b. middle piece
   c. body
   d. tail

True or false

9. _____ The testes perform two primary functions: spermatogenesis and secretion of hormones.

10. _____ Testosterone is secreted by the anterior pituitary.

11. _____ The urogenital triangle surrounds the anus.

12. _____ *Capacitation* refers to the release of enzymes contained within the acrosome.

13. _____ *Sustentacular cells* and *efferent ductules* are synonymous.

14. _____ The bulbourethral glands are a supporting structure of the male reproductive system.

15. _____ Testosterone is sometimes referred to as "the anabolic hormone."

Labeling—match each term with its corresponding number on the following sagittal section of the pelvis depicting placement of male reproductive organs.

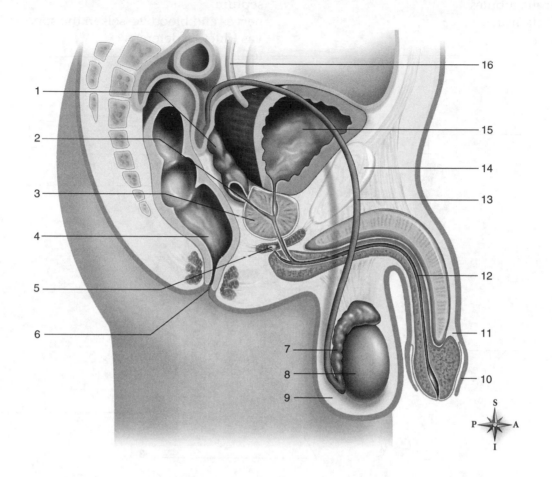

_____ urinary bladder

_____ epididymis

_____ rectum

_____ seminal vesicle

_____ foreskin (prepuce)

_____ vas (ductus) deferens

_____ bulbourethral (Cowper) gland

_____ anus

_____ scrotum

_____ penis

_____ prostate gland

_____ testis

_____ urethra

_____ ejaculatory duct

_____ pubic symphysis

_____ ureter

Labeling—using the terms provided, label the following tubules of the testis and epididymis.

seminiferous tubules
tunica albuginea
epididymis
lobule

septum
nerves and blood vessels in the spermatic cord
vas (ductus) deferens
testis

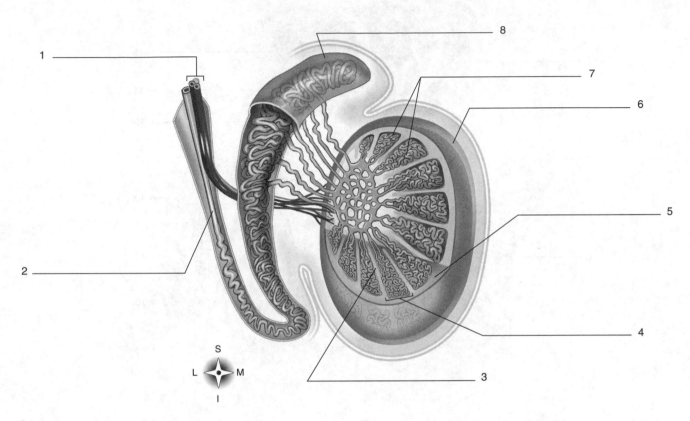

If you had difficulty with this section, review pages 1043-1051.

II—REPRODUCTIVE DUCTS AND ACCESSORY REPRODUCTIVE GLANDS

Multiple Choice—select the best answer.

16. Which of the following is *not* a function of the epididymis?
    a. a duct through which sperm travel on their journey to the exterior of the body
    b. production of spermatozoa
    c. maturation of spermatozoa
    d. secretion of a portion of seminal fluid

17. The ejaculatory ducts are formed by the union of the:
    a. seminal vesicles and ampulla.
    b. vas deferens and urethra.
    c. seminal vesicles and vas deferens.
    d. seminal vesicles and urethra.

18. Which of the following accessory reproductive glands produce(s) a secretion rich in fructose?
    a. seminal vesicles
    b. prostate
    c. bulbourethral gland
    d. Cowper glands

19. Which of the following accessory glands secrete(s) an alkaline substance?
    a. seminal vesicles
    b. bulbourethral gland
    c. all of the above
    d. none of the above

20. The most common cancer in American men is cancer of the:
    a. testes.
    b. prostate.
    c. penis.
    d. bladder.

True or false

21. _____ The duct of the vas deferens is an extension of the tail of the epididymis.

22. _____ Sperm may be stored in the vas deferens for up to a month with no loss of fertility.

23. _____ A vasectomy is a procedure intended to render a man sterile.

24. _____ Prostate-specific antigen (PSA) is always elevated in the blood of men with prostate cancer.

▶ *If you had difficulty with this section, review pages 1051-1054.*

III—SUPPORTING STRUCTURES, SEMINAL FLUID, AND MALE FERTILITY

Multiple Choice—select the best answer.

25. The greatest amount of seminal fluid is secreted by the:
    a. prostate.
    b. testes.
    c. seminal vesicles.
    d. epididymis.

26. Elevation of the testes is caused by contraction of the:
    a. dartos fascia and muscle.
    b. cremaster muscle.
    c. corpora cavernosa.
    d. corpus spongiosum.

27. Functional sterility results when sperm count falls below:
    a. 5 million/mL of semen.
    b. 25 million/mL of semen.
    c. 100 million/mL of semen.
    d. 500 million/mL of semen.

28. Which of the following factors related to sperm does *not* affect male fertility?
    a. size
    b. shape
    c. texture
    d. motility

True or false

29. _____ The urethra lies within the corpora cavernosa.

30. _____ The terminal end of the corpus spongiosum forms the glans penis.

31. _____ *Emission* and *ejaculation* are synonymous terms.

Labeling—using the terms provided, label the following parts of the penis.

corpus cavernosum
bulb
glans penis
bulbourethral gland
deep artery
openings of ejaculatory ducts
prostate

urethra
crus penis
corpus spongiosum
foreskin (prepuce)
external urinary meatus
bladder
opening of bulbourethral gland

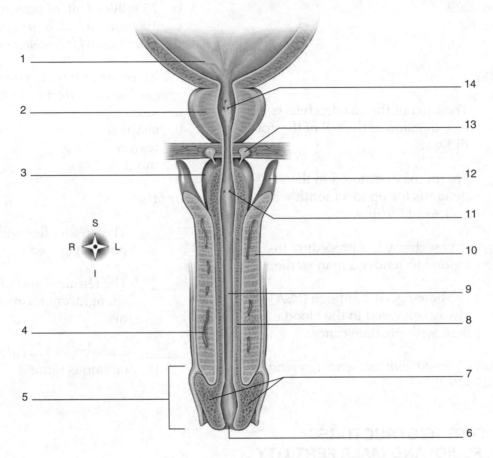

▶ *If you had difficulty with this section, review pages 1053-1057.*

IV—MECHANISMS OF DISEASE

Fill in the blanks.

32. Decreased sperm production is called
    _____.

33. Testes normally descend into the scrotum
    about _____ before birth.

34. If a baby is born with undescended testes,
    a condition called _____
    results.

35. A common noncancerous condition of the
    prostate in older men is known as
    _____ _____
    _____.

36. _____ is a condition in
    which the foreskin fits so tightly over the
    glans that it cannot retract.

37. Failure to achieve an erection of the penis
    is called _____ or _____
    _____.

38. An accumulation of fluid in the scrotum is known as a _____.

39. An _____
_____ results when the intestines push through the weak area of the abdominal wall that separates the abdominopelvic cavity from the scrotum.

▶ *If you had difficulty with this section, review pages 1057-1059.*

Crossword Puzzle

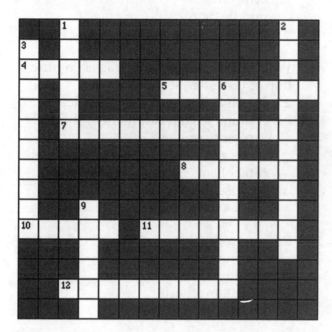

Across
4. Male organ of copulation
5. Accessory reproductive gland
7. Provide protection for germ cells (two words)
8. Sex cell
10. Ejaculate from the penis
11. Male sex hormone
12. Reproductive organs

Down
1. Sex glands where reproductive cells are formed
2. Androgen
3. Genital duct
6. Mature male gametes
9. Male gonads

APPLYING WHAT YOU KNOW

40. Trent is an infant who was born with undescended testes. What is the clinical term for his condition? How easily is this diagnosed? What can Trent's doctor do to treat his condition? How serious is his condition if left untreated? What are his chances of normal testicular and sexual development?

41. John noticed an unusual swelling of his scrotum. What possible conditions may he be experiencing? Also, he did notice that the swelling occurred after a day of heavy lifting while moving out of his apartment. Based on this detail, which condition is he more likely to be experiencing? Describe the anatomy of this condition. How will the doctor treat John?

DID YOU KNOW

- The testes produce approximately 50 million sperm per day. Every 2 to 3 months they produce enough cells to populate the entire earth.

- Men reach the peak of their sexual powers in their late teens or early twenties, and then begin to slowly decline. Women, however, do not reach their sexual peak until their late twenties or early thirties, and then remain at this level through their late fifties or early sixties.

ONE LAST QUICK CHECK

Multiple Choice—select the best answer.

42. The testes are suspended outside the body cavity to do which of the following?
    a. protect them from trauma
    b. keep them cooler
    c. keep them supplied with a greater number of blood vessels
    d. protect them from infection

43. What is the removal of the foreskin from the glans penis called?
    a. vasectomy
    b. sterilization
    c. circumcision
    d. ligation

44. The testes are surrounded by a tough membrane called the:
    a. ductus deferens.
    b. tunica albuginea.
    c. septum.
    d. seminiferous membrane.

45. The _____ lie(s) near the septa that separate the lobules.
    a. ductus deferens
    b. sperm
    c. interstitial cells
    d. nerves

46. Sperm are found in the walls of the:
    a. seminiferous tubule.
    b. interstitial cells.
    c. septum.
    d. blood vessels.

47. The scrotum provides an environment that is approximately _____ for the testes.
    a. the same as the body temperature
    b. 5° C warmer than the body temperature
    c. 3° C warmer than the body temperature
    d. 3° C cooler than the body temperature

48. The _____ produce(s) testosterone.
    a. seminiferous tubules
    b. prostate gland
    c. bulbourethral glands
    d. interstitial cells

49. The part of the sperm that contains genetic information that will be inherited is the:
    a. tail.
    b. acrosome.
    c. middle piece.
    d. head.

50. Which one of the following is *not* a function of testosterone?
    a. It causes deepening of the voice.
    b. It promotes development of the male accessory organs.
    c. It has a stimulatory effect on protein catabolism.
    d. It causes greater muscular development and strength.

51. Sperm production is called:
    a. spermatogonia.
    b. spermatids.
    c. spermatogenesis.
    d. spermatocyte.

52. The section of the sperm that contains enzymes that enable it to break down the covering of the ovum and permit entry should contact occur is the:
    a. acrosome.
    b. middle piece.
    c. tail.
    d. stem.

Matching—insert the letter in the space next to the appropriate description.

a. epididymis
b. vas deferens
c. ejaculatory duct
d. prepuce
e. seminal vesicles
f. prostate gland
g. Cowper glands
h. corpus spongiosum
i. semen
j. spermatic cord

53. _____ continuation of ducts that start in the epididymis

54. _____ erectile tissue

55. _____ also known as *bulbourethral*

56. _____ narrow tube that lies along the top of and behind the testes

57. _____ doughnut-shaped gland beneath the bladder

58. _____ union of the vas deferens with the ducts from the seminal vesicles

59. _____ mixture of sperm and secretions of accessory sex glands

60. _____ contributes 60% of the seminal fluid volume

61. _____ removed during circumcision

62. _____ enclose the vas deferens, blood vessels, lymphatics, and nerves

CHAPTER 35

Female Reproductive System

The female reproductive system is truly extraordinary and diverse. It produces ova, receives the penis and sperm during intercourse, is the site of conception, houses and nourishes the embryo during the prenatal development, and nourishes the infant after birth.

Because of its diversity, the physiology of the female is generally considered to be more complex than that of the male. Much of the activity of this system revolves around the menstrual cycle and the monthly preparation that the female undergoes for a possible pregnancy.

The organs of this system are divided into essential organs and accessory organs of reproduction. The essential organs of the female are the ovaries. Just as with the male, the essential organs of the female are referred to as the *gonads*. The gonads of the female produce ova and are responsible for producing hormones necessary for the appearance of the secondary sex characteristics.

The menstrual cycle of the female typically covers a period of 28 days. Each cycle consists of three phases: menstrual period, postmenstrual phase, and premenstrual phase. Changes in the blood levels of the hormones that are responsible for the menstrual cycle also cause physical and emotional changes in the female. A knowledge of these phenomena and the female system are necessary to complete your understanding of the reproductive system.

I—OVERVIEW OF THE FEMALE REPRODUCTIVE SYSTEM

Multiple Choice—select the best answer.

1. Which of the following is *not* an accessory organ of reproduction in women?
   a. ovaries
   b. uterus
   c. vagina
   d. vulva

2. The term that refers to the external female genitalia is:
   a. vagina.
   b. vulva.
   c. perineum.
   d. urogenital triangle.

True or false

3. _____ Ova are the female gametes.

4. _____ An episiotomy is associated with the perineum.

Labeling—match each term with its corresponding number on the following frontal section of the female pelvic organs.

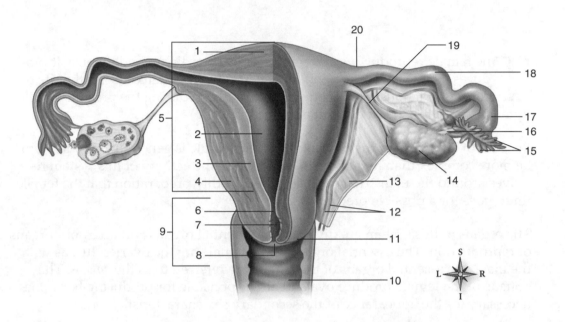

_____ broad ligament

_____ fundus of uterus

_____ external os of vaginal cervix

_____ endometrium

_____ fimbriae

_____ fornix of vagina

_____ myometrium

_____ internal os of cervix

_____ uterine artery and vein

_____ ampulla of uterine tube

_____ isthmus of uterine tube

_____ cervical canal

_____ cervix of uterus

_____ uterine body cavity

_____ ovarian ligament

_____ vagina

_____ ovary

_____ infundibulopelvic ligament

_____ body of uterus

_____ infundibulum of uterine tube

Labeling—match each term with its corresponding number on the following sagittal section of the pelvis showing the female reproductive organs.

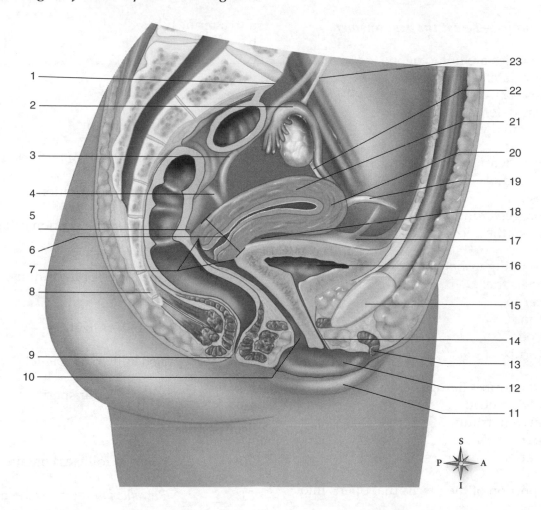

_____ suspensory ligament (of uterine tube)

_____ rectouterine pouch (of Douglas)

_____ labium majus

_____ uterine tube

_____ uterosacral ligament

_____ cervix

_____ fornix of vagina

_____ urethra

_____ coccyx

_____ anus

_____ ovarian ligament

_____ vagina

_____ sacral promontory

_____ ureter

_____ vesicouterine pouch

_____ labium minus

_____ urinary bladder

_____ fundus of uterus

_____ round ligament

_____ clitoris

_____ pubic symphysis

_____ parietal peritoneum

_____ body of uterus

▶ *If you had difficulty with this section, review pages 1063-1066.*

II—OVARIES, UTERUS, UTERINE TUBES, AND VAGINA

Multiple Choice—select the best answer.

5. The ovaries are homologous to the male:
    a. prostate.
    b. testes.
    c. vas deferens.
    d. seminal vesicle.

6. Cells of ovarian tissue secrete:
    a. estradiol.
    b. estrone.
    c. progesterone.
    d. all of the above.

7. The bulging upper component of the uterus is the:
    a. cervix.
    b. fundus.
    c. body.
    d. fornix.

8. The innermost lining of the uterus is the:
    a. endometrium.
    b. myometrium.
    c. perimetrium.
    d. parietal peritoneum.

9. The portion of the uterus that opens into the vagina is the:
    a. internal os.
    b. external os.
    c. fornix.
    d. cervix.

10. The fringelike projections of the uterine tubes are called the:
    a. isthmus.
    b. ampulla.
    c. infundibulum.
    d. fimbriae.

Matching—insert the letter of the correct structure in the blank next to the description.

a. uterine tubes
b. uterus
c. vagina

11. _____ isthmus

12. _____ myometrium

13. _____ terminal end of birth canal

14. _____ site of menstruation

15. _____ intermediate portion called the *ampulla*

16. _____ consists of body, fundus, and cervix

17. _____ site of fertilization

18. _____ also known as *oviduct*

19. _____ receptacle for sperm

True or false

20. _____ Ovarian follicles contain oocytes.

21. _____ *Retroflexion* refers to the normal position of the uterus in relation to the vagina and urinary bladder.

22. _____ The afterbirth is also referred to as the *fornix*.

23. _____ The "G spot" is an "erotic zone" described by Dr. Grafenberg.

▶ *If you had difficulty with this section, review pages 1066-1072.*

III—VULVA

Multiple Choice—select the best answer.

24. The female organ that is homologous to the penile structure in the male is the:
    a. labia minora.
    b. labia majora.
    c. clitoris.
    d. vulva.

25. The area between the labia minora is the:
    a. vulva.
    b. vestibule.
    c. mons pubis.
    d. "G spot."

26. Which of the following is *not* a structure of the vulva?
    a. vagina
    b. labia majora
    c. urinary meatus
    d. clitoris

27. The Bartholin's glands are homologous to the male:
    a. epididymis.
    b. bulbourethral glands.
    c. seminal vesicles.
    d. prostate gland.

28. The external genitals of the female may be referred to collectively as the:
    a. mons pubis.
    b. labia majora.
    c. greater vestibule.
    d. pudendum.

Labeling—match each term with its corresponding number on the following diagram of the external female genitals (genitalia).

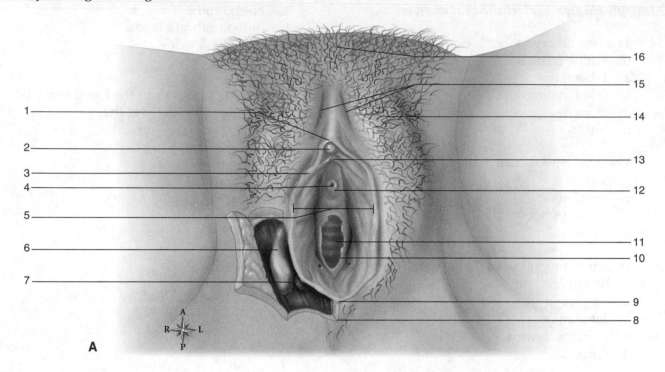

posterior commissure (of labia)

clitoris (glans)

vestibule

mons pubis

labium minus

vestibular bulb

pudendal fissure

opening of lesser vestibular (Skene) gland

external urinary meatus

greater vestibular gland

frenulum (of labia)

labium majus

orifice of vagina

hymen

frenulum (of clitoris)

foreskin (prepuce)

Labeling—match each term with its corresponding number on the following diagram of the vulva.

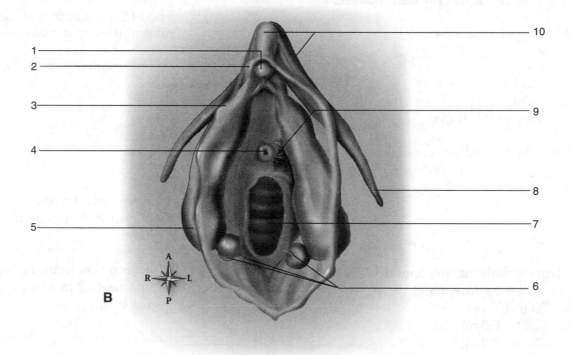

clitoris (glans)

labium minus

external urinary meatus

greater vestibular glands and ducts (Bartholin gland)

orifice of vagina

bulb of the vestibule

foreskin (prepuce)

lesser vestibular glands and ducts (Skene gland)

crus clitoris

corpus cavernosum

▶ *If you had difficulty with this section, review pages 1072-1074.*

IV—FEMALE REPRODUCTIVE CYCLE

Multiple Choice—select the best answer.

29. Menses occurs on days _____ of a new cycle.
    a. 1 to 5
    b. 1 to 14
    c. 6 to 14
    d. none of the above

30. Ovulation usually occurs on cycle day _____ of a 28-day cycle.
    a. 1
    b. 7
    c. 14
    d. 28

31. Menstrual discharge generally does not clot and is approximately:
    a. 30 to 100 mL.
    b. 100 to 350 mL.
    c. 300 to 550 mL.
    d. 500 to 600 mL.

32. Which of the following hormones triggers ovulation?
    a. estrogen
    b. progesterone
    c. luteinizing hormone (LH)
    d. follicle-stimulating hormone (FSH)

33. The average age at which menopause occurs is:
    a. 40 years.
    b. 45 to 50 years.
    c. 55 to 60 years.
    d. 60 to 65 years.

True or false

34. _____ The time of ovulation can be easily predicted by simply knowing the length of a previous cycle.

35. _____ Cyclical changes in the ovaries result from cyclical changes in the amounts of gonadotropins secreted by the anterior pituitary.

36. _____ Contraceptive pills and implants function by preventing ovulation.

37. _____ The first menstrual flow is known as the *climacteric*.

38. _____ The LH surge occurs at the beginning of the menstrual cycle.

▶ *If you had difficulty with this section, review pages 1074-1082.*

V—BREASTS

True or false

39. _____ The larger the breasts, the greater the amount of glandular tissue present.

40. _____ Milk secretion from the breasts begins about 3 or 4 hours after giving birth.

41. _____ Milk ejection is stimulated by oxytocin.

42. _____ Human milk provides active immunity to the offspring in the form of maternal antibodies.

▶ *If you had difficulty with this section, review pages 1082-1086.*

VI—MECHANISMS OF DISEASE

Matching—choose the correct response.

a. amenorrhea
b. dysmenorrhea
c. exogenous infection
d. dysfunctional uterine bleeding (DUB)
e. myoma
f. vaginitis
g. sexually transmitted disease (STD)
h. premenstrual syndrome (PMS)
i. pelvic inflammatory disease (PID)
j. Pap smear
k. endometriosis
l. leukorrhea

43. _____ often occurs from STDs or from a "yeast infection"

44. _____ benign tumor of smooth muscle and fibrous connective tissue; also known as a *fibroid tumor*

45. _____ absence of normal menstruation

46. _____ collection of symptoms that regularly occur in many women during the premenstrual phase

47. _____ acute or chronic inflammation caused by pathogens which spread up from vagina (complication of STI organism)

48. _____ venereal disease (broad term)

49. _____ results from pathogenic organisms transmitted from another person; e.g., STD

50. _____ painful menstruation

51. _____ whitish discharge

52. _____ results from a hormonal imbalance rather than from an infection or disease condition

53. _____ screening test for cervical cancer

54. _____ characterized by displaced uterine tissue

▶ *If you had difficulty with this section, review pages 1086-1093.*

Crossword Puzzle

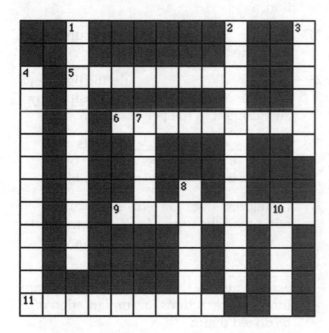

Across
5. Female sex hormone
6. Release of ovum
9. Secretion of milk
11. Climacteric

Down
1. Fallopian tube (two words)
2. Menarche
3. Lower portion of birth canal
4. Lining of uterus
7. External genitalia
8. Womb
10. Female gonad

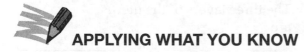

APPLYING WHAT YOU KNOW

55. Prior to having children, Lorena used oral contraceptives to prevent an unwanted pregnancy with her husband. Describe the physiologic mechanism of action of oral contraceptives. After having three children by the age of 35, the couple decided that Lorena would have a tubal ligation. Describe how this procedure prevents pregnancy.

56. Harlean contracted gonorrhea. By the time she made an appointment to see her doctor, it had spread to her abdominal organs. How is this possible when gonorrhea is a disease of the reproductive system?

DID YOU KNOW

- During menstruation, the sensitivity of a woman's middle finger is reduced.

- During pregnancy, the uterus expands to 500 times its normal size.

- There are an estimated 925,000 daily occurrences of STI transmission and 550,000 daily pregnancies worldwide.

ONE LAST QUICK CHECK

Matching—select the best answer for the descriptions.

a. salpingitis
b. vulva
c. Kegel
d. dysmenorrhea
e. *Candida albicans*
f. G spot
g. ovary
h. endometriosis
i. climacteric
j. fibroids

57. _____ essential organ of reproduction

58. _____ external reproductive organ

59. _____ yeast infection

60. _____ benign tumors of uterine tissue

61. _____ inflammation of the uterine tube

62. _____ erotic zone

63. _____ exercise to reduce stress incontinence

64. _____ menopause

65. _____ displaced endometrial tissue

66. _____ menstrual cramps

Fill in the blanks.

67. The _____ _____ phase occurs between ovulation and the onset of the menses.

68. _____ stimulates breast alveoli to secrete milk.

69. _____ stimulates breast alveoli to eject milk.

70. Sexual cell division is known as _____.

71. Immediately after ovulation, cells of the ruptured follicle enlarge and become transformed into the _____ _____.

72. A fold of mucous membrane known as the _____ forms a border around the external opening of the vagina, partially closing the orifice.

73. _____ is marked by the passage of 1 full year without menstruation.

74. The _____ occurs on days 1 to 5 of a new cycle.

75. _____ uterine ligaments hold the uterus in its normal position by anchoring it in the pelvic cavity.

76. The _____ permits exchange of materials between the offspring's blood and the maternal blood.

77. Development of the fetus in a location other than the uterus is referred to as an _____ pregnancy.

78. _____ is secreted each month by the corpus luteum to calm uterine contractions for implantation of a fertilized ovum.

79. The three layers of the uterus are _____, _____, and _____.

80. Damage to muscle fibers of the levator ani may result in urinary or fecal _____.

81. _____ is the failure to conceive after 1 year of regular unprotected intercourse.

CHAPTER 36

Growth and Development

Millions of fragile microscopic sperm swim against numerous obstacles to reach the ova and create a new life. At birth, the newborn will fill his lungs with air and cry lustily, signaling to the world that he is ready to begin the cycle of life. This cycle will be marked by ongoing changes, periodic physical growth, and continuous development.

This chapter reviews the more significant events that occur in the normal growth and development of an individual from conception to death. Realizing that each person is unique, we nonetheless can discover amid all the complexities of humanity some constants that are understandable and predictable.

A knowledge of human growth and development is essential in understanding the commonalties that influence individuals as they pass through the cycle of life.

I—A NEW HUMAN LIFE

Multiple Choice—select the best answer.

1. Which of the following processes reduces the number of chromosomes in each daughter cell to half the number present in the parent cell?
   a. mitosis
   b. meiosis
   c. prophase
   d. telophase

2. Forty-six chromosomes per body cell is known as the _____ number of chromosomes.
   a. haploid
   b. diploid
   c. tetrad
   d. both a and c

3. Each primary spermatocyte undergoes meiotic division I to form:
   a. four haploid secondary spermatocytes.
   b. four diploid secondary spermatocytes.
   c. one diploid secondary spermatocyte.
   d. two haploid secondary spermatocytes.

4.   A mature follicle ready to burst open from the ovary's surface is a:
      a.   graafian follicle.
      b.   theca cell.
      c.   zygote.
      d.   first polar body.

5.   Fertilization occurs in the:
      a.   ovary.
      b.   fallopian tubes.
      c.   uterus.
      d.   vagina.

6.   The phenomenon of "crossing over" takes place during:
      a.   meiosis I only.
      b.   meiosis II only.
      c.   both meiosis I and meiosis II.
      d.   both meiosis and mitosis.

True or false

7.   _____ Sex cells contain 23 chromosomes and are therefore referred to as *diploid*.

8.   _____ The process of "crossing over" allows for almost infinite variety to the genetic makeup of an individual.

9.   _____ Completion of meiosis II in the released oocyte requires the head of a sperm cell to enter the oocyte.

10.   _____ *Zygote* is the term used to describe the ovulated ovum that is awaiting fertilization.

11.   _____ *Insemination* and *fertilization* are synonymous terms.

12.   _____ The ovum can live for up to 3 days.

13.   _____ During oogenesis, the cytoplasm is not equally divided among daughter cells.

14.   _____ Sperm cells can live in the female reproductive tract for up to 3 days.

▶ *If you had difficulty with this section, review pages 1096-1103.*

II—PRENATAL PERIOD

Multiple Choice—select the best answer.

15.   About 3 days after fertilization, the zygote forms into a solid mass of cells called a(n):
      a.   morula.
      b.   blastocyst.
      c.   inner cell mass.
      d.   embryo.

16.   The outer wall of the blastocyst is referred to as the:
      a.   yolk sac.
      b.   trophoblast.
      c.   chorion.
      d.   morula.

17.   The "bag of waters" is also called the:
      a.   amniotic sac.
      b.   yolk sac.
      c.   chorion.
      d.   placenta.

18.   Which of the following is *not* a primary germ layer?
      a.   ectoderm
      b.   exoderm
      c.   endoderm
      d.   mesoderm

19.   By which month of fetal development are all organ systems formed and functioning?
      a.   second
      b.   third
      c.   fourth
      d.   fifth

True or false

20.   _____ Placental tissue secretes large amounts of human chorionic gonadotropin (hCG) early in pregnancy.

21.   _____ The yolk sac plays a critical role in the nutrition of the developing human offspring.

22. _____ The process by which the primary germ layers develop into many different kinds of tissues is called *organogenesis*.

23. _____ The blastocyst is a hollow ball of cells.

24. _____ Division of the cells of the zygote is called *cleavage*.

Labeling—using the terms provided, label the following parts of the diagram depicting fertilization and implantation.

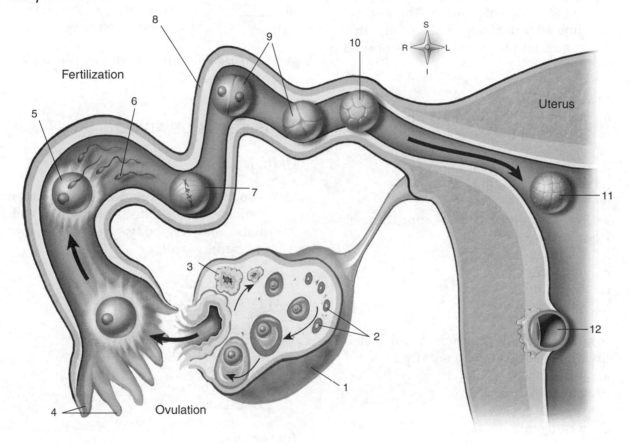

_____ implantation
_____ developing follicles
_____ morula
_____ spermatozoa
_____ corpus luteum
_____ uterine (fallopian) tube

_____ blastocyst
_____ ovary
_____ fimbriae
_____ discharged ovum
_____ first mitosis
_____ divided zygote

▶ *If you had difficulty with this section, review pages 1103-1114.*

III—BIRTH, OR PARTURITION, AND THE POSTNATAL PERIOD

Multiple Choice—select the best answer.

25. Stage two of labor is best described as the:
    a. onset of contractions until uterine dilation is complete.
    b. expulsion of the placenta through the vagina.
    c. time of maximum cervical dilation until the baby exits through the vagina.
    d. time after the baby exits through the vagina and the cervix regains normal aperture.

26. Fraternal twins:
    a. are also called *identical twins*.
    b. arise from the same zygote.
    c. arise from two different sperm and two different ova.
    d. arise from a single sperm.

27. The period of infancy lasts approximately from birth to:
    a. 4 weeks.
    b. 6 months.
    c. 12 months.
    d. 18 months.

28. A rare, inherited condition in which an individual appears to age rapidly is:
    a. senescence.
    b. progeria.
    c. preeclampsia.
    d. teratogenia.

29. Birth weight generally triples by:
    a. 6 months.
    b. 12 months.
    c. 18 months.
    d. 24 months.

True or false

30. _____ A cesarean section is a surgical procedure that delivers a newborn through an incision in the abdomen and uterine wall.

31. _____ When a single zygote divides early in its development and forms two separate individuals, it is referred to as *identical twinning*.

32. _____ Stage one of labor usually lasts from a few minutes to an hour.

33. _____ Neonates have both a lumbar and thoracic curve to their spines.

34. _____ Girls experience adolescent growth spurt before boys do.

▶ *If you had difficulty with this section, review pages 1114-1120.*

IV—EFFECTS OF AGING

Multiple Choice—select the best answer.

35. A sound exercise program throughout life could reduce the effects of aging in which of the following body systems?
    a. cardiovascular
    b. skeletal
    c. muscular
    d. all of the above

36. Clouding of the lens of the eye is called:
    a. presbyopia.
    b. myopia.
    c. glaucoma.
    d. cataract.

True or false

37. _____ The number of functioning nephron units in the kidneys decreases by almost 50% between the ages of 30 and 75.

38. _____ Progesterone therapy may be used to relieve some symptoms of menopause.

▶ *If you had difficulty with this section, review pages 1120-1124.*

V—MECHANISMS OF DISEASE

Matching—select the best answer for the descriptions.

a. placenta previa
b. tubal pregnancy
c. preeclampsia
d. spontaneous abortion
e. stillbirth
f. birth defects
g. puerperal fever
h. mastitis
i. teratogens
j. abruptio placentae

39. _____ pregnancy-induced hypertension

40. _____ placenta grows too close to the cervical opening

41. _____ miscarriage

42. _____ common type of ectopic pregnancy

43. _____ breast inflammation

44. _____ congenital abnormalities

45. _____ separation of placenta from uterine wall

46. _____ childbed fever

▶ *If you had difficulty with this section, review pages 1124-1129.*

Crossword Puzzle

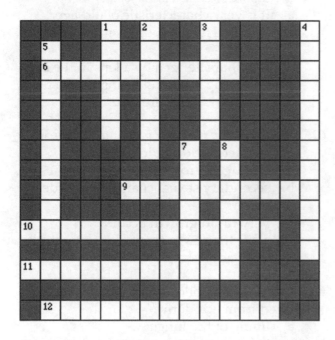

Across
6. Study of individual development before birth
9. Hollow ball that implants itself in the uterus
10. Conception
11. Birth
12. Process where germ layers develop into various tissues

Down
1. Solid mass formed by zygote
2. First 4 weeks of infancy
3. Fertilized ovum
4. Attachment of fertilized ovum in uterus
5. Older adulthood
7. Length of pregnancy
8. Develops from the trophoblast

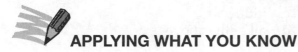

APPLYING WHAT YOU KNOW

47. John is 70 years old. He has always enjoyed food and has a hearty appetite. Lately, however, he has complained that food "just doesn't taste as good anymore." What might be a possible explanation?

48. Gary and Harry were identical twins. Christine gave birth to a baby boy and identified Gary as the father of the child on the birth certificate. Paternity testing later revealed that both twins were the father. How is this possible?

DID YOU KNOW

- A 3-week-old embryo is no larger than a sesame seed. A 1-month-old fetus's body is no heavier than an envelope and a sheet of paper. Its hand is no bigger than a teardrop.

- Between the ages of 30 and 70, a nose may lengthen and widen by as much as half an inch and the ears may be a quarter-inch longer because cartilage is one of the few tissues that continues to grow as we age.

ONE LAST QUICK CHECK

Matching—choose the correct term for the appropriate description.

a.   placenta
b.   gestation
c.   antenatal
d.   histogenesis
e.   C-section
f.   endoderm
g.   zygote
h.   parturition
i.   embryonic phase
j.   ultrasonogram

49. _____   fertilized ovum

50. _____   inside germ layer

51. _____   before birth

52. _____   length of pregnancy

53. _____   structural "anchor" during pregnancy

54. _____   process of birth

55. _____   surgical procedure in which a newborn is delivered through an incision in the abdomen and uterine wall

56. _____   study of how the primary germ layers develop into many different kinds of tissues

57. _____   fertilization until the end of the eighth week of gestation

58. _____   monitors progress of developing fetus

Multiple Choice—select the best answer.

59. Degenerative changes in the urinary system that accompany old age include which of the following?
    a.   decreased capacity of the bladder and the inability to empty or void completely
    b.   decrease in the number of nephrons
    c.   less blood flow through the kidneys
    d.   all of the above

60. Any hardening of the arteries is referred to as which of the following?
    a.   angioma
    b.   atherosclerosis
    c.   angina
    d.   arteriosclerosis
    e.   all of the above

61. Which of the following is characteristic of the disorder called *presbyopia*?
    a.   It is very characteristic of old age.
    b.   If causes farsightedness in some individuals.
    c.   It is characterized by a lens in the eye becoming hard and losing its elasticity.
    d.   All of the above are true.

62. Which of the following events, if any, is *not* characteristic of adolescence?
    a.   closure of growth plates
    b.   secondary sexual characteristics develop
    c.   very rapid growth occurs
    d.   all of the above events are characteristic of adolescence

63. Which of the following structures is derived from ectoderm?
    a.   lining of the lungs
    b.   brain
    c.   kidneys
    d.   all of the above

Matching—select the best answer from the list of descriptions.

a. older adulthood
b. study of aging
c. Hutchinson-Gilford disease
d. fat accumulation in arteries
e. secondary sexual characteristics

64. _____ atherosclerosis

65. _____ adolescence

66. _____ senescence

67. _____ progeria

68. _____ gerontology

CHAPTER 37

Genetics and Heredity

Look around your classroom and you will notice various combinations of hair color, eye color, body size, skin tone, hair texture, gender, etc. Everyone has unique body features and this phenomenon alerts us to the marvel of genetics. Independent units, called *genes*, are responsible for the inheritance of biological traits. Genes determine the structure and function of the human body by producing specific regulatory enzymes. Some genes are dominant and some are recessive. Dominant genes produce traits that appear in the offspring and recessive genes have traits that do not appear in the offspring when they are masked by a dominant gene.

Gene therapy is one of the latest advances of science. This revolutionary branch of medicine combines current technology with genetic research to unlock the secrets of the human body. Daily discoveries into the prevention, diagnosis, treatment, and cure of diseases and disorders are being revealed as a result of genetic therapy. A knowledge of genetics is necessary to understand the basic mechanism by which traits are transmitted from parents to offspring.

I—THE SCIENCE OF GENETICS, CHROMOSOMES AND GENES, GENE EXPRESSION

Multiple Choice—select the best answer.

1. When its genetic codes are being expressed, DNA is in a threadlike form called:
   a. mRNA.
   b. chromosomes.
   c. chromatin.
   d. tRNA.

2. Each DNA molecule can be called either a chromatin strand or a:
   a. gene.
   b. genome.
   c. chromosome.
   d. gamete.

3. A person with a genotype expressed as *AA* is said to be:
   a. heterozygous recessive.
   b. heterozygous dominant.
   c. homozygous recessive.
   d. homozygous dominant.

4. Both males and females need at least:
   a. one normal Y chromosome.
   b. two normal X chromosomes.
   c. one normal X chromosome.
   d. two normal Y chromosomes.

5. The entire collection of genetic material in each typical cell of the human body is called the:
   a. genome.
   b. chromosome.
   c. genotype.
   d. phenotype.

6. Mutations are caused:
   a. spontaneously.
   b. by mutagens.
   c. by environmental agents that damage DNA.
   d. all of the above.

7. Red-green color blindness is an example of an X-linked recessive condition. If X is normal, X1 is recessive, and Y is normal, an individual with the genotype XX1 will be a:
   a. normal male.
   b. color-blind male.
   c. normal female and a carrier.
   d. normal female and not a carrier.

8. The scientific study of genetics began in the:
   a. 16th century.
   b. 17th century.
   c. 18th century.
   d. 19th century.

True or false

9. _____ Each of the 23 pairs of chromosomes always appear to be nearly identical to each other.

10. _____ The manner in which genotype is expressed is termed *phenotype*.

11. _____ *Sickle-cell trait* and *sickle-cell anemia* are synonymous terms.

12. _____ Normal males have the sex chromosome combination XX, whereas normal females have the sex chromosome combination XY.

13. _____ X-linked recessive traits appear much more frequently in males than in females.

14. _____ Statistical evidence supports the notion that having sexual intercourse on the day of ovulation increases the probability of conceiving a male.

15. _____ Each cell of the body, except gametes, contains 46 pairs of chromosomes.

16. _____ A person whose genotype is heterozygous for albinism will express the abnormal phenotype of albinism.

▶ *If you had difficulty with this section, review pages 1131-1141.*

II—MEDICAL GENETICS, PREVENTION AND TREATMENT OF GENETIC DISEASES

Multiple Choice—select the best answer.

17. Trisomy and monosomy result from:
    a. an error in meiosis called *disjunction*.
    b. an error in meiosis called *nondisjunction*.
    c. single-gene abnormality.
    d. chromosome breakage.

18. Trisomy 21 is also called:
    a. Klinefelter syndrome.
    b. Down syndrome.
    c. Turner syndrome.
    d. cystic fibrosis.

19. A person with the sex chromosomes XXY is afflicted with:
    a. Klinefelter syndrome.
    b. Down syndrome.
    c. Turner syndrome.
    d. cystic fibrosis.

20. Which of the following is *not* a recessive X-linked genetic disease?
    a. hemophilia
    b. red-green color blindness
    c. sickle-cell anemia
    d. cleft palate

21. Which of the following abnormal genes are linked to some form of cancer?
    a. codominant genes
    b. tumor suppressor genes
    c. oncogenes
    d. recessive genes

22. A grid used to determine the mathematical probability of inheriting genetic traits is called:
    a. a pedigree.
    b. a Punnett square.
    c. amniocentesis.
    d. a chorionic villus sampling.

23. Which of the following genetic diseases can be treated to some degree, if diagnosed early?
    a. PKU
    b. Turner syndrome
    c. Klinefelter syndrome
    d. all of the above

24. In gene replacement therapy:
    a. genetically altered cells are introduced into the body.
    b. genetic disease is treated by inducing an alteration in metabolism.
    c. synthetic hormones are used to relieve symptoms.
    d. genes that specify production of abnormal, disease-causing proteins are replaced by normal or "therapeutic" genes.

25. Disorders that involve trisomy or monosomy can be detected after a _____ is produced.
    a. genotype
    b. phenotype
    c. karyotype
    d. polytype

26. Cells that display distinct chromosomes during collection via amniocentesis and chorionic villus sampling are in:
    a. prophase.
    b. metaphase.
    c. anaphase.
    d. telophase.

True or false

27. _____ *Congenital disorders* and *inherited disorders* are synonymous terms.

28. _____ Sickle-cell trait is milder than sickle-cell anemia.

29. _____ Parkinson disease is linked to an error in the nuclear DNA.

30. _____ A pedigree is a chart that illustrates genetic relationships in a family over several generations.

31. _____ Xeroderma pigmentosum is characterized by the inability of skin cells to repair genetic damage caused by the (UV) radiation in sunlight.

32. _____ Cystic fibrosis is a blood-clotting disorder.

33. _____ Cleft palate is a recessive X-linked disorder.

34. _____ Chorionic villus sampling is a procedure newer than amniocentesis.

35. _____ "Genes are not there to cause disease."

▶ *If you had difficulty with this section, review pages 1141-1151.*

Crossword Puzzle

Across

2. Having half of the normal chromosomes
8. Triplet of autosomes
9. Entire collection of genetic material in each cell
10. Grid used to predict genetic traits (two words)

Down

1. Used to identify chromosomal disorders
3. Having a characteristic pair of chromosomes
4. Presence of one autosome
5. Equal effect of different dominant genes
6. Genotype with two identical forms of a gene
7. One of the 44 chromosomes (excluding sex chromosomes)

APPLYING WHAT YOU KNOW

36. Deb's mother has a dominant gene for dark skin color. Her father has a dominant gene for light skin color. What color will Deb's skin most likely be?

37. Mr. and Mrs. Mihm both carry recessive genes for cystic fibrosis. Using your knowledge of the Punnett square, estimate the probability of one of their offspring inheriting this condition.

DID YOU KNOW

- Scientists estimate that they could fill a 1000-volume encyclopedia with the coded instructions in the DNA of a single human cell if the instructions could be translated into English.

- Identical twins do not have identical fingerprints. No two sets of prints are alike, including those of identical twins.

ONE LAST QUICK CHECK

Multiple Choice—select the best answer.

38. Independent assortment of chromosomes ensures:
    a. each offspring from a single set of parents is genetically unique.
    b. at meiosis each gamete receives the same number of chromosomes.
    c. that the sex chromosomes always match.
    d. an equal number of males and females are born.

39. Which of the following statements is *not* true of a pedigree?
    a. They are useful to genetic counselors in predicting the possibility of producing offspring with genetic disorders.
    b. They may allow a person to determine his or her likelihood of developing a genetic disorder later in life.
    c. They indicate the occurrence of those family members affected by a trait, as well as carriers of the trait.
    d. All of the above are true of a pedigree.

40. The genes that cause albinism are:
    a. codominant.
    b. dominant.
    c. recessive.
    d. AA.

41. During meiosis, matching pairs of chromosomes line up and exchange genes from their location to the same location on the other side; a process called:
    a. gene linkage.
    b. crossing over.
    c. cross-linkage.
    d. genetic variation.

42. When a sperm cell unites with an ovum, a _____ is formed.
    a. zygote
    b. chromosome
    c. gamete
    d. none of the above

43. DNA molecules can also be called:
    a. a chromatin strand.
    b. a chromosome.
    c. a and b.
    d. none of the above.

44. Sex-linked traits:
    a. show up more often in females than in males.
    b. are nonsexual traits carried on sex chromosomes.
    c. are the result of genetic mutation.
    d. all of the above.

45. If a person has only X chromosomes, that person is:
    a. missing essential proteins.
    b. abnormal.
    c. female.
    d. male.

46. A karyotype:
    a. can detect trisomy.
    b. is useful for diagnosing a tubal pregnancy.
    c. is frequently used as a tool in gene augmentation therapy.
    d. can detect the presence of oncogenes.

47. Which of the following pairs is mismatched?
    a. osteogenesis imperfecta—dominant
    b. Turner syndrome—trisomy
    c. PKU—recessive
    d. cystic fibrosis—recessive

Completion—using the terms below, complete the following statements.

a. cystic fibrosis
b. males
c. phenylketonuria
d. carrier
e. genome
f. females
g. dominant
h. oncogenes
i. karyotype
j. Tay-Sachs disease
k. amniocentesis
l. hemophilia

48. Abnormal genes called _____ are believed to be related to cancer.

49. Fetal tissue may be collected by a procedure called _____.

50. An abnormal accumulation of phenylalanine results in _____.

51. The entire collection of genetic material in each cell is called the _____.

52. _____ is caused by recessive genes in chromosome pair seven.

53. A _____ is a person who has a recessive gene that is not expressed.

54. Absence of an essential lipid-producing enzyme may result in the recessive condition _____.

55. _____ is a recessive X-linked disorder characterized as a blood clotting disorder.

56. A gene capable of masking the effects of a recessive gene for the same trait is a _____ gene.

Fill in the blanks.

57. Each gene in a chromosome contains a genetic code that the cell transcribes to a _____ molecule.

58. The analysis of all mRNA codes actually transcribed from the human genome is known as _____.

59. The shorter segment of a chromosome is called the _____ _____ and the longer segment is called the _____ _____.

60. The most well-known chromosomal disorder is trisomy 21 or _____ _____.

61. To get therapeutic genes to cells that need them, researchers use genetically altered _____ as carriers.

62. An _____ is often used in genomics to show the overall physical structure of a chromosome.

Answer Key

CHAPTER 1

Anatomy and Physiology and Characteristics of Life
1. b, p. 5
2. c, p. 5
3. a, p. 5
4. b, p. 6
5. c, p. 6

Levels of Organization
6. d, p. 7
7. a, p. 7
8. c, p. 8
9. c, p. 9
10. c, p. 9
11. d, p. 8
12. e, p. 8
13. a, p. 8
14. c, p. 8
15. b, p. 8
16. a, p. 9
17. a, p. 9
18. a, p. 9
19. b, p. 9
20. b, p. 9
21. e, p. 9
22. e, p. 9
23. d, p. 9
24. d, p. 9
25. e, p. 9
26. c, p. 9

Anatomical Position, Body Cavities, Body Regions, Anatomical Terms, and Body Planes
27. b, p. 10
28. a, p. 11
29. a, p. 10
30. d, p. 13
31. c, p. 11
32. c, p. 10
33. b, p. 11
34. b, p. 16
35. c, p. 16
36. d, p. 13
37. inferior, p. 15
38. anterior, p. 15
39. lateral, p. 15
40. proximal, p. 15
41. superficial, p. 15
42. equal, p. 16
43. anterior and posterior, p. 16
44. upper and lower, p. 16
45. frontal, p. 16
46. a, p. 10
47. b, p. 11
48. a, p. 11
49. a, p. 11
50. a, p. 10
51. a, p. 10

Homeostasis and Homeostatic Mechanisms of Control
52. a, p. 19
53. d, p. 20
54. a, p. 21
55. b, p. 22
56. f, p. 21
57. f, p. 23
58. t, p. 21
59. t, p. 23

Mechanisms of Disease
60. b, p. 25
61. e, p. 25
62. a, p. 25
63. d, p. 25
64. c, p. 25
65. f, p. 25
66. h, p. 25
67. i, p. 25
68. g, p. 25
69. j, p. 25
70. pathophysiology, p. 25
71. homeostasis, p. 25
72. mutated, p. 25
73. parasite, p. 25
74. tumors, p. 27
75. self-immunity, p. 27

Applying What You Know

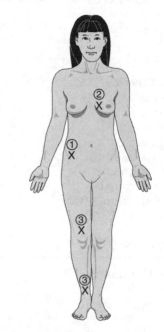

76. #1 on diagram
77. #2 on diagram
78. #3 on diagram

One Last Quick Check
79. a, p. 19
80. d, p. 14
81. d, p. 16
82. a, p. 5
83. b, p. 14
84. d, p. 11
85. d, p. 15
86. d, p. 13
87. a, p. 13
88. c, p. 15

Fill in the Blanks
89. eponyms, p. 6
90. bilateral symmetry, p. 10
91. medullary, p. 15
92. apical, p. 15
93. DNA, p. 17
94. hormones, p. 19

95. homeostatic control mechanisms, p. 20
96. feed-forward, p. 22
97. intrinsic control, p. 23
98. gerontology, p. 24
99. bacteria, p. 26
100. genetic factor, p. 27

Diagrams

Directions and Planes of the Body
1. superior
2. proximal
3. posterior (dorsal)
4. anterior (ventral)
5. inferior
6. sagittal plane
7. frontal plane
8. lateral

Body Cavities
1. cranial
2. spinal
3. thoracic
4. pleural
5. mediastinum
6. diaphragm
7. abdominal
8. abdominopelvic
9. pelvic

CHAPTER 2

Basic Chemistry
1. c, p. 35
2. c, p. 36
3. c, p. 36
4. d, p. 37
5. c, p. 37
6. c, p. 38
7. b, p. 38
8. a, p. 40
9. t, p. 36
10. t, p. 36
11. f, p. 39
12. f, p. 39
13. t, p. 40
14. oxygen
15. calcium
16. potassium
17. sodium
18. magnesium
19. iron
20. selenium

Metabolism
21. a, p. 41
22. d, p. 41
23. b, p. 41
24. c, p. 41
25. e, p. 42

Inorganic Molecules
26. d, p. 43
27. d, p. 43
28. c, p. 44
29. b, p. 44
30. c, p. 45
31. t, p. 44
32. t, p. 45
33. t, p. 44
34. t, p. 43
35. f, p. 43

Organic Molecules
36. c, p. 46
37. d, p. 46
38. c, p. 51
39. a, p. 52
40. c, p. 51
41. b, p. 49
42. c, p. 57
43. d, p. 55
44. a, p. 55
45. f, p. 50
46. t, p. 51
47. f, p. 53
48. t, p. 52
49. t, p. 51
50. t, p. 50

Applying What You Know
51. (A) Basement (B) Increasing ventilation or sealing the basement floors
52. Unsaturated fats can often form a solid mass at higher temperatures. Review pages 48 and 49 for more information.

One Last Quick Check
53. e, p. 37
54. b, p. 57
55. g, p. 37
56. a, p. 36
57. i, p. 46
58. f, p. 55
59. h, p. 43
60. c, p. 44
61. b, p. 46
62. c, p. 48
63. a, p. 51
64. c, p. 48
65. b, p. 46
66. c, p. 48
67. a, p. 51
68. b, p. 44
69. a, p. 44
70. b, p. 44
71. b, p. 44
72. a, p. 44

CHAPTER 3

Functional Anatomy of Cells
1. b, p. 70
2. d, p. 72
3. b, p. 73
4. d, p. 77
5. a, p. 74
6. a, p. 78
7. b, p. 78
8. f, p. 70
9. t, p. 72
10. f, p 78
11. t, p. 77
12. f, p. 69
13. a, p. 69
14. d, p. 69
15. b, p. 69
16. f, p. 69
17. c, p. 69
18. h, p. 69
19. g, p. 69
20. e, p. 69

Cytoskeleton
21. cytoskeleton, p. 79
22. microfilaments, p. 80
23. microtubules, p. 80
24. centrosome, p. 80
25. microvilli, cilia, flagella, p. 82
26. gap junctions, p. 84
27. desmosomes, p. 83

Applying What You Know
28. (a) CD 36 (b) LDL (c) stroke, diabetes, cancer, muscular dystrophy
29. mitochondria

One Last Quick Check
30. b, p. 82
31. c, p. 83
32. b, p. 83
33. b, p. 73
34. b, p. 70
35. e, p. 67
36. d, p. 67
37. b, p. 67
38. a, p. 67
39. c, p. 67
40. composite, p. 68
41. hydrophilic, p. 70
42. signal transduction, p. 72
43. peroxisomes, p. 69
44. nucleus, p. 78
45. integral membrane proteins, p. 72

Diagrams

Cell Anatomy
1. centrosome
2. smooth endoplasmic reticulum
3. rough endoplasmic reticulum
4. nuclear envelope
5. nucleolus
6. microvilli
7. Golgi apparatus
8. cilia
9. mitochondria
10. ribosomes

CHAPTER 4

Movement of Substances Through Cell Membranes
1. d, p. 101
2. b, p. 92
3. c, p. 101
4. a, p. 94
5. b, p. 97
6. f, p. 96
7. t, p. 97
8. t, p. 100
9. t, p. 91
10. f, p. 96
11. b, p. 94
12. a, p. 94
13. c, p. 95
14. d, p. 91
15. e, p. 99

Cell Metabolism
16. b, p. 102
17. d, p. 102
18. a, p. 103
19. d, p. 103
20. b, p. 104
21. b, p. 102
22. t, p. 105
23. t, p. 102
24. f, p. 102
25. t, p. 108
26. t, p. 106
27. f, p. 105
28. b, p. 106
29. c, p. 106
30. a, p. 105

Applying What You Know
31. diffusion
32. shrink

One Last Quick Check
33. a, p. 98
34. b, p. 91
35. d, p. 92
36. a, p. 103

37. c, p. 105
38. b, p. 97
39. c, p. 97
40. c, p. 97
41. a, p. 101
42. b, p. 94
43. a, p. 95
44. b, p. 95
45. f, p. 100
46. c, p. 103
47. h, p. 103
48. e, p. 100
49. g, p. 96
50. d, p. 92
51. i, p. 105
52. a, p 92

Diagrams

Cellular Respiration
1. glucose
2. acetyl-CoA
3. citric acid cycle
4. mitochondrion
5. ATP
6. O_2
7. H_2O
8. aerobic
9. anaerobic
10. transition
11. pyruvic acid
12. lactic acid

CHAPTER 5

Protein Synthesis and Cell Growth
1. d, p. 114
2. a, p. 115
3. b, p. 116
4. b, p. 117
5. c, p. 116
6. d, p. 116
7. a, p. 114
8. e, p. 116
9. a, p. 117
10. c, p. 117
11. d, p. 117
12. f, p. 116
13. b, p. 118

Cell Reproduction
14. enzyme (all others refer to cell reproduction)
15. end phase (all others refer to anaphase)
16. telophase (all others refer to meiosis)
17. mitosis (all others refer to meiosis)
18. interphase (all others are phases of mitosis)

19. a, p. 123
20. b, p. 124
21. b, p. 124
22. d, p. 123
23. c, p. 123
24. telophase, p. 124
25. anaphase, p. 124
26. metaphase, p. 124
27. interphase, p. 124
28. prophase, p. 124

Mechanisms of Disease
29. t, p. 126
30. t, p. 127
31. t, p. 126
32. f, p. 127
33. t, p. 127
34. Genes are responsible for all of our healthy attributes or conditions such as sex, hair color, eyes, etc. Genetic disorders are pathological conditions caused by mistakes, or mutations, in a cell's genetic code. Abnormal genes often cause a specific disease that can be identified just weeks after conception and can many times be treated prior to delivery.
35. When a broken arm is immobilized in a cast for a long period, muscles that move the arm often atrophy. Because the muscles are temporarily out of use, muscle cells decrease in size. Dan's arm will return to normal as he begins to use his arm more and returns to the level of exercise that he had prior to the fracture.

One Last Quick Check
36. a, p. 116
37. a, p. 122
38. d, p. 124
39. d, p. 116
40. c, p. 124
41. b, p. 116
42. c, p. 116
43. a, p. 124
44. a, p. 117
45. c, p. 119
46. uracil (RNA contains the base uracil, not DNA)
47. thymine (the others refer to RNA)
48. interphase (the others refer to translation)

49. prophase (the others refer to anaphase)
50. gene (the others refer to stages of cell division)
51. obligatory base pairing, p. 115
52. proteome, p. 119
53. double helix, p. 114
54. meiosis, p. 124
55. gametes, p. 124

Diagrams

DNA Molecule
1. hydrogen bonds
2. sugar
3. phosphate
4. cytosine
5. guanine
6. adenine
7. thymine

Mitosis
1. prophase
2. metaphase
3. anaphase
4. telophase

CHAPTER 6

Principal Types of Tissues
1. b, p. 132
2. c, p. 132
3. d, p. 132
4. b, p. 134
5. b, p. 132
6. a, p. 132
7. t, p. 132
8. t, p. 134
9. f, p. 132
10. t, p. 132

Epithelial Tissue
11. d, p. 135
12. b, p. 140
13. b, p. 138
14. b, p. 137
15. d, p. 138
16. b, p. 141
17. a, p. 142
18. d, p. 142
19. a, p. 138
20. t, p. 135
21. f, p. 136
22. f, p. 141
23. b, p. 138
24. e, p. 138
25. d, p. 138
26. h, p. 139
27. a, p. 138
28. c, p. 138

Connective Tissue
29. a, p. 144
30. c, p. 143
31. b, p. 145
32. d, p. 144
33. c, p. 148
34. d, p. 150
35. a, p. 150
36. b, p. 150
37. a, p. 151
38. d, p. 146
39. t, p. 145
40. t, p. 150
41. f, p. 150
42. f, p. 151
43. t, p. 143
44. f, p. 147

Muscle Tissue
45. b, p. 152
46. c, p. 153
47. a, p. 154
48. b, p. 152
49. c, p. 152
50. c, p. 152

Nervous Tissue
51. d, p. 154
52. b, p. 154
53. c, p. 154
54. a, p. 154
55. e, p. 154

Tissue Repair
56. regeneration, p. 154
57. keloid, p. 154
58. phagocytic, p. 154
59. connective, p. 154
60. nerve, p. 154

Body Membranes
61. a, p. 155
62. b, p. 156
63. f, p. 156
64. t, p. 157

Tumors and Cancer
65. slowly, p. 158
66. are not, p. 158
67. papilloma, p. 159
68. sarcoma, p. 159
69. oncologist, p. 159
70. cytotoxic, p. 160

Applying What You Know
71. Too lean. Holly should be in the 20–22% range to be considered normal. Holly's obsession may put her at risk for other disease conditions because of the stress to her body of being "too lean."

72. Modalities—medical imaging, biopsy, and blood tests Tissues—epithelial, connective, and muscle

One Last Quick Check
73. squamous, p. 136
74. cuboidal, p. 136
75. columnar, p. 136
76. simple squamous, p. 136
77. simple cuboidal, p. 136
78. simple columnar, p. 136
79. stratified squamous, p. 136
80. pseudostratified columnar, p. 136
81. a, p. 132
82. d, p. 140
83. b, p. 143
84. c, p. 145
85. c, p. 147
86. b, p. 152
87. a, p. 156
88. c, p. 156
89. c, p. 132
90. g, p. 135
91. e, p. 137
92. l, p. 139
93. a, p. 142
94. j, p. 144
95. i, p. 146
96. h, p. 152
97. k, p. 157
98. b, p. 157
99. f, p. 158
100. d, p. 159

Diagrams

Tissue #1 is simple cuboidal epithelium
1. basement membrane
2. cell nuclei
3. cuboidal epithelial cells
4. lumen of tubule

Tissue #2 is simple columnar epithelial
1. goblet cells
2. columnar epithelial cell

Tissue #3 is pseudostratified columnar ciliated epithelium
1. columnar cell
2. basement membrane
3. cilia

Tissue#4 is stratified squamous (keratinized) epithelium
1. stratified squamous epithelium
2. keratinized layer
3. basal cells
4. dermis

5. basement membrane

Tissue #5 is adipose
1. storage area for fat
2. plasma membrane
3. nucleus of adipose

Tissue #6 is collagenous dense regular fibrous connective
1. fibroblast
2. collagenous fibers

Tissue #7 is compact bone
1. osteon (Haversian system)

Tissue #8 is skeletal muscle
1. cross striations of muscle cell
2. nuclei of muscle cell
3. muscle fiber

Tissue #9 is cardiac muscle
1. nucleus
2. intercalated disks

Tissue #10 is nervous
1. nerve cell body
2. axon
3. dendrites

CHAPTER 7

Skin Function and Structure
1. b, p. 172
2. a, p. 174
3. d, p. 174
4. d, p. 174
5. a, p. 174
6. d, p. 177
7. b, p. 173
8. c, p. 177
9. b, p. 178
10. c, p. 178
11. f, p. 172
12. t, p. 177
13. t, p. 179
14. f, p. 176
15. t, p. 178

Functions of the Skin
16. d, p. 181
17. d, p. 182
18. c, p. 183
19. a, p. 182
20. b, p. 184
21. f, p. 183
22. f, p. 182
23. t, p. 184

Appendages of the Skin
24. b, p. 185
25. a, p. 186
26. c, p. 188
27. b, p. 187
28. d, p. 186

29. t, p. 185
30. f, p. 185
31. t, p. 187
32. t, p. 186
33. t, p. 186

Mechanisms of Disease
34. f, p. 189
35. c, p. 189
36. a, p. 190
37. b, p. 190
38. g, p. 190
39. h, p. 190
40. d, p. 190
41. e, p. 190
42. Fever or febrile, p. 191
43. Heat exhaustion, p. 191
44. Heat stroke, p. 192
45. Frostbite c, p. 192

Burns
46. a, p. 192
47. b, p. 193
48. f, p. 192
49. t, p. 193
50. c, p. 193
51. a, p. 193
52. d, p. 193
53. b, p. 193
54. e, p. 193

Applying What You Know
55. 46%
56. fingerprints
57. It is theorized that adults who had more than two blistering sunburns before the age of 20 have a greater risk of developing melanoma than someone who experienced no burns.
    Bernie's exposure may have been during his youth or adolescence.

One Last Quick Check
58. a, p. 177
59. d, p. 187
60. b, p. 178
61. d, p. 193
62. b, p. 188
63. c, p. 190 and A & P Connect
64. c, p. 186
65. b, p. 181
66. a, p. 176
67. a, p. 174
68. c, p. 178
69. b, p. 177
70. e, p. 186
71. f, p. 185
72. g, p. 186
73. a, p. 176

74. d, p. 187
75. h, p. 187
76. i, p. 189
77. j, p. 190

Diagrams

Skin
1. epidermis
2. dermis
3. hypodermis
4. blood vessels
5. lamellar (Pacini) corpuscle
6. sweat gland
7. subcutaneous adipose tissue
8. reticular layer of dermis
9. papillary layer of dermis
10. arrector pili muscle
11. root of hair
12. hair follicle
13. sebaceous gland
14. sweat gland
15. sweat duct
16. dermal papillae
17. shaft of hair
18. opening of sweat duct
19. sulcus
20. ridges of dermal papillae
21. nerve fibers
22. sweat duct
23. friction ridge
24. sulcus
25. dermo-epidermal junction

Rule of Nines
1. 4.5%
2. 4.5%
3. 18%
4. 4.5%
5. 1%
6. 9%
7. 9%
8. 4.5%
9. 4.5%
10. 18%
11. 4.5%
12. 9%
13. 9%

CHAPTER 8

Types of Bones
1. f, p. 203
2. k, p. 203
3. h, p. 202
4. e, p. 202
5. d, p. 202
6. i, p. 201
7. j, p. 203
8. c, p. 201
9. a, p. 202
10. b, p. 203

11. g, p. 201

Bone Tissue Structure, Bone Marrow, and Regulation of Blood Calcium Levels
12. d, p. 203
13. b, p. 204
14. c, p. 204
15. b, p. 206
16. b, p. 208
17. c, p. 208
18. t, p. 204
19. f, p. 207
20. t, p. 207
21. t, p. 208
22. f, p. 200
23. f, p. 207

Bone Development, Remodeling, and Repair
24. b, p. 210
25. d, p. 210
26. a, p. 210
27. b, p. 213
28. b, p. 214
29. t, p. 210
30. f, p. 210
31. f, p. 213
32. t, p. 213
33. t, p. 212

Cartilage
34. b, p. 214
35. c, p. 215
36. b, p. 217
37. f, p. 214
38. t, p. 215
39. t, p. 215

Mechanisms of Disease
40. Chondrosarcoma, p. 216
41. Osteosarcoma, p. 216
42. Osteoporosis, p. 216
43. Paget's disease, p. 218
44. Osteomyelitis, p. 218

Applying What You Know
45. (a) Osteoporosis
    (b) DXA—dual energy x-ray absorptiometry scan or bone density (RA) imagery of the wrist
    (c) hormonal therapy (HRT), bone-building nonhormonal drugs such as Fosamax or Miacalcin, vitamin (D) and mineral (calcium) therapy, and weight-bearing exercises.
46. The bones are responsible for the majority of our blood cell formation. Her disease condition might be inhibiting the production of blood cells.
47. Epiphyseal cartilage is present only while a child is still growing. It becomes bone in adulthood. It is particularly vulnerable to fractures in childhood and preadolescence.
48. Ms. Strickland's surgeon most likely used a synthetic skeletal repair material called "vitos" which facilitates fracture repairs. Unlike metal stabilizers, vitos "patches" degrade naturally in the body following surgery and do not require surgical removal.

One Last Quick Check
49. support, protection, movement, mineral storage, and hematopoiesis, p. 200
50. medullary cavity, p. 203
51. articular cartilage, p. 202
52. endosteum, p. 203
53. hematopoiesis, p. 200
54. red bone marrow, p. 207
55. periosteum, p. 202
56. long, short, flat, irregular, and sesamoid, p. 200
57. calcium, p. 208
58. hyaline, p. 214
59. d, p. 206
60. b, p. 201
61. e, p. 201
62. a, p. 202
63. c, p. 214
64. i, p. 207
65. f, p. 204
66. j, p. 204
67. g, p. 214
68. h, p. 204

Diagrams

Long Bone
1. epiphysis
2. diaphysis
3. epiphysis
4. periosteum
5. yellow marrow
6. endosteum
7. medullary cavity
8. compact bone
9. red marrow cavities
10. epiphyseal line
11. spongy bone
12. articular cartilage

Cross-Section of Cancellous and Compact Bone
1. osteons (Haversian systems)
2. periosteum (inner layer)
3. periosteum (outer layer)
4. trabeculae
5. compact bone
6. cancellous (spongy) bone
7. medullary (marrow) cavity
8. transverse (Volkmann) canals
9. central (Haversian) canals
10. endosteum

CHAPTER 9

Divisions of the Skeleton
1. a, p. 226
2. a, p. 224
3. b, p. 224
4. a, p. 226
5. b, p. 226
6. b, p. 226
7. a, p. 226
8. b, p. 226
9. a, p. 226
10. b, p. 226

The Skull
11. c, p. 238
12. d, p. 238
13. a, p. 239
14. c, p. 226
15. a, p. 240
16. b, p. 241
17. f, p. 226
18. t, p. 241
19. t, p. 237
20. f, p. 243
21. t, p. 232

Sternum and Ribs
22. e, p. 248
23. c, p. 248
24. a, p. 248
25. d, p. 248
26. f, p. 248
27. b, p. 248
28. g, p. 248

The Appendicular Skeleton/ Upper Extremity
29. b, p. 250
30. d, p. 251
31. d, p. 251
32. t, p. 251
33. f, p. 254
34. t, p. 251
35. f, p. 254

The Appendicular Skeleton/ Lower Extremity
36. b, p. 255
37. a, p. 255
38. a, p. 255
39. c, p. 260
40. f, p. 255
41. f, p. 257
42. f, p. 260
43. f, p. 260

Skeletal Differences in Men and Women
44. b, p. 262
45. a, p. 262
46. a, p. 262
47. b, p. 262
48. a, p. 262
49. b, p. 262

Cycle of Life: Mechanisms of Disease
50. b, p. 265
51. c, p. 264
52. f, p. 265
53. t, p. 265

Applying What You Know
54. Bill could have possibly injured his humerus and his ulna.
55. (a) High heels cause a forward thrust to the body which forces an undue amount of weight on the heads of the metatarsals. (b) Metatarsals, tarsals, and phalanges

One Last Quick Check
56. coxal (all others refer to the spine)
57. axial (all others refer to the appendicular skeleton)
58. maxilla (all others refer to the cranial bones)
59. ribs (all others refer to the shoulder girdle)
60. vomer (all others refer to the bones of the middle ear)
61. ulna (all others refer to the coxal bone)
62. ethmoid (all others refer to the hand and wrist)
63. nasal (all others refer to cranial bones)
64. anvil (all others refer to the cervical vertebra)
65. c, p. 233
66. g, p. 248
67. j, l, m, k, p. 256
68. n, p. 257
69. i, p. 253
70. a, p. 232
71. p, p. 260
72. b, d, p. 234
73. f, p. 235
74. h, q, p. 251
75. o, t, p. 257
76. r, p. 233
77. s, e, p. 238
78. simple fracture, p. 264
79. otitis media, p. 265
80. scoliosis, p. 265

Diagrams

Anterior View of Skull
1. glabella
2. ethmoid bone
3. sphenoid bone
4. nasal bone
5. vomer
6. mental foramen of mandible
7. mandible
8. maxilla
9. perpendicular plate of ethmoid bone
10. optic foramen of sphenoid bone
11. parietal bone
12. frontal bone

Floor of Cranial Cavity
1. crista galli
2. cribriform plate
3. superior orbital fissure
4. optic foramen
5. foramen ovale
6. foramen lacerum
7. foramen spinosum
8. internal acoustic meatus
9. jugular foramen
10. foramen magnum
11. occipital bone
12. parietal bone
13. petrous portion of the temporal bone
14. temporal bone
15. sella turcica
16. greater wing
17. lesser wing
18. sphenoid bone
19. ethmoid bone
20. frontal bone

Skull Viewed from Below
1. incisive foramen
2. zygomatic process of maxilla
3. zygomatic arch
4. temporal bone
5. styloid process
6. foramen ovale
7. carotid canal
8. mastoid process
9. stylomastoid foramen
10. mastoid foramen
11. parietal bone
12. foramen magnum
13. occipital bone
14. occipital condyle
15. jugular foramen
16. foramen lacerum
17. vomer
18. lateral pterygoid plate of sphenoid
19. zygomatic process of temporal bone
20. medial pterygoid plate of sphenoid
21. temporal process of zygomatic bone
22. horizontal plate of palatine bone
23. palatine process of maxilla
24. hard palate

Skull Viewed from the Right Side
1. squamous suture
2. parietal bone
3. lambdoid suture
4. temporal bone
5. occipital bone
6. external acoustic meatus
7. condyloid process of mandible
8. mastoid process of temporal bone
9. styloid process
10. pterygoid process of sphenoid bone
11. coronoid process of mandible
12. mandible
13. mental foramen of mandible
14. maxilla
15. zygomatic bone
16. nasal bone
17. lacrimal bone
18. ethmoid bone
19. sphenoid bone
20. frontal bone
21. coronal suture

Bones of the Left Orbit
1. optic canal of sphenoid bone
2. superior orbital fissure of sphenoid bone
3. ethmoid bone
4. lacrimal bone
5. maxilla
6. inferior orbital fissure
7. infraorbital foramen
8. zygomatic bone
9. sphenoid bone

10. frontal bone
11. supraorbital foramen of the frontal bone
12. supraorbital margin of the frontal bone

The Vertebral Column
1. thoracic curvature
2. intervertebral foramina
3. sacral curvature
4. atlas
5. axis
6. cervical curvature
7. lumbar curvature
8. coccyx
9. sacrum
10. lumbar vertebrae
11. thoracic vertebrae
12. cervical vertebrae

Vertebrae Atlas
1. transverse process
2. transverse foramen
3. anterior arch
4. facet for dens of axis
5. vertebral foramen
6. superior articular facet for occipital condyle
7. posterior arch

Cervical Vertebra
1. spinous process
2. lamina
3. pedicle
4. transverse foramen
5. transverse process
6. superior articular facet
7. vertebral foramen

Lumbar Vertebra
1. spinous process
2. lamina
3. transverse process
4. pedicle
5. superior articular facet
6. vertebral foramen

Axis
1. spinous process
2. transverse process
3. transverse foramen
4. dens
5. superior articular facet
6. vertebral foramen

Thoracic Vertebra
1. spinous process
2. lamina
3. transverse process
4. pedicle
5. superior articular facet
6. inferior articular facet
7. vertebral foramen

Thoracic Cage
1. costosternal articulation
2. true ribs
3. false ribs
4. floating ribs
5. costal cartilage
6. xiphoid process
7. body
8. manubrium
9. sternum
10. clavicle

Scapula Anterior View
1. superior angle
2. superior border
3. coracoid process
4. acromion
5. supraglenoid tubercle
6. glenoid cavity
7. infraglenoid tubercle
8. lateral (axillary) border
9. inferior angle
10. medial (vertebral) border
11. costal surface

Posterior View
1. acromion
2. coracoid process
3. spine
4. superior border
5. medial angle
6. medial (vertebral) border
7. inferior angle
8. posterior (dorsal) surface
9. lateral (axillary) border
10. glenoid cavity

Lateral View
1. coracoid process
2. glenoid cavity
3. infraglenoid tubercle
4. lateral (axillary) border
5. inferior angle

Bones of the Arm Anterior View
1. greater tubercle
2. lesser tubercle
3. intertubercular groove
4. deltoid tuberosity
5. humerus
6. lateral epicondyle
7. capitulum
8. trochlea
9. medial epicondyle
10. coronoid fossa
11. head
12. trochlear notch
13. head of radius
14. radial tuberosity
15. radius
16. styloid process of radius

17. styloid process of ulna
18. ulna
19. coronoid process
20. olecranon process

Posterior View
1. head
2. anatomical neck
3. surgical neck
4. humerus
5. olecranon fossa
6. medial epicondyle
7. trochlea
8. lateral epicondyle
9. greater tubercle
10. coronoid process
11. ulna
12. styloid process of ulna
13. styloid process of radius
14. radius
15. radial tuberosity
16. neck
17. head of radius
18. olecranon process

Bones of the Hand and Wrist
1. trapezoid
2. trapezium
3. scaphoid
4. radius
5. ulna
6. lunate
7. triquetrum
8. capitate
9. pisiform
10. hamate
11. distal phalanx
12. middle phalanx
13. proximal phalanx
14. metacarpal bone
15. hamate
16. capitate
17. pisiform
18. triquetrum
19. lunate
20. ulna
21. radius
22. scaphoid
23. trapezium
24. trapezoid

Coxal Bone
1. ilium
2. anterior superior iliac spine
3. anterior inferior iliac spine
4. margin of acetabulum
5. acetabulum
6. obturator foramen
7. pubis
8. ischial tuberosity
9. ischium
10. ischial spine

11. posterior inferior iliac spine
12. posterior superior iliac spine
13. iliac crest

Bones of the Thigh and Leg
1. greater trochanter
2. lateral epicondyle
3. medial epicondyle
4. femur
5. lesser trochanter
6. intertrochanteric line
7. neck
8. head
9. lateral condyle
10. head of fibula
11. fibula
12. lateral malleolus
13. medial malleolus
14. tibia
15. crest
16. tibial tuberosity
17. medial condyle
18. intercondylar eminence

Foot
1. phalanges
2. metatarsal bones
3. tarsal bones
4. cuneiform bones
5. navicular bone
6. talus
7. calcaneus
8. cuboid

CHAPTER 10

Classification of Joints
1. b, p. 272
2. a, p. 272
3. a, p. 272
4. c, p. 274
5. c, p. 274
6. d, p. 274
7. c, p. 276
8. d, p. 275
9. t, p. 274
10. f, p. 275
11. t, p. 275
12. t, p. 272
13. f, p. 274
14. f, p. 272
15. f, p. 275
16. t, p. 276
17. a, p. 274
18. a, p. 272
19. b, p. 276
20. c, p. 272
21. c, p. 272
22. a, p. 274
23. b, p. 275
24. c, p. 272
25. b, p. 272

26. b, p. 274
27. a, p. 272
28. b, p. 274
29. d, p. 275
30. c, p. 274
31. b, p. 276
32. e, p. 275
33. d, p. 275
34. c, p. 276
35. a, p. 276
36. a, p. 276
37. f, p. 275

Representative Synovial Joints
38. c, p. 277
39. b, p. 281
40. b, p. 281
41. a, p. 282
42. d, p. 286
43. c, p. 285
44. b, p. 282
45. c, p. 293

Types and Range of Movement at Synovial Joints
46. e, p. 286
47. c, p. 291
48. f, p. 292
49. g, p. 291
50. b, p. 291
51. d, p. 291
52. a, p. 291
53. h, p. 292
54. i, p. 292
55. j, p. 291

Mechanisms of Disease
56. arthroscopy, p. 294
57. osteoarthritis or degenerative joint disease, p. 293
58. arthritis, p. 295
59. gouty arthritis, p. 295
60. sprain, p. 295

Applying What You Know
61. (a) Nodular swelling, joint pain, tenderness, aching, stiffness, and limited motion. Systemic symptoms may also include fever, anemia, weight loss, profound fatigue, and possible pericarditis.
    (b) Small joints of the hand, wrist, and feet progressing often to the larger joints.
62. (a) Gouty arthritis
    (b) Swelling, tenderness, and pain, typically in the joints of the fingers, wrists, elbows, ankles, and knees.

(c) Allopurinol (Zyloprim) is the drug of choice to treat this disease.

One Last Quick Check
63. diarthroses
64. synarthrotic
65. diarthrotic
66. ligaments
67. articular cartilage
68. least movable
69. largest
70. 2
71. mobility
72. pivot
73. t, p. 275
74. f, p. 272
75. f, p. 293
76. t, p. 278
77. t, p. 291
78. t, p. 291
79. f, p. 292
80. f, p. 292
81. f, p. 295
82. t, p. 282

Diagrams

Synovial Joint
1. bone
2. periosteum
3. blood vessel
4. nerve
5. articular cartilage
6. joint cavity
7. joint capsule
8. articular cartilage
9. synovial membrane

Shoulder Joint
1. coracoid process of scapula
2. glenoid cavity
3. superior transverse ligament of scapula
4. articular cartilage of glenoid cavity
5. scapula
6. glenoidal lip (labrum)
7. humerus
8. head of humerus
9. articular cartilage of humerus
10. bursa
11. tendon of long head of biceps brachii muscle
12. synovial cavity

Hip Joint
1. acetabular labrum
2. head
3. articular capsule
4. greater trochanter
5. femur

6. lesser trochanter
7. articular capsule
8. transverse acetabular ligament
9. ligamentum teres
10. articular cavity
11. acetabulum
12. ilium

Knee Joint Anterior View

1. lateral condyle of femur
2. lateral meniscus
3. fibular collateral (lateral) ligament
4. transverse ligament of knee
5. fibula
6. tibia
7. tibial tuberosity
8. tibial collateral (medial) ligament
9. medial meniscus
10. anterior cruciate ligament (ACL)
11. medial condyle of femur
12. posterior cruciate ligament (PCL)
13. femur

Knee Joint Posterior View

1. femur
2. ligament of Wrisberg
3. medial condyle
4. medial meniscus
5. tibial collateral (medial) ligament
6. posterior cruciate ligament
7. tibia
8. fibula
9. fibular collateral (lateral) ligament
10. lateral meniscus
11. lateral condyle
12. anterior cruciate ligament

Vertebrae

1. lamina
2. anterior longitudinal ligament
3. body of vertebra
4. intervertebral disk
5. posterior longitudinal ligament
6. ligamentum flavum
7. intervertebral foramen
8. supraspinous ligament
9. interspinous ligament
10. spinous process

CHAPTER 11

Skeletal Muscle Structure

1. c, p. 302

2. d, p. 304
3. a, p. 302
4. a, p. 306
5. d, p. 306
6. a, p. 306
7. f, p. 305
8. t, p. 305
9. t, p. 305
10. f, p. 307
11. t, p. 306

How Muscles Are Named

12. c, p. 309
13. a, p. 308
14. f, p. 309
15. e, p. 309
16. g, p. 311
17. b, p. 309
18. d, p. 309

Important Skeletal Muscles: Muscles of the Face and Neck

19. b, p. 312
20. e, p. 312
21. a, p. 312
22. c, p. 312
23. f, p. 314
24. d, p. 312

Important Skeletal Muscles: Trunk Muscles

25. t, p. 317
26. t, p. 317
27. f, p. 321
28. t, p. 315
29. t, p. 321

Important Skeletal Muscles: Upper Limb Muscles

30. a, p. 325
31. c, p. 322
32. a, p. 327
33. d, p. 327
34. f, p. 326
35. t, p. 331
36. t, p. 325
37. t, p. 324
38. f, p. 327

Important Skeletal Muscles: Lower Limb Muscles

39. d, p. 339
40. a, p. 339
41. c, p. 337
42. d, p. 340
43. a, p. 339
44. t, p. 340
45. f, p. 333
46. f, p. 339

Applying What You Know

47. (a) Carpal tunnel syndrome
(b) The wrist, hand, and fingers are affected due to tenosynovitis. Pain may radiate to the forearm and shoulder. (c) Injections of anti-inflammatory agents or surgical removal of tissue pressing on median nerve.
48. deltoid area
49. See Tables 11-3 and 11-13 to 11-19

One Last Quick Check

50. c, a, b, p. 324
51. a, p. 340
52. a, b, p. 340
53. a, p. 327
54. c, p. 333
55. b, f, p. 340
56. a, p. 333
57. a, d, p. 324
58. b, p. 333
59. b, p. 327
60. a, p. 314
61. b, p. 322
62. d, a, p. 333
63. d, p. 305
64. b, p. 305
65. a, p. 306
66. e, p. 306
67. c, p. 306

Diagrams

Facial Muscles Lateral View

1. epicranial aponeurosis
2. temporalis
3. occipitofrontalis (occipital portion)
4. masseter
5. sternocleidomastoid
6. depressor anguli oris
7. orbicularis oris
8. buccinator
9. zygomaticus major
10. orbicularis oculi
11. corrugator supercilii
12. occipitofrontalis (frontal portion)

Muscles of the Thorax

1. external intercostals
2. diaphragm
3. central tendon of diaphragm
4. internal intercostals

Muscles of the Trunk and Abdominal Wall

1. linea alba
2. rectus abdominis
3. external oblique
4. internal ligament

5. internal oblique
6. transverse abdominis
7. rectus abdominis

Muscles Acting on the Shoulder Girdle
1. trapezius
2. seventh cervical vertebra
3. rhomboid major
4. rhomboid minor
5. levator scapulae
6. pectoralis minor (cut)
7. subscapularis
8. latissimus dorsi
9. serratus anterior
10. latissimus dorsi (cut)
11. pectoralis minor
12. teres major
13. teres minor
14. subscapularis

Rotator Cuff Muscles
1. clavicle
2. acromion process
3. infraspinatus
4. greater tubercle
5. teres minor
6. intertubercular (bicipital) groove
7. humerus
8. subscapularis
9. lesser tubercle
10. supraspinatus
11. coracoid process

Muscles that Move the Upper Arm
1. deltoid (cut)
2. coracobrachialis
3. pectoralis major
4. serratus anterior
5. deltoid
6. thoracolumbar fascia
7. latissimus dorsi
8. teres major
9. infraspinatus
10. rhomboideus major
11. teres minor
12. rhomboideus minor
13. supraspinatus
14. levator scapulae

Muscles of the Upper Arm
1. triceps brachii
2. brachioradialis
3. brachialis
4. biceps brachii (long head)
5. pectoralis major
6. deltoid
7. clavicle
8. biceps brachii
9. radius

10. pronator teres
11. ulna
12. brachialis
13. triceps brachii
14. teres major
15. coracobrachialis

Muscles that Act on the Forearm
1. coracoid process
2. supraglenoid tuberosity
3. biceps brachii (long head)
4. biceps brachii (short head)
5. radial tuberosity
6. olecranon process of ulna
7. triceps brachii (medial head)
8. triceps brachii: lateral (short head)
9. triceps brachii (long head)
10. posterior surface of humerus; lateral intermuscular septum
11. infraglenoid tubercle
12. coracoid process
13. coracobrachialis
14. medial surface of humerus
15. medial epicondyle of humerus
16. pronator teres
17. lateral surface of radius
18. coronoid process of ulna
19. brachialis
20. humerus (distal half)

Muscles of the Forearm
1. pronator teres
2. palmaris longus
3. flexor pollicis brevis (superficial)
4. opponens pollicis (deep)
5. flexor digiti minimi
6. abductor digiti minimi
7. flexor carpi ulnaris
8. flexor carpi radialis
9. palmar interosseus
10. pronator quadratus
11. flexor digitorum profundus
12. supinator
13. brachioradialis
14. flexor digitorum superficialis
15. extensor carpi ulnaris (cut)
16. extensor pollicis brevis
17. extensor pollicis longus
18. abductor pollicis longus
19. extensor carpi radialis brevis
20. extensor carpi radialis longus
21. supinator (deep)

Muscles of the Thigh
1. tensor fasciae latae
2. iliotibial tract

3. vastus lateralis
4. vastus medialis
5. rectus femoris
6. sartorius
7. gracilis
8. iliopsoas
9. adductor brevis
10. adductor longus
11. adductor magnus
12. fibula
13. tibia
14. pectineus

Muscles of the Lower Leg
1. soleus
2. extensor digitorum longus
3. fibularis peroneus brevis
4. tibialis anterior
5. tibia
6. gastrocnemius
7. calcaneal tendon (Achilles tendon)
8. calcaneus

CHAPTER 12

Function of Skeletal Muscle Tissue
1. b, p. 348
2. a, p. 348
3. a, p. 350
4. d, p. 348
5. c, p. 352
6. a, p. 350
7. c, p. 348
8. a, p. 352
9. c, p. 348
10. b, p. 353
11. t, p. 352
12. f, p. 348
13. f, p. 350
14. t, p. 352
15. t, p. 350
16. t, p. 357
17. f, p. 348
18. f, p. 358
19. t, p. 357
20. t, p. 359

Function of Skeletal Muscle Organs
21. d, p. 360
22. d, p. 362
23. a, p. 360
24. d, p. 366
25. a, p. 363
26. c, p. 364
27. c, p. 364
28. f, p. 358
29. t, p. 366
30. t, p. 361
31. f, p. 363

Function of Cardiac and Smooth Muscle Tissue

32. c, p. 368
33. b, p. 368
34. b, p. 368
35. c, p. 368
36. a, p. 368
37. c, p. 368
38. a, p. 369
39. b, p. 368
40. a, p. 368
41. c, p. 369

Mechanisms of Disease

42. myalgia, p. 372
43. myoglobin, p. 372
44. poliomyelitis, p. 372
45. muscular dystrophy, p. 373
46. myasthenia gravis, p. 373

Applying What You Know

47. Linda may have more slow and intermediate fibers than fast fibers. The former are conducive to long races rather than short ones.
48. Muscles in a dead body may be stiff because individual muscle fibers ran out of the ATP required to "turn off" a muscle contraction.

One Last Quick Check

49. a, p. 366
50. b, p. 366
51. b, p. 364
52. d, p. 356
53. a, p. 368
54. d, p. 361
55. f, p. 356
56. t, p. 360
57. t, p. 362
58. t, p. 361
59. t, p. 373
60. t, p. 370
61. t, p. 368
62. t, p. 365
63. f, p. 348

Diagrams

Structure of Skeletal Muscle

1. tendon
2. bone
3. muscle fiber (muscle cell)
4. sarcoplasmic reticulum
5. Z disk
6. thin filament
7. thick filament
8. sarcomere
9. myofibril
10. T tubule

11. fascicle
12. endomysium
13. perimysium
14. epimysium
15. muscle
16. fascia

Neuromuscular Junction and Skeletal Muscle Cell

1. motor neuron fiber
2. Schwann cell
3. sarcoplasm
4. acetylcholine (Ach) receptor sites
5. synaptic cleft
6. motor endplate
7. synaptic vesicles (containing Ach)
8. myelin sheath
9. sarcomere
10. sarcolemma
11. mitochondria
12. T tubule
13. sarcoplasmic reticulum
14. triad
15. myofibril

Motor Unit

1. myelin sheath
2. Schwann cell
3. neuromuscular junction
4. nucleus
5. muscle fibers
6. myofibrils
7. motor neuron

Cardiac Muscle Fiber

1. intercalated disks
2. sarcomere
3. sarcolemma
4. myofibril
5. mitochondrion
6. sarcoplasmic reticulum
7. T tubule
8. diad
9. nucleus

CHAPTER 13

Organization of the Nervous System

1. c, p. 382
2. f, p. 382
3. a, p. 383
4. h, p. 383
5. g, p. 383
6. b, p. 382
7. d, p. 383
8. e, p. 383

Cells of the Nervous System

9. b, p. 385

10. a, p. 384
11. d, p. 387
12. a, p. 384
13. c, p. 386
14. d, p. 386
15. a, p. 384
16. c, p. 386
17. c, p. 387
18. b, p. 388
19. a, p. 390
20. c, p. 390
21. d, p. 391

Nerves and Tracts

22. c, p. 392
23. b, p. 392
24. b, p. 392
25. d, p. 392
26. c, p. 392

Repair of Nerve Fibers

27. t, p. 392
28. t, p. 392
29. f, p. 392

Nerve Impulses

30. a, p. 393
31. b, p. 393
32. b, p. 394
33. a, p. 394
34. t, p. 393
35. f, p. 395
36. f, p. 394

Action Potential

37. b, p. 398
38. b, p. 396
39. c, p. 398
40. b, p. 398
41. t, p. 395
42. f, p. 397
43. t, p. 396
44. t, p. 404

Synaptic Transmission

45. c, p. 400
46. b, p. 400
47. a, p. 403
48. f, p. 399
49. t, p. 403
50. t, p. 401

Neurotransmitters

51. d, p. 404
52. b, p. 405
53. c, p. 408
54. c, p. 410
55. d, p. 399
56. f, p. 408
57. t, p. 410

Mechanisms of Disease
58. multiple sclerosis, p. 411
59. glioma, p. 411
60. glioblastoma multiforme, p. 411
61. multiple neurofibromatosis, p. 412
62. glia, p. 411

Applying What You Know
63. (a) Multiple sclerosis
    (b) CNS (c) Myelin loss and demyelination of the white matter in the CNS (d) No known cure
    (e) Cause is thought to be related to autoimmunity and viral infections.
64. CNS damage is most often permanent. Since the damage is suspected to involve the spinal cord—which is part of the CNS—the prognosis for repair is not good.

One Last Quick Check
65. presynaptic, p. 400
66. neurotransmitter, p. 406
67. communicate, p. 404
68. specifically, p. 404
69. pain, p. 410
70. sensory, p. 390
71. ganglion, p. 392
72. telodendria, p. 388
73. a, p. 388
74. b, p. 384
75. b, p. 384
76. a, p. 390
77. a, p. 390
78. b, p. 386
79. b, p. 385
80. a, p. 390
81. b, p. 386
82. a, p. 390

Diagrams

Typical Neuron
1. telodendria
2. synaptic knobs
3. node of Ranvier
4. axon collateral
5. myelin sheath
6. Schwann cell
7. axon
8. axon hillock
9. nucleus
10. cell body (soma)
11. mitochondrion
12. Golgi apparatus
13. dendrite

Myelinated Axon
1. node of Ranvier
2. neurilemma (sheath of Schwann cell)
3. neurofibrils, microfilaments and microtubules
4. plasma membrane of axon
5. myelin sheath
6. nucleus of Schwann cell

Classification of Neurons
1. multipolar neuron
2. bipolar neuron
3. (pseudo) unipolar neuron

Reflex Arc
1. gray matter
2. interneuron
3. sensory neuron axon
4. cell body
5. spinal nerve
6. motor neuron axon
7. white matter
8. dendrite
9. synapse

Chemical Synapse
1. motor neuron cell body
2. axon of presynaptic neuron
3. axon of motor neuron
4. synaptic knobs
5. action potential
6. voltage-gated Ca++ channels
7. synaptic cleft
8. stimulus-gated Na+ channels
9. neurotransmitters
10. synaptic knob
11. voltage-gated Na+ channels
12. voltage-gated K+ channels

CHAPTER 14

Coverings of the Brain and Spinal Cord
1. a, p. 421
2. c, p. 422
3. b, p. 423
4. c, p. 421

Cerebrospinal Fluid
5. c, p. 424
6. a, p. 424
7. d, p. 424
8. d, p. 424
9. t, p. 424
10. f, p. 426 and A&P Connect

The Spinal Cord
11. b, p. 428
12. d, p. 428
13. a, p. 428
14. c, p. 428
15. b, p. 428
16. d, p. 428
17. c, p. 428
18. a, p. 428
19. e, p. 428

The Brain
20. b, p. 429
21. d, p. 431
22. a, p. 432
23. b, p. 436
24. d, p. 436
25. c, p. 437
26. b, p. 443
27. a, p. 438
28. b, p. 444
29. a, p. 442
30. t, p. 432
31. f, p. 434
32. f, pp. 433, 446
33. t, p. 437
34. t, p. 438

Somatic Sensory and Motor Pathways
35. c, p. 449
36. c, p. 449
37. a, p. 451
38. t, p. 450
39. f, p. 450

Mechanisms of Disease
40. d, p. 453
41. b, p. 452
42. a, p. 452
43. c, p. 453

Applying What You Know
44. hydrocephalus
45. (a) dementia
    (b) Alzheimer disease

One Last Quick Check
46. e, p. 431
47. d, pp. 444, 445
48. a, p. 434
49. d, p. 434
50. e, p. 443
51. b, p. 440
52. c, p. 440
53. d, p. 434
54. c, p. 437
55. d, p. 426
56. d, p. 435

Diagrams

Coverings of the Brain
1. superior sagittal sinus (of dura)
2. periosteum
3. subdural space
4. skull

5. falx cerebri
6. pia mater
7. muscle
8. skin
9. subarachnoid space
10. arachnoid mater
11. dura mater
12. periosteum
13. one functional layer

Fluid Spaces of the Brain
1. cerebral hemisphere
2. anterior horn of lateral ventricle
3. interventricular foramen
4. third ventricle
5. inferior horn of lateral ventricle
6. fourth ventricle
7. pons
8. central canal of spinal cord
9. cerebellum
10. cerebral aqueduct
11. posterior horn of lateral ventricle

Flow of Cerebrospinal Fluid and the Layers of the Brain
1. arachnoid villus
2. choroid plexus of lateral ventricle
3. superior sagittal sinus
4. interventricular foramen
5. choroid plexus of third ventricle
6. cerebral aqueduct
7. choroid plexus of fourth ventricle
8. median foramen
9. central canal of spinal cord
10. dura mater
11. cisterna magna
12. lateral foramen
13. cerebral cortex
14. subarachnoid space
15. arachnoid layer
16. falx cerebri (dura mater)
17. pia mater

Spinal Cord
1. cervical enlargement
2. lumbar enlargement
3. end of spinal cord
4. cauda equina
5. filum terminale
6. lateral column
7. posterior column
8. anterior column
9. gray commissure
10. gray matter
11. posterior median sulcus
12. central canal

13. dorsal (posterior) nerve root
14. dorsal root ganglion
15. spinal nerve
16. ventral (anterior) nerve root
17. lateral column
18. posterior column
19. anterior column
20. white columns (funiculi)
21. anterior median fissure

Spinal Cord Tracts
1. tectospinal
2. vestibulospinal
3. reticulospinal
4. anterior corticospinal
5. rubrospinal
6. lateral corticospinal
7. fasciculus gracilis
8. fasciculus cuneatus
9. posterior spinocerebellar
10. lateral spinothalamic
11. anterior spinocerebellar
12. spinotectal
13. anterior spinothalamic

Left Hemisphere of Cerebrum
1. central sulcus
2. superior frontal gyrus
3. frontal lobe
4. lateral fissure
5. temporal lobe
6. occipital lobe
7. parietooccipital sulcus
8. parietal lobe
9. postcentral gyrus

Cerebral Cortex
1. precentral gyrus
2. premotor area
3. prefrontal area
4. motor speech (Broca) area
5. transverse gyrus
6. auditory association area
7. primary auditory area
8. sensory speech (Wernicke) area
9. visual cortex
10. visual association area
11. somatic sensory association area
12. primary taste area
13. postcentral gyrus

CHAPTER 15

Spinal Nerves
1. a, p. 464
2. c, p. 466
3. a, p. 466
4. b, p. 468
5. a, p. 468
6. t, p. 466

7. t, p. 466
8. f, p. 472
9. f, p. 471
10. t, p. 468

Cranial Nerves
11. g, p. 476
12. a, p. 475
13. j, p. 478
14. h, p. 478
15. b, p. 475
16. e, p. 476
17. i, p. 478
18. c, p. 475
19. d, p. 475
20. f, p. 476
21. l, p. 480
22. k, p. 480

Somatic Motor Nervous System
23. b, p. 481
24. a, p. 483
25. a, p. 481

Applying What You Know
26. The two nerves that might possibly be involved are cranial nerve IX (glossopharyngeal) and cranial nerve X (vagus). Both nerves are mixed, meaning that they contain axons of sensory and motor neurons.
27. (a) Herpes zoster or shingles (b) Varicella zoster virus or chickenpox (c) It attacks a dermatome (T-4) and symptoms occur in that region. (d) His immunologic protective mechanism may have become diminished due to the stress.

One Last Quick Check
28. a, p. 473
29. d, p. 478
30. a, p. 478
31. c, p. 476
32. vestibulocochlear, p. 478
33. trigeminal, p. 476
34. diabetes mellitus, p. 464
35. voluntary, p. 481
36. skeletal, p. 481
37. phrenic and phrenic, p. 468
38. a, p. 473
39. b, p. 471
40. a, p. 479
41. b, p. 472
42. b, p. 464
43. a, p. 475

44. b, p. 468
45. b, p. 466
46. b, p. 472
47. a, p. 480

Diagrams

Spinal Nerves
1. cervical vertebrae
2. brachial plexus
3. thoracic vertebrae
4. lumbar vertebrae
5. sacrum
6. coccyx
7. filum terminale
8. coccygeal nerve
9. sacral nerves
10. sacral plexus
11. lumbar nerves
12. lumbar plexus
13. cauda equina
14. dura mater
15. thoracic nerves
16. cervical nerves
17. cervical plexus

Cranial Nerves
1. trochlear nerve
2. optic nerve
3. oculomotor nerve
4. abducens nerve
5. facial nerve
6. vestibulocochlear nerve
7. vagus nerve
8. accessory nerve
9. hypoglossal nerve
10. glossopharyngeal nerve
11. trigeminal nerve
12. olfactory nerve

Patellar Reflex
1. gray matter
2. spinal cord
3. motor neuron
4. quadriceps muscle (effector)
5. patellar tendon
6. patella
7. stretch receptor
8. sensory neuron
9. dorsal root ganglion

CHAPTER 16

Autonomic Nervous System
1. c, p. 490
2. d, p. 492
3. b, p. 496
4. a, p. 500
5. b, p. 500
6. f, p. 490
7. t, p. 490
8. t, p. 490

9. f, p. 501
10. t, p. 492
11. autonomic nerves, ganglia and plexuses, p. 490
12. preganglionic, p. 490
13. collateral, p. 492
14. ramus, p. 491
15. norepinephrine, p. 494
16. short and then long, p. 492
17. adrenergic, p. 494
18. characteristics of the receptor, p. 496
19. nicotinic, p. 497
20. quickly, p. 497

Functions of the Autonomic Nervous System
21. t, p. 498
22. f, p. 498
23. t, p. 499
24. t. p. 499
25. f, p. 501

Applying What You Know
26. (1) Sympathetic
    (2a) Muscular—skeletal muscles faster
    (2b) Circulatory—stronger heartbeat, dilated blood vessels
    (2c) Respiratory—dilated bronchi
    (2d) Digestive—increased blood sugar levels
    (3) Dysfunction of the sympathetic effectors and perhaps even the ANS itself.
27. Biofeedback

One Last Quick Check
28. d, p. 489
29. e, p. 489
30. f, p. 490
31. b, p. 489
32. a, p. 490
33. c, p. 491
34. c, p. 494
35. b, p. 491
36. b, p. 492
37. d, p. 492
38. b, p. 498
39. a, p. 498
40. a, p. 498
41. b, p. 498
42. a, p. 498
43. b, p. 498
44. a, p. 498
45. a, p. 498
46. b, p. 498
47. b, p. 498

Diagram

Autonomic Conduction Path
1. axon of somatic motor neuron
2. collateral ganglion
3. postganglionic neuron's axon
4. sympathetic ganglion
5. axon of preganglionic sympathetic neuron

CHAPTER 17

Sensory Receptors
1. b, p. 506
2. d, p. 507
3. a, p. 511
4. b, p. 508
5. a, p. 507
6. f, p. 507
7. t, p. 508
8. f, p. 507
9. t, p. 512
10. t, p. 507

The Sense of Smell and the Sense of Taste
11. b, pp. 514, 516
12. d, p. 513
13. c, p. 516
14. b, p. 517
15. t, p. 514
16. f, p. 514
17. t, p. 515
18. f, p. 516

Sense of Hearing and Balance: The Ear
19. a, p. 519
20. c, p. 519
21. d, p. 520
22. d, p. 523
23. b, p. 522
24. b, p. 523
25. d, p. 522
26. t, p. 520
27. f, p. 519
28. t, p. 521
29. t, p. 520
30. f, p. 524

Vision: The Eye
31. c, p. 526
32. a, p. 526
33. a, p. 527
34. d, p. 528
35. d, p. 529
36. a, p. 526
37. c, p. 525
38. a, p. 530
39. c, p. 530

40. a, p. 526
41. f, p. 524
42. f, p. 525
43. t, p. 525
44. t, p. 526
45. f, p. 533
46. t, p. 532
47. t, p. 527
48. t, p. 530
49. f, p. 530
50. f, p. 531

Mechanisms of Disease
51. c, p. 534
52. a, p. 534
53. d, p. 534
54. e, p. 535
55. b, p. 535
56. f, p. 535
57. c, p. 535
58. e, p. 536
59. f, p. 536
60. a, p. 536
61. j, p. 536
62. b, p. 536
63. h, p. 536
64. g, p. 537
65. i, p. 537
66. d, p. 537

Applying What You Know
67. The eustachian tube connects the throat to the middle ear and provides a perfect pathway for the spread of infection.
68. (a) Legally blind
(b) 20/200
(c) myopia
(d) concave contact lenses or glasses

One Last Quick Check
69. a, p. 519
70. b, p. 520
71. a, p. 517
72. c, p. 524
73. b, p. 526
74. b, p. 513
75. d, p. 528
76. b, p. 526
77. d, p. 516
78. a, p. 518
79. t, p. 519
80. f, p. 537
81. t, p. 536
82. f, p. 523
83. t, p. 535
84. t, p. 526
85. t, p. 528
86. t, p. 514
87. t, p. 508

88. t, p. 523

Diagrams

Midsagittal Section of the Nasal Area
1. olfactory bulb
2. fibers of olfactory nerve
3. cribriform plate of ethmoid bone
4. olfactory tract
5. olfactory recess
6. nasopharynx
7. palate
8. nasal cavity
9. frontal bone

The Ear
1. malleus
2. incus
3. stapes
4. auditory ossicles
5. auditory tube
6. round window
7. vestibule
8. cochlea
9. cochlear nerve
10. vestibular nerve
11. vestibulocochlear (acoustic) nerve
12. facial nerve
13. oval window
14. semicircular canals
15. inner ear
16. tympanic membrane
17. middle ear
18. temporal bone
19. external acoustic meatus
20. auricle (pinna)
21. external ear

The Eye
1. pupil
2. lens
3. lacrimal caruncle
4. optic disk
5. optic nerve
6. central artery and vein
7. fovea centralis
8. macula
9. posterior chamber
10. sclera
11. choroid
12. retina
13. ciliary body
14. lower lid
15. iris
16. anterior chamber
17. cornea

Extrinsic Muscles of the Right Eye
1. superior oblique

2. medial rectus
3. superior rectus
4. optic nerve
5. levator palpebrae superioris (cut)
6. lateral rectus
7. inferior oblique
8. trochlea

Lacrimal Apparatus
1. lacrimal caruncle
2. lacrimal canals
3. lacrimal sac
4. nasolacrimal duct
5. puncta
6. lacrimal ducts
7. lacrimal gland

CHAPTER 18

Organization of the Endocrine System and Hormones
1. a, p. 546
2. c, p. 546
3. d, p. 547
4. c, p. 546
5. a, p. 548
6. d, p. 548
7. c, p. 547
8. a, p. 552
9. c, p. 553
10. b, p. 550
11. t, p. 546
12. t, p. 547
13. f, p. 548
14. f, p. 555
15. t, p. 546
16. b, p. 553
17. a, p. 553
18. a, p. 553
19. a, p. 553
20. a, p. 553
21. b, p. 553
22. b, p. 553
23. b, p. 553

Prostaglandins
24. b, p. 557
25. c, p. 557
26. paracrine, p. 556
27. autocrine, p. 556
28. seminal vesicles, p. 557
29. immunity, p. 557
30. peristalsis, p. 557

Applying What You Know
31. Prostaglandins F (PGFs)
32. In the presence of an injury, prostaglandins may be synthesized and released into surrounding tissue fluid. They may serve as an in-

flammatory agent and may cause swelling, redness, and pain. Aspirin is a COX inhibitor that reduces the effect of prostaglandins in the body.

One Last Quick Check
33. endocrine reflexes, p. 553
34. kidneys, p. 550
35. antagonism, p. 550
36. endocytosis, p. 552
37. amount, p. 551
38. signal transduction, p. 546
39. hyposection, p. 555
40. second messenger, p. 552
41. calcium, p. 552
42. pituitary, p. 554
43. d, p. 557
44. e, p. 557
45. a, p. 556
46. b, p. 556
47. c, p. 557
48. a, p. 547
49. c, p. 548
50. d, p. 550
51. b, p. 550
52. a, p. 550

Diagrams

Endocrine Glands
1. pineal
2. parathyroids
3. testes (male)
4. ovaries (female)
5. pancreas (islets)
6. adrenals
7. thymus
8. thyroid
9. pituitary
10. hypothalamus

Target Cell Concept
1. target
2. receptors
3. nontarget cells
4. hormone
5. capillary

CHAPTER 19

Pituitary Gland
1. b, p. 564
2. a, p. 567
3. d, p. 569
4. c, p. 566
5. b, p. 569
6. a, p. 567
7. d, p. 566
8. c, p. 567
9. e, p. 567
10. h, p. 566

11. g, p. 570
12. f, p. 566
13. i, p. 567
14. b, p. 570

Pineal, Thyroid, and Parathyroid Glands
15. b, p. 572
16. b, p. 572
17. b, p. 572
18. b, p. 576
19. c, p. 576
20. t, p. 575
21. f, p. 575
22. t, p. 574
23. t, p. 571
24. f, p. 572

Adrenal Glands
25. b, p. 578
26. d, p. 578
27. a, p. 578
28. t, p. 577
29. f, p. 587
30. t, p. 578

Pancreatic Islets
31. c, p. 582
32. a, p. 582
33. t, p. 582
34. f, p. 582
35. b, p. 581
36. c, p. 581
37. a, p. 581
38. d, p. 581

Other Endocrine Glands and Tissues
39. a, p. 585
40. b, p. 585
41. c, p. 585
42. f, p. 585
43. f, p. 586
44. t, p. 586

Mechanisms of Disease
45. e, p. 587
46. h, p. 587
47. a, p. 587
48. c, p. 588
49. f, p. 588
50. g, p. 588
51. b, p. 588
52. d, p. 588

Applying What You Know
53. (a) hCG is high during early pregnancy (b) placenta (c) It forms on the lining of the uterus as an interface between the circulatory systems of the mother and the

developing child. It is a temporary endocrine gland.
54. (a) Diabetes mellitus (b) inadequate amount or abnormal type of insulin (c) insulin

One Last Quick Check
55. a, p. 578
56. c, p. 587
57. d, p. 587
58. c, p. 566
59. d, p. 571
60. d, p. 570
61. b, p. 585
62. d, p. 580
63. d, p. 581
64. b, p. 580
65. j, p. 588
66. g, p. 571
67. h, p. 588
68. i, p. 566
69. b, p. 587
70. f, p. 585
71. a, p. 587
72. d, p. 571
73. e, p. 587
74. c, p. 578

Diagrams

Major Endocrine Glands
1. pineal
2. parathyroids
3. testes (male)
4. ovaries (female)
5. pancreas (islets)
6. adrenals
7. thymus
8. thyroid
9. pituitary
10. hypothalamus

Location and Structure of Pituitary Gland
1. optic chiasma
2. infundibulum
3. pituitary diaphragm
4. pituitary gland (hypophysis)
5. nasal cavity
6. brainstem
7. hypothalamus
8. pineal gland
9. thalamus
10. pars anterior
11. pars intermedia
12. adenohypophysis
13. sella turcica (of sphenoid bone)
14. neurohypophysis
15. infundibulum
16. mammillary body

17. third ventricle
18. optic chiasma

Structure of Thyroid and Parathyroid Glands
1. epiglottis
2. hyoid bone
3. larynx (thyroid cartilage)
4. superior parathyroid glands
5. thyroid gland
6. inferior parathyroid glands
7. trachea

CHAPTER 20

Composition of Blood and Red Blood Cells
1. a, p. 599
2. a, p. 600
3. c, p. 600
4. b, p. 601
5. d, p. 603
6. t, p. 600
7. f, p. 604
8. t, p. 604
9. f, p. 604
10. f, p. 602

White Blood Cells and Platelets
11. d, p. 605
12. i, p. 606
13. b, p. 607
14. c, p. 607
15. f, p. 607
16. h, p. 606
17. j, p. 606
18. g, p. 609

19. a, p. 605
20. e, p. 606

Blood Types
21. b, p. 610
22. a, p. 610
23. d, p. 610
24. t, p. 610
25. f, p. 610
26. f, p. 610

Blood Plasma
27. t, p. 613
28. t, p. 613
29. f, p. 613

Blood Clotting
30. b, p. 614
31. d, p. 617
32. c, p. 617

Mechanisms of Disease
33. Polycythemia, p. 619
34. Aplastic anemia, p. 620
35. pernicious anemia, p. 620
36. sickle cell anemia or thalassemia, p. 620
37. Leukopenia, p. 620
38. thrombus, p. 622
39. embolus, p. 622
40. Hemophilia, p. 622

Applying What You Know
41. Theoretically, infused red blood cells and elevation of hemoglobin levels after transfusion should increase oxygen consumption and muscle performance during exercise. In practice, however, the advantage appears to be minimal.
42. No. If Mrs. Shearer were a negative Rh factor and her husband were a positive Rh factor, it would set up the strong possibility of erythroblastosis fetalis.
43. Both procedures assist the clotting process.

One Last Quick Check
44. b, p. 621
45. b, p. 619
46. a, p. 606
47. a, p. 613
48. d, p. 613
49. a, p. 607
50. a, p. 622
51. d, p. 610
52. c, p. 602
53. b, p. 615
54. d, p. 606
55. f, p. 619
56. h, p. 613
57. a, p. 607
58. g, p. 621
59. c, p. 608
60. b, p. 613
61. e, p. 612
62. i, p. 601
63. j, p. 606
64. l, p. 620
65. k, p. 600

Diagrams

Human Blood Cells

BODY CELL		FUNCTION
Erythrocyte		Oxygen and carbon dioxide transport
Neutrophil		Immune defense (phagocytosis)
Eosinophil		Defense against parasites
Basophil		Inflammatory response and heparin secretion
B lymphocyte		Antibody production (precursor of plasma cells)
T lymphocyte		Cellular immune response
Monocyte		Immune defenses (phagocytosis)
Thrombocyte		Blood clotting

Blood Typing

Recipient's blood		Reactions with donor's blood			
RBC antigens	Plasma antibodies	Donor type O	Donor type A	Donor type B	Donor type AB
None (Type O)	Anti-A Anti-B				
A (Type A)	Anti-B				
B (Type B)	Anti-A				
AB (Type AB)	(none)				

 Normal blood   Agglutinated blood

CHAPTER 21

Heart
1. b, p. 634
2. c, p. 635
3. a, p. 638
4. a, p. 638
5. d, p. 638
6. d, p. 640
7. c, p. 640
8. d, p. 637
9. d, p. 638
10. b, p. 642
11. Trace the Blood Flow, p. 639, tricuspid (3) pulmonary veins (7) pulmonary arteries (6) mitral (9) vena cava (1) right ventricle (4) aorta (12) pulmonary semilunar valve (5) left ventricle (10) right atrium (2) left atrium (8) aortic semilunar valve (11)
12. echocardiography, p. 639
13. Troponins test and creatine kinase (CK), p. 635
14. inhibitory or depressor, p. 642
15. cardiopulmonary resuscitation (CPR), p. 630

Blood Vessels
16. d, p. 642
17. c, p. 644
18. e, p. 646
19. g, p. 647
20. f, p. 644
21. b, p. 645
22. a, p. 644
23. t, p. 645
24. f, p. 643
25. t, p. 648
26. f, p. 643

Major Blood Vessels
27. d, p. 647
28. c, p. 647
29. b, p. 647
30. d, p. 662
31. b, p. 666
32. b, p. 666
33. a, p. 667
34. d, p. 647
35. systemic circulation, p. 647
36. cerebral arterial circle, p. 651
37. veins, p. 658
38. hepatic portal system, p. 663
39. ascites, p. 664
40. (a) umbilical arteries, p. 666
(b) umbilical vein, p. 666
41. veins, p. 661

Mechanisms of Disease
42. i, p. 672
43. b, p. 671
44. d, p. 671
45. e, p. 671
46. a, p. 670
47. c, p. 672
48. f, p. 673
49. g, p. 673
50. j, p. 672
51. h, p. 672
52. l, p. 669
53. k, p. 669

Applying What You Know
54. Congestive heart failure. Left-sided heart failure often leads to right-sided heart failure. The combination of both problems may require a transplant, implant, or may lead to death.
55. coronary bypass surgery
56. Cardiac enzymes usually increase over the next few hours following a heart attack. These elevations suggest that Mr. Wertz may have had a myocardial infarction with resulting heart muscle damage.

One Last Quick Check
57. c, p. 639
58. d, p. 669
59. c, p. 634
60. d, p. 638
61. b, p. 673
62. b, p. 670
63. g, p. 651
64. a, p. 671
65. i, p. 665
66. c, p. 666
67. f, p. 672
68. b, p. 673
69. h, p. 647
70. d, p. 672
71. e, p. 639
72. j, p. 670

Diagrams

Heart
1. aorta
2. superior vena cava
3. right atrium
4. left AV (mitral) valve
5. right AV (tricuspid) valve
6. chordae tendineae
7. right ventricle
8. interventricular septum
9. papillary muscle
10. left ventricle
11. right ventricle
12. pulmonary veins
13. right atrium
14. openings to coronary arteries
15. pulmonary trunk
16. aortic semilunar valve
17. left atrium

Blood Vessels
1. valve
2. endothelium (tunica intima)
3. basement membrane (tunica intima)
4. smooth muscle (tunica media)
5. fibrous connective (tunica externa)
6. endothelium (tunica intima)
7. basement membrane (tunica intima)
8. internal elastic membrane
9. smooth muscle (tunica media)
10. fibrous connective tissue (tunica externa)
11. internal elastic membrane

Veins
1. right brachiocephalic
2. right subclavian
3. superior vena cava
4. right pulmonary
5. small cardiac
6. inferior vena cava
7. hepatic
8. hepatic portal
9. superior mesenteric
10. median cubital (basilic)
11. common iliac
12. external iliac
13. femoral
14. great saphenous
15. small saphenous
16. fibular
17. anterior tibial
18. posterior tibial
19. venous dorsal arch
20. digital
21. popliteal
22. femoral
23. digital
24. internal iliac
25. common iliac
26. inferior mesenteric
27. splenic
28. long thoracic
29. basilic
30. great cardiac
31. cephalic
32. axillary

33. left subclavian
34. left brachiocephalic
35. internal jugular
36. external jugular
37. facial
38. angular
39. occipital

Arteries
1. right common carotid
2. right subclavian
3. brachiocephalic
4. right coronary
5. axillary
6. brachial
7. superior mesenteric
8. abdominal aorta
9. common iliac
10. internal iliac (hypogastric)
11. external iliac
12. deep medial circumflex femoral
13. descending branch of lateral circumflex femoral
14. deep artery of thigh
15. popliteal
16. anterior tibial
17. peroneal
18. posterior tibial
19. arcuate
20. dorsal pedis
21. femoral
22. perforating arteries
23. digital
24. superficial palmar arch
25. deep palmar arch
26. ulnar
27. radial
28. inferior mesenteric
29. celiac
30. renal
31. splenic
32. aorta
33. left coronary
34. pulmonary
35. arch of aorta
36. left subclavian
37. left common carotid
38. external carotid
39. internal carotid
40. facial
41. occipital

Fetal Circulation
1. aortic arch
2. abdominal aorta
3. common iliac arteries
4. internal iliac arteries
5. umbilical arteries
6. fetal umbilicus
7. umbilical cord
8. fetal side of placenta

9. maternal side of placenta
10. umbilical vein
11. hepatic portal vein
12. ductus venosus
13. inferior vena cava
14. foramen ovale
15. superior vena cava
16. ascending aorta
17. pulmonary trunk
18. ductus arteriosus

Hepatic Portal Circulation
1. inferior vena cava
2. stomach
3. gastric vein
4. spleen
5. pancreatic vein
6. splenic vein
7. gastroepiploic vein
8. descending colon
9. inferior mesenteric vein
10. small intestine
11. appendix
12. ascending colon
13. superior mesenteric vein
14. pancreas
15. duodenum
16. hepatic portal vein
17. liver
18. hepatic veins

CHAPTER 22

Hemodynamics and the Heart as a Pump
1. b, p. 684
2. b, p. 683
3. a, p. 686
4. b, p. 686
5. a, p. 689
6. t, p. 689
7. f, p. 684
8. f, p. 686
9. t, p. 689
10. t, p. 689

Circulation and Blood Pressure
11. d, p. 690
12. c, p. 692
13. b, p. 693
14. d, p. 694
15. d, p. 695
16. a, p. 692
17. b, p. 707
18. c, p. 710
19. b, p. 695
20. d, p. 697
21. f, p. 692
22. t, p. 692
23. t, p. 692
24. t, p. 698
25. f, p. 701

26. t, p. 703
27. t, p. 706
28. t, p. 708
29. f, p. 710
30. t, p. 700

Mechanisms of Disease
31. septic shock, p. 714
32. cardiogenic shock, p. 714
33. anaphylaxis; anaphylactic shock, p. 714
34. neurogenic shock, p. 714
35. low blood volume, p. 714
36. toxic shock syndrome, p. 714

Applying What You Know
37. (a) Hypovolemic shock (b) The body might respond by increasing the heart rate, decreasing the urine output and decreasing available fluids to the tissues.
38. (a) heart block (b) artificial pacemaker

One Last Quick Check
39. c, p. 714
40. a, p. 714
41. c, p. 714
42. c, p. 701
43. a, p. 714
44. a, p. 701
45. (a) sinoatrial (SA) node (b) atrioventricular (AV) node (c), AV bundle (bundle of His) (d) subendocardial branches (Purkinje fibers), p. 683
46. ECG and EKG, p. 685
47. cardiac cycle, p. 687
48. residual volume, p. 689
49. cardiac output, p. 691
50. epinephrine, p. 695
51. Starling's law of the capillaries, p. 703
52. e, p. 682
53. k, p. 683
54. a, p. 686
55. b, p. 712
56. c, p. 712
57. g, p. 706
58. i, p. 689
59. d, p. 694
60. h, p. 700
61. f, p. 700
62. j, p. 706
63. l, p. 710

Diagram

ECG Strip Recording
1. atrial depolarization

2. ventricular depolarization (and atrial repolarization)
3. ventricular repolarization

Pulse Points
1. superficial temporal artery
2. facial artery
3. carotid artery
4. brachial artery
5. radial artery
6. femoral artery
7. popliteal artery
8. posterior tibial artery
9. dorsalis pedis artery

CHAPTER 23

Lymphatic Vessels, Lymph, and Circulation of Lymph
1. c, p. 723
2. b, p. 726
3. a, p. 725
4. d, p. 725
5. c, p. 726
6. b, p. 727
7. a, p. 726
8. t, p. 723
9. f, p. 723
10. t, p. 724
11. t, p. 725
12. t, p. 725
13. t, p. 725
14. t, p. 724

Lymph Nodes
15. b, p. 729
16. d, p. 729
17. a, p. 731
18. c, p. 732
19. f, p. 729
20. t, p. 728

Lymphatic Drainage of the Breast
21. a, p. 733
22. c, p. 732

Tonsils, Thymus, and Spleen
23. a, p. 733
24. c, p. 735
25. c, p. 734
26. f, p. 734
27. f, p. 735
28. t, p. 736

Mechanisms of Disease
29. Lymphoma, p. 739
30. acute otitis media, p. 738
31. blood poisoning, p. 738
32. filarial, p. 738
33. Hodgkin and non-Hodgkin, p. 739

Applying What You Know
34. (a) Yes (b) Yes (c) The spleen destroys old blood cells and platelets. Preventing this will allow Ms. Langston to preserve her own supply and avoid anemia.
35. Baby Wilson had no means of producing T cells, thus making him susceptible to several diseases. Isolation was a means of controlling his exposure to these diseases.

One Last Quick Check
36. b, p. 733
37. c, p. 736
38. c, p. 736
39. a, p. 734
40. c, p. 736
41. a, p. 735
42. a, p. 734
43. t, p. 725
44. t, p. 726
45. t, p. 727
46. f, p. 728
47. t, p. 738
48. f, p. 733
49. f, p. 735
50. f, p. 736

Diagrams

Principal Organs of the Lymphatic System
1. tonsils
2. cervical lymph node
3. right lymphatic duct
4. superficial cubital (supratrochlear) lymph nodes
5. aggregated lymphoid nodules (Peyer patches) in intestinal wall
6. red bone marrow
7. inguinal lymph node
8. cisterna chyli
9. spleen
10. thoracic duct
11. axillary lymph node
12. thymus gland
13. entrance of thoracic duct into subclavian vein

Lymph Node
1. afferent lymph vessel
2. capsule
3. efferent lymph vessel
4. hilum
5. medullary cords
6. cortical nodules
7. sinuses
8. germinal center

Lymphatic Drainage of Breast
1. supraclavicular nodes
2. interpectoral (Rotter) nodes
3. midaxillary nodes
4. lateral axillary (brachial) nodes
5. subscapular nodes
6. anterior axillary (pectoral) nodes
7. parasternal nodes
8. subclavicular nodes

CHAPTER 24

Innate Immunity
1. d, p. 746
2. c, p. 748
3. a, p. 753
4. a, p. 752
5. b, p. 752
6. f, p. 746
7. t, p. 748
8. f, p. 755
9. f, p. 755
10. t, p. 753

Adaptive Immunity
11. b, p. 756
12. b, p. 756
13. d, p. 756
14. a, p. 758
15. b, p. 763
16. b, p. 760
17. c, p. 758
18. b, p. 764
19. b, p. 761
20. b, p. 765
21. immunoglobulin, p. 758
22. IgM, p. 760
23. cowpox virus, p. 763
24. attenuated, p. 763
25. active immunity, p. 768
26. tumor markers, p. 766
27. PSA, p. 766
28. adaptive immune, p. 766
29. natural passive, p. 760
30. artificial active, p. 760

Mechanisms of Disease
31. c, p. 774
32. a, p. 774
33. b, p. 774
34. e, p. 772
35. d, p. 773

Applying What You Know
36. (a) Passive acquired immunity (b) active artificial immunity (c) Active immunity usually lasts longer than passive.

37. (a) AIDS (b) azidothymidine (AZT) and dideoxyinosine (DDI)

One Last Quick Check
38. a, p. 764
39. d, p. 774
40. b, p. 755
41. d, p. 758
42. b, p. 762
43. d, p. 762
44. c, p. 760
45. allergy, p. 772
46. antihistamines, p. 772
47. pus, p. 752
48. lymphotoxin, p. 765
49. specific immunity, p. 746
50. inflammatory response, p. 749
51. f, p. 774
52. t, p. 774
53. t, p. 772
54. f, p. 774
55. f, p. 765

Diagram

T Cell Development
1. stem cell
2. T-cell
3. sensitized T-cell

4. memory cell
5. effector T-cell

CHAPTER 25

Selye's Concept of Stress
1. b, p. 785
2. b, p. 783
3. b, p. 785
4. b, p. 784
5. d, p. 784
6. f, p. 786
7. f, p. 791
8. t, p. 786
9. f, p. 784
10. t, p. 786
11. c, p. 784
12. e, p. 786
13. d, p. 786
14. f, p. 784
15. b, p. 786
16. a, p. 784

Some Current Concepts About Stress
17. c, p. 788
18. d, p. 789
19. b, p. 790
20. t, p. 788
21. f, p. 790
22. f, p. 790

23. t, p. 791
24. f, p. 792
25. t, p. 788

Applying What You Know
26. (a) Stress (b) See Figure 25-6, p. 789 (c) Immune diseases, decreased quality of life, ulcers, hypertension, chemical dependency, impaired relationships, and loss of contact with reality.
27. (a) Sympathetic (b) No, digestion decreases under the influence of the sympathetic nervous system.

One Last Quick Check
28. General adaptation syndrome, p. 784
29. exhaustion, p. 786
30. corticotropin-releasing hormone, p. 788
31. fight or flight reaction, pp. 787, 788
32. Psychophysiology, p. 791
33. f, p. 792
34. t, p. 783
35. t, p. 790
36. f, p. 784
37. t, p. 783
38. t, p. 788

Stress-Related Diseases and Conditions

TARGET ORGAN OR SYSTEM	DISEASE OR CONDITION
Cardiovascular system	Coronary artery disease Hypertension Stroke Disturbances of heart rhythm
Muscles	Tension headaches Muscle contraction backache
Connective tissues	Rheumatoid arthritis (autoimmune disease) Related inflammatory diseases of connective tissue
Pulmonary system	Asthma (hypersensitivity reaction) Hay fever (hypersensitivity reaction) Changes in breathing patterns
Immune system	Immunosuppression or immune deficiency Autoimmune diseases
Gastrointestinal system	Ulcer Irritable bowel syndrome Diarrhea Nausea and vomiting Ulcerative colitis
Genitourinary system	Diuresis Impotence (erectile dysfunction) Loss of libido (sexual desire)
Skin	Eczema Neurodermatitis Acne
Endocrine system	Diabetes mellitus Amenorrhea
Central nervous system	Fatigue and lethargy Type A behavior Overeating Depression Insomnia

CHAPTER 26

Upper Respiratory Tract
1. a, p. 799
2. c, p. 799
3. d, p. 801
4. c, p. 802
5. a, p. 804
6. f, p. 799
7. f, p. 802
8. t, p. 803
9. f, p. 805
10. t, p. 805

Lower Respiratory Tract
11. a, p. 808
12. b, p. 809
13. c, p. 812
14. d, p. 815
15. f, p. 807
16. f, p. 808
17. t, p. 808
18. f, p. 812
19. f, p. 812
20. t, p. 809
21. f, p. 815
22. t, p. 809
23. t, p. 810
24. f, p. 814

Mechanisms of Disease
25. d, p. 818
26. g, p. 818
27. b, p. 817
28. a, p. 817
29. c, p. 817
30. f, p. 816
31. e, p. 816
32. h, p. 816

Applying What You Know
33. (a) epiglottis
    (b) *Haemophilus influenzae* type B
    (c) yes
34. (a) croup
    (b) no
35. During the day Mr. Gorski's cilia are paralyzed because of his heavy smoking. They use the time when Mr. Gorski is asleep to sweep accumulations of mucus and bacteria toward the pharynx. When Mr. Gorski awakens, these collections are waiting to be eliminated.

One Last Quick Check
36. a, p. 802
37. b, p. 803
38. a, p. 802
39. a, p. 799
40. a, p. 799
41. b, p. 803
42. b, p. 817
43. c, p. 805
44. a, p. 816
45. b, p. 816
46. a, p. 799
47. air distributor, p. 799
48. gas exchanger, p. 799
49. filters, p. 799
50. warms, p. 799
51. humidifies, p. 799
52. nose, p. 799
53. pharynx, p. 799
54. larynx, p. 799
55. trachea, p. 799
56. bronchi, p. 799
57. lungs, p. 799
58. alveoli, p. 809
59. Exchange, p. 809
60. respiratory membrane, p. 814
61. surface, p. 814

Diagrams

Respiratory System
1. upper respiratory tract
2. lower respiratory tract
3. bronchioles
4. bronchioles
5. capillary
6. alveolar sac
7. alveoli
8. alveolar duct
9. left and right primary bronchi
10. trachea
11. larynx
12. laryngopharynx
13. oropharynx
14. nasopharynx
15. pharynx
16. nasal cavity

Divisions of the Pharynx and Nearby Structures
1. lingual tonsil
2. hyoid bone
3. vocal cords
4. trachea
5. esophagus
6. laryngopharynx
7. epiglottis
8. oropharynx
9. palatine tonsil
10. uvula
11. soft palate
12. nasopharynx
13. opening of the auditory (eustachian) tube
14. pharyngeal tonsil (adenoids)

Paranasal Sinuses
1. sphenoid sinus
2. maxillary sinus
3. lacrimal sac
4. ethmoid air cells
5. superior nasal concha of ethmoid
6. middle nasal concha of ethmoid
7. inferior concha
8. oral cavity
9. maxillary sinus
10. sphenoid sinus
11. frontal sinus
12. ethmoid air cells
13. frontal sinus

Lobes and Fissures of the Lungs
1. first rib
2. right superior lobe
3. right primary bronchus
4. horizontal fissure
5. right middle lobe
6. oblique fissure
7. seventh rib
8. right inferior lobe
9. sternum (xiphoid process)
10. left inferior lobe
11. oblique fissure
12. body of sternum
13. left primary bronchus
14. left superior lobe
15. sternum (manubrium)
16. trachea

CHAPTER 27

Pulmonary Ventilation
1. b, p. 826
2. c, p. 826
3. b, p. 828
4. c, p. 834
5. d, p. 835
6. d, p. 836
7. d, p. 824
8. d, p. 835
9. a, p. 824
10. d, p. 826
11. t, p. 826
12. f, p. 834
13. t, p. 835
14. t, p. 836
15. t, p. 835

Pulmonary Gas Exchange
16. a, p. 838
17. d, p. 840
18. c, p. 839
19. a, p. 840

20. t, p. 835
21. t, p. 838
22. f, p. 840
23. t, p. 838

Blood Transportation of Gases and Systemic Gas Exchange
24. d, p. 842
25. b, p. 844
26. d, p. 846
27. c, p. 843
28. t, p. 842
29. f, p. 844
30. f, p. 846
31. t, p. 847

Regulation of Breathing
32. d, p. 848
33. b, p. 849
34. f, p. 848
35. t, p. 849

Mechanisms of Disease
36. COPD; chronic obstructive pulmonary disease, p. 854
37. Bronchitis, p. 854
38. Emphysema, p. 854
39. Asthma, p. 854

Applying What You Know
40. (a) obstructive pulmonary disorders (b) COPD which may include bronchitis, emphysema, and asthma (c) They obstruct inspiration and expiration. The primary difficulty is in emptying their lungs adequately which creates a buildup of CO_2 in the lungs.
41. The "diving reflex" was responsible for this phenomenon. It is a protective response of the body to cold water immersion that slows the metabolism and tissue requirements to enable survival.

One Last Quick Check
42. d, p. 824
43. c, p. 844
44. c, p. 843
45. b, p. 828
46. d, p. 834
47. d, p. 834
48. d, p. 834
49. e, p. 834
50. c, p. 834
51. a, p. 835
52. f, p. 836
53. d, p. 838

54. b, p. 842
55. i, p. 836
56. j, p. 849
57. g, p. 851
58. h, p. 849

Diagrams

Pulmonary Volumes
1. total lung capacity (TLC)
2. inspiratory reserve volume (IRV)
3. tidal volume (TV)
4. expiratory reserve volume (ERV)
5. residual volume (RV)
6. vital capacity (VC)

Respiratory Centers of Brainstem
1. limbic system (emotional responses)
2. PRG
3. apneustic center
4. pons
5. central chemoreceptors
6. DRG
7. VRG
8. medullary rhythmicity area
9. medulla
10. respiratory muscles
11. stretch receptors in lungs and thorax
12. aortic chemoreceptors and baroreceptors
13. carotid chemoreceptors and baroreceptors
14. cortex (voluntary control)

CHAPTER 28

Overview of the Digestive System
1. c, p. 862
2. b, p. 864
3. t, p. 862
4. f, p. 864
5. a, p. 863
6. a, p. 863
7. a, p. 863
8. b, p. 863
9. b, p. 863
10. b, p. 863
11. b, p. 863
12. b, p. 863
13. a, p. 863
14. a, p. 863

Mouth and Pharynx
15. d, p. 865
16. b, p. 868
17. c, p. 868

18. d, p. 869
19. b, p. 870
20. t, p. 868
21. f, p. 866
22. f, p. 868
23. t, p. 870
24. f, p. 865

Esophagus and Stomach
25. b, p. 870
26. d, p. 873
27. c, p. 873
28. t, p. 873
29. t, p. 871
30. t, p. 874

Small Intestine, Large Intestine, Appendix, and Peritoneum
31. c, p. 875
32. b, p. 876
33. a, p. 879
34. b, p. 881
35. f, p. 878
36. f, p. 880
37. t, p. 879
38. t, p. 880

Liver, Gallbladder, and Pancreas
39. b, p. 882
40. d, p. 882
41. b, p. 884
42. a, p. 884
43. t, p. 882
44. f, p. 884
45. t, p. 886
46. t, p. 886

Mechanisms of Disease
47. d, p. 894
48. g, p. 893
49. f, p. 893
50. e, p. 888
51. i, p. 892
52. a, p. 888
53. h, p. 894
54. b, p. 888
55. c, p. 894
56. k, p. 888
57. j, p. 888

Applying What You Know
58. (a) cholelithiasis (b) jaundice (c) obstruction of the bile flow into the duodenum (d) cholecystectomy or ultrasound lithotripsy
59. pylorospasm

One Last Quick Check
60. d, p. 868
61. a, p. 868

62. c, p. 869
63. d, p. 869
64. d, p. 888
65. a, p. 868
66. c, p. 875
67. b, p. 868
68. c, p. 870
69. c, p. 875
70. a, p. 884
71. b, p. 876
72. d, p. 886
73. c, p. 882
74. f, p. 878
75. f, p. 879
76. t, p. 870
77. t, p. 864
78. t, p. 870
79. t, p. 864
80. t, p. 881
81. t, p. 862
82. f, p. 872

Diagrams

Digestive Organs
1. parotid gland
2. submandibular salivary gland
3. pharynx
4. esophagus
5. diaphragm
6. transverse colon
7. hepatic flexure of colon
8. ascending colon
9. ileum
10. cecum
11. vermiform appendix
12. rectum
13. anal canal
14. sigmoid colon
15. descending colon
16. splenic flexure of colon
17. spleen
18. stomach
19. liver
20. trachea
21. larynx
22. sublingual salivary gland
23. tongue
24. common hepatic duct
25. cystic duct
26. gallbladder
27. duodenum
28. pancreas
29. stomach
30. spleen
31. liver

Tooth
1. crown
2. neck
3. root
4. bone
5. cementum
6. periodontal membrane
7. periodontal ligament
8. root canal
9. gingiva (gum)
10. pulp cavity with nerves and vessels
11. dentin
12. enamel
13. cusp

Stomach
1. esophagus
2. gastroesophageal opening
3. lower esophageal sphincter (LES)
4. cardia
5. lesser curvature
6. pylorus
7. pyloric sphincter
8. duodenal bulb
9. duodenum
10. rugae
11. greater curvature
12. mucosa
13. submucosa
14. oblique muscle layer
15. circular muscle layer
16. longitudinal muscle layer
17. muscularis
18. serosa
19. body of stomach
20. fundus

Wall of Small Intestine
1. mesentery
2. serosa
3. muscularis
4. longitudinal muscle
5. circular muscle
6. submucosa
7. mucosa
8. plica (fold)

Divisions of Large Intestine
1. superior mesenteric artery
2. hepatic (right colic) flexure
3. ascending colon
4. cecum
5. rectum
6. superior rectal artery and vein
7. sigmoid colon
8. sigmoid artery and vein
9. descending colon
10. inferior mesenteric artery and vein
11. splenic (left colic) flexure
12. transverse colon

Liver
1. inferior vena cava
2. right lobe
3. gallbladder
4. round ligament
5. falciform ligament
6. left lobe
7. right lobe proper
8. common hepatic duct
9. hepatic portal vein
10. inferior vena cava
11. caudate lobe
12. falciform ligament
13. hepatic artery
14. left lobe
15. quadrate lobe
16. gallbladder

Common Bile Duct and Its Tributaries
1. corpus (body) of gallbladder
2. neck of gallbladder
3. cystic duct
4. liver
5. minor duodenal papilla
6. accessory pancreatic duct
7. major duodenal papilla
8. duodenum
9. sphincter muscles
10. pancreas
11. superior mesenteric artery and vein
12. pancreatic duct
13. common bile duct
14. common hepatic duct
15. right and left hepatic ducts

CHAPTER 29

Digestion
1. b, p. 904
2. a, p. 904
3. b, p. 910
4. a, p. 910
5. b, p. 912
6. b, p. 907
7. c, p. 912
8. f, p. 905
9. f, p. 907
10. t, p. 908
11. f, p. 909
12. t, p. 913
13. f, p. 907
14. t, p. 910

Secretion and Control of Digestive Gland Secretion
15. b, p. 914
16. b, p. 914
17. d, p. 916
18. d, p. 920
19. t, p. 916
20. t, p. 918
21. f, p. 919

22. t, p. 914

Absorption and Elimination
23. b, p. 921
24. b, p. 924
25. c, p. 923
26. f, p. 921
27. t, p. 921
28. f, p. 924
29. f, p. 922
30. t, p. 914

Applying What You Know
31. (a) pain in the abdomen with possible hemorrhage
    (b) duodenum or possibly the stomach

(c) *Helicobacter pylori* bacterium and hyperacidity
(d) drugs that reduce hydrochloric acid formation and antibiotics to kill the bacteria
32. Replacement of fluids should focus on large amounts of cool, diluted, or isotonic fluids.

One Last Quick Check
33. a, p. 912
34. c, p. 907
35. a, p. 907
36. d, p. 904
37. c, p. 913

38. c, p. 910
39. a, p. 913
40. b, p. 918
41. d, p. 913
42. c, p. 913
43. b, p. 907
44. a, p. 916
45. d, p. 908
46. c, p. 908
47. f, p. 908
48. t, p. 904
49. t, p. 920
50. t, p. 906
51. t, p. 917
52. f, p. 910

Diagrams

Chemical Digestion

DIGESTIVE JUICES AND ENZYMES		SUBSTANCE DIGESTED (OR HYDROLYZED)	RESULTING PRODUCT*
Saliva			
Amylase (ptyalin)		Starch (polysaccharide)	Maltose (disaccharide)
Gastric Juice			
Protease (pepsin)** plus hydrochloric acid		Proteins	Partially digested proteins
Pancreatic Juice			
Proteases (e.g., trypsin)†		Proteins (intact or partially digested)	Peptides and **amino acids**
Lipases		Fats emulsified by bile	**Fatty acids, monoglycerides, and glycerol**
Amylase		Starch	Maltose
Nucleases		Nucleic acids (DNA, RNA)	Nucleotides
Intestinal Enzymes‡			
Peptidases		Peptides	**Amino acids**
Sucrase		Sucrose (cane sugar)	**Glucose** and **fructose**§ (monosaccharides)
Lactase		Lactose (milk sugar)	**Glucose** and **galactose** (monosaccharides)
Maltase		Maltose (malt sugar)	**Glucose**
Nucleotidases and phosphatases		Nucleotides	Nucleosides

*Substances in **boldface type** are end products of digestion (that is, completely digested nutrients ready for absorption).
**Secreted in inactive form (pepsinogen); activated by low pH (hydrochloric acid)
†Secreted in inactive form (trypsinogen); activated by enterokinase, an enzyme in the intestinal brush border.
‡Brush-border enzymes.
§Glucose is also called *dextrose*; fructose is also called *levulose*.

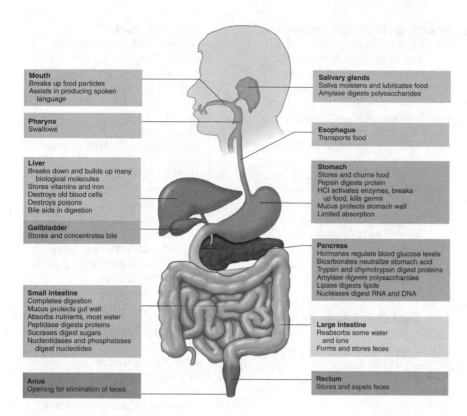

Mouth
Breaks up food particles
Assists in producing spoken
  language

Pharynx
Swallows

Liver
Breaks down and builds up many
  biological molecules
Stores vitamins and iron
Destroys old blood cells
Destroys poisons
Bile aids in digestion

Gallbladder
Stores and concentrates bile

Small intestine
Completes digestion
Mucus protects gut wall
Absorbs nutrients, most water
Peptidase digests proteins
Sucrases digest sugars
Nucleotidases and phosphatases
  digest nucleotides

Anus
Opening for elimination of feces

Salivary glands
Saliva moistens and lubricates food
Amylase digests polysaccharides

Esophagus
Transports food

Stomach
Stores and churns food
Pepsin digests protein
HCl activates enzymes, breaks
  up food, kills germs
Mucus protects stomach wall
Limited absorption

Pancreas
Hormones regulate blood glucose levels
Bicarbonates neutralize stomach acid
Trypsin and chymotrypsin digest proteins
Amylase digests polysaccharides
Lipase digests lipids
Nucleases digest RNA and DNA

Large intestine
Reabsorbs some water
  and ions
Forms and stores feces

Rectum
Stores and expels feces

CHAPTER 30

Overview of Nutrition and Metabolism
1. a, p. 933
2. d, p. 932
3. t, p. 932
4. f, p. 934

Carbohydrates
5. a, p. 934
6. b, p. 934
7. c, p. 935
8. a, p. 935
9. a, p. 935 and A&P Connect
10. b, p. 936
11. d, p. 942
12. b, p. 942
13. t, p. 940
14. t, p. 936
15. f, p. 936
16. f, p. 940
17. t, p. 943
18. t, p. 942
19. f, p. 945
20. t, p. 943
21. t, p. 944
22. f, p. 945
23. f, p. 934
24. t, p. 937
25. t, p. 939
26. f, p. 939
27. f, p. 942

Lipids
28. a, p. 946
29. c, p. 946
30. a, p. 947
31. c, p. 948
32. d, p. 946
33. f, p. 947
34. t, p. 947
35. t, p. 948
36. t, p. 947
37. t, p. 948

Proteins
38. b, p. 949
39. b, p. 949
40. d, p. 950
41. f, p. 949
42. t, p. 949
43. t, p. 950
44. f, p. 950
45. t, p. 949

Vitamins and Minerals
46. b, p. 952
47. a, p. 953
48. c, p. 953
49. f, p. 952
50. t, p. 953
51. t, p. 953
52. f, p. 952

Metabolic Rate and Mechanisms for Regulating Food Intake
53. b, p. 955
54. c, p. 956
55. c, p. 958
56. b, p. 958
57. f, p. 957
58. t, p. 959
59. t, p. 958
60. f, p. 957
61. f, p. 955

Mechanisms of Disease
62. b, p. 961
63. e, p. 963
64. a, p. 961
65. f, p. 963
66. d, p. 962
67. c, p. 962
68. g, p. 963

Applying What You Know
69. weight loss and anorexia nervosa
70. Iron would be the first mineral of choice. It is found in meat, eggs, vegetables, and legumes.
    Copper sources which might also help the anemia would be seafood, organ meats, and legumes.

One Last Quick Check
71. b, p. 936
72. a, p. 942
73. c, p. 942
74. c, p. 958
75. b, p. 958
76. d, p. 934
77. a, p. 947
78. bile (all others refer to carbohydrate metabolism)
79. amino acids (all others refer to fat metabolism)
80. M (all others refer to vitamins)
81. iron (all others refer to protein metabolism)
82. insulin (all others tend to increase blood glucose)
83. folic acid (all others are minerals)
84. ascorbic acid (all others refer to the B-complex vitamins)
85. a, p. 934
86. c, p. 948
87. d, p. 953
88. e, p. 953
89. a, p. 935

90. e, p. 953
91. a, p. 935
92. b, p. 947
93. b, p. 946

CHAPTER 31

Anatomy of the Urinary System
1. d, p. 971
2. c, p. 972
3. c, p. 973
4. b, p. 976
5. d, p. 976
6. c, p. 980
7. c, p. 979
8. a, p. 980
9. f, p. 972
10. f, p. 973
11. t, p. 975
12. t, p. 979
13. f, p. 973
14. t, p. 976
15. f, p. 972

Physiology of the Urinary System
16. b, p. 982
17. a, p. 982
18. d, p. 982
19. a, p. 984
20. c, p. 986
21. d, p. 990
22. c, p. 994
23. d, p. 992
24. c, p. 991
25. t, p. 984
26. f, p. 984
27. t, p. 987
28. t, p. 982
29. f, p. 983
30. f, p. 983
31. t, p. 984
32. f, p. 982
33. f, p. 992
34. f, p. 992
35. t, p. 983

Mechanisms of Disease
36. i, p. 994
37. c, p. 994
38. f, p. 996
39. g, p. 994
40. k, p. 995
41. a, p. 995
42. h, p. 996
43. j, p. 996
44. b, p. 994
45. d, p. 996
46. e, p. 996
47. l, p. 995

Applying What You Know
48. Hemorrhage causes a drop in blood pressure, which decreases the urine output and can eventually lead to kidney failure.
49. Stage I—Often asymptomatic because healthy nephrons compensate for the ones destroyed by disease
Stage 2—Renal insufficiency; BUN increases, polyuria and dehydration may occur
Stage 3—Uremia; high BUN, loss of kidney function, oliguria, edema, hypertension, and eventual death if an artificial kidney or transplant not available.

One Last Quick Check
50. b, p. 997
51. d, p. 996
52. a, p. 989
53. c, p. 976
54. c, p. 984
55. b, p. 976
56. c, p. 973
57. b, p. 979
58. a, p. 972
59. b, p. 974
60. e, p. 994
61. c, p. 994
62. f, p. 995
63. d, p. 975
64. j, p. 994
65. h, p. 994
66. a, p. 976
67. g, p. 996
68. i, p. 974
69. b, p. 975
70. k, p. 996

Diagrams

Kidney
1. interlobular arteries
2. renal column
3. renal sinus
4. hilum
5. renal pelvis
6. renal papilla of pyramid
7. ureter
8. medulla
9. medullary pyramid
10. major calyces
11. minor calyces
12. cortex
13. capsule (fibrous)

Nephron
1. proximal convoluted tubule (PCT)
2. renal corpuscle
3. distal convoluted tubule (DCT)
4. arcuate artery and vein
5. papilla of renal pyramid
6. thin ascending limb of Henle loop (tALH)
7. Henle loop
8. descending limb of Henle loop
9. thick ascending limb of Henle loop (TAL)
10. vasae rectae
11. collecting duct (CD)
12. peritubular capillaries
13. juxtamedullary nephron
14. interlobular artery and vein
15. afferent arteriole
16. efferent arteriole
17. cortical nephron

Male Urinary Bladder
1. ureter
2. opening of ureter
3. rugae
4. prostate gland
5. external urinary sphincter
6. bulbourethral gland
7. prostatic urethra
8. internal urethral sphincter
9. opening of ureter
10. trigone
11. smooth muscle (detrusor)
12. cut edge of peritoneum

CHAPTER 32

Overview of Fluid and Electrolyte Balance
1. c, p. 1005
2. c, p. 1006
3. a, p. 1006
4. b, p. 1006
5. d, p. 1008
6. d, p. 1009
7. c, p. 1007
8. f, p. 1004
9. t, p. 1006
10. t, p. 1009
11. f, p. 1005
12. t, p. 1010
13. f, p. 1009
14. t, p. 1007

Mechanisms that Maintain Homeostasis of Total Fluid Volume
15. d, p. 1010
16. c, p. 1010
17. f, p. 1010
18. t, p. 1012

Regulation of Water and Electrolyte Levels in Plasma, Interstitial Fluid, and Intracellular Fluid
19. a, p. 1013
20. c, p. 1012
21. c, p. 1014
22. c, p. 1016
23. t, p. 1015
24. f, p. 1015
25. t, p. 1016
26. t, p. 1016

Regulation of Sodium and Potassium Levels in Body Fluids
27. f, p. 1017
28. t, p. 1018
29. t, p. 1018
30. f, p. 1013
31. t, p. 1018

Mechanisms of Disease
32. a, p. 1019
33. d, p. 1020
34. e, p. 1020
35. b, p. 1019
36. c, p. 1019
37. t, p. 1019
38. f, p. 1020
39. t, p. 1020
40. f, p. 1020

Applying What You Know
41. Ms. Titus could not accurately measure water intake created by foods or catabolism, nor could she measure output created by lungs, skin, or the intestines.
42. Jack's body contained more water. Obese people have a lower water content than slender people.

One Last Quick Check
43. inside, p. 1005
44. extracellular, p. 1005
45. extracellular, p. 1005
46. lower, p. 1004
47. more, p. 1004
48. decreases, p. 1004
49. a, p. 1005
50. d, p. 1005
51. c, p. 1009
52. e, p. 1009
53. d, p. 1019
54. c, p. 1010
55. b, p. 1020
56. d, p. 1009
57. a, p. 1015
58. a, p. 1006
59. d, p. 1009
60. t, p. 1006
61. t, p. 1015
62. t, p. 1017

CHAPTER 33

Mechanisms that Control pH of Body Fluids
1. c, p. 1026
2. a, p. 1026
3. b, p. 1027
4. d, p. 1027
5. c, p. 1026
6. a, p. 1027
7. c, p. 1027
8. t, p. 1026
9. f, p. 1027
10. t, p. 1027
11. f, p. 1026
12. t, p. 1027
13. t, p. 1028

Buffer Mechanisms for Controlling pH of Body Fluids
14. a, p. 1030
15. c, p. 1030
16. t, p. 1031
17. f, p. 1032
18. t, p. 1028
19. f, p. 1031
20. t, p. 1030

Respiratory and Urinary Mechanisms of pH Control
21. d, p. 1032
22. b, p. 1032
23. b, p. 1034
24. a, p. 1032
25. c, p. 1035
26. t, p. 1032
27. f, p. 1033
28. t, p. 1035
29. f, p. 1030
30. t, p. 1032

Mechanisms of Disease
31. f, p. 1036
32. e, p. 1036
33. a, p. 1036
34. b, p. 1036
35. g, p. 1036
36. c, p. 1037
37. d, p. 1038

Applying What You Know
38. Normal saline contains chloride ions, which replace bicarbonate ions and thus relieve the bicarbonate excess that occurs during severe vomiting.
39. Most citrus fruits, although acid-tasting, are fully oxidized with the help of buffers during metabolism and have little effect on acid-base balance. Cranberry juice is one of the few exceptions.

One Last Quick Check
40. a, p. 1032
41. c, p. 1032
42. a, p. 1033
43. d, p. 1026
44. a, p. 1036
45. d, p. 1038
46. d, p. 1030
47. a, p. 1029
48. g, p. 1026
49. c, p. 1026
50. h, p. 1028
51. e, p. 1037
52. f, p. 1038
53. a, p. 1036
54. b, p. 1036
55. d, p. 1031

CHAPTER 34

Male Reproductive Organs
1. a, p. 1045
2. b, p. 1046
3. c, p. 1046
4. d, p. 1047
5. c, p. 1048
6. a, p. 1048
7. a, p. 1049
8. c, p. 1050
9. t, p. 1048
10. f, p. 1048
11. f, p. 1046
12. t, p. 1050
13. f, p. 1047
14. f, p. 1046
15. t, p. 1049

Reproductive Ducts and Accessory Reproductive Glands
16. b, p. 1051
17. c, p. 1052
18. a, p. 1053
19. c, pp. 1053, 1054
20. b, p. 1053
21. t, p. 1051
22. t, p. 1052
23. t, p. 1052
24. f, p. 1053

Supporting Structures, Seminal Fluid, and Male Fertility
25. c, p. 1053
26. b, p. 1054

27. b, p. 1055
28. c, p. 1055
29. f, p. 1055
30. t, p. 1055
31. f, p. 1055

Mechanisms of Disease
32. oligospermia, p. 1057
33. 2 months, p. 1057
34. cryptorchidism, p. 1057
35. benign prostatic hypertrophy, p. 1058
36. Phimosis, p. 1058
37. impotence; erectile dysfunction, p. 1058
38. hydrocele, p. 1058
39. inguinal hernia, p. 1058

Applying What You Know
40. (a) cryptorchidism (b) easily detected by palpation of the scrotum (c) surgery or testosterone injections (d) early detection results in normal testicular and sexual development.
41. (a) hydrocele or inguinal hernia (b) inguinal hernia (c) Swelling of the scrotum occurs when the intestine pushes through the weak area of the abdominal wall that separates the abdominopelvic cavity from the scrotum. (d) external supports or surgical repair

One Last Quick Check
42. b, p. 1054
43. c, p. 1055 and A&P Connect
44. b, p. 1047
45. c, p. 1047
46. a, p. 1047
47. d, p. 1054
48. d, p. 1049
49. d, p. 1050
50. c, p. 1049
51. c, p. 1048
52. a, p. 1050
53. b, p. 1051
54. h, p. 1058
55. g, p. 1054
56. a, p. 1051
57. f, p. 1053
58. c, p. 1052
59. i, p. 1055
60. e, p. 1053
61. d, p. 1055 and A&P Connect
62. j, p. 1051

Diagrams

Male Pelvis—Sagittal Section
1. seminal vesicle
2. ejaculatory duct
3. prostate gland
4. rectum
5. bulbourethral (Cowper) gland
6. anus
7. epididymis
8. testis
9. scrotum
10. foreskin (prepuce)
11. penis
12. urethra
13. vas (ductus) deferens
14. pubic symphysis
15. urinary bladder
16. ureter

Tubules of Testis and Epididymis
1. nerves and blood vessels in the spermatic cord
2. vas (ductus) deferens
3. septum
4. lobule
5. tunica albuguinea
6. testis
7. seminiferous tubules
8. epididymis

Penis
1. bladder
2. prostate
3. bulb
4. deep artery
5. foreskin (prepuce)
6. external urinary meatus
7. glans penis
8. corpus spongiosum
9. urethra
10. corpus cavernosum
11. opening of bulbourethral gland
12. crus penis
13. bulbourethral gland
14. openings of ejaculatory ducts

CHAPTER 35

Overview of the Female Reproductive System
1. a, p. 1064
2. b, p. 1065
3. t, p. 1064
4. t, p. 1065

Ovaries, Uterus, Uterine Tubes, and Vagina
5. b, p. 1066
6. d, p. 1068
7. b, p. 1068
8. a, p. 1069
9. b, p. 1070
10. d, p. 1070
11. a, p. 1070
12. b, p. 1069
13. c, p. 1072
14. b, p. 1070
15. a, p. 1070
16. b, p. 1068
17. a, p. 1071
18. a, p. 1070
19. c, p. 1072
20. t, p. 1067
21. f, p. 1068
22. f, p. 1068
23. t, p. 1072

Vulva
24. c, p. 1074
25. b, p. 1073
26. a, p. 1071
27. b, p. 1074
28. d, p. 1072

Female Reproductive Cycle
29. a, p. 1075
30. c, p. 1076
31. a, p. 1075
32. c, p. 1076
33. b, p. 1081
34. f, p. 1076
35. t, p. 1076
36. t, p. 1080
37. f, p. 1081
38. f, p. 1076

Breasts
39. f, p. 1082
40. f, p. 1084
41. t, p. 1084
42. f, p. 1085

Mechanisms of Disease
43. f, p. 1088
44. e, p. 1088
45. a, p. 1086
46. h, p. 1088
47. i, p. 1088
48. g, p. 1088
49. c, p. 1088
50. b, p. 1086
51. l, p. 1088
52. d, p. 1086
53. j, p. 1090
54. k, p. 1089

Applying What You Know

55. (a) Contraceptive pills contain synthetic progesterone-like compounds such as progestin, sometimes combined with synthetic estrogens. By sustaining a high blood concentration of these substances, contraceptive pills prevent the monthly development of a follicle. With no ovum to be expelled, ovulation does not occur, and therefore pregnancy cannot occur.

(b) Tubal ligation involves tying a piece of suture material around each uterine tube in two places, then cutting the tube between these two points. Sperm and eggs are thus prevented from meeting. This procedure is a surgical sterilization.

56. The uterine tubes are not attached to the ovaries and infections can exit at this area and enter the abdominal cavity.

One Last Quick Check

57. g, p. 1064
58. b, p. 1065
59. e, p. 1088
60. j, p. 1088
61. a, p. 1088
62. f, p. 1072
63. c, p. 1072
64. i, p. 1081
65. h, p. 1089
66. d, p. 1086
67. premenstrual or postovulatory, p. 1076
68. Prolactin, p. 1084
69. Oxytocin, p. 1084
70. meiosis, p. 1074
71. corpus luteum, p. 1075
72. hymen, p. 1072
73. Menopause, p. 1081
74. menses or menstrual period, p. 1075
75. Eight, p. 1068
76. placenta, p. 1070
77. ectopic, p. 1066
78. relaxin, p. 1068
79. endometrium, myometrium, and perimetrium (parietal peritoneum), p. 1069
80. incontinence, p. 1072
81. infertility, p. 1081

Diagrams

Female Pelvic Organs

1. fundus of uterus
2. uterine body cavity
3. endometrium
4. myometrium
5. body of uterus
6. internal os of cervix
7. cervical canal
8. external os of vaginal cervix
9. cervix of uterus
10. vagina
11. fornix of vagina
12. uterine artery and vein
13. broad ligament
14. ovary
15. fimbriae
16. infundibulopelvic ligament
17. infundibulum of uterine tube
18. ampulla of uterine tube
19. ovarian ligament
20. isthmus of uterine tube

Sagittal Section of Female Pelvis

1. sacral promontory
2. uterine tube
3. ureter
4. uterosacral ligament
5. rectouterine pouch (of Douglas)
6. cervix
7. fornix of vagina
8. coccyx
9. anus
10. vagina
11. labium majus
12. labium minus
13. clitoris
14. urethra
15. pubic symphysis
16. urinary bladder
17. parietal peritoneum
18. vesicouterine pouch
19. round ligament
20. fundus of uterus
21. body of uterus
22. ovarian ligament
23. suspensory ligament (of uterine tube)

External Female Genitals (Genitalia)

1. foreskin (prepuce)
2. clitoris (glans)
3. labium minus
4. external urinary meatus
5. vestibule
6. vestibular bulb
7. greater vestibular gland
8. mons pubis
9. pudendal fissure
10. labium majus
11. frenulum (of clitoris)
12. opening of lesser vestibular (Skene) gland
13. orifice of vagina
14. hymen
15. frenulum (of labia)
16. posterior commissure (of labia)

Vulva

1. clitoris (glans)
2. foreskin (prepuce)
3. labium minus
4. external urinary meatus
5. bulb of the vestibule
6. greater vestibular glands and ducts (Bartholin glands)
7. orifice of vagina
8. crus clitoris
9. lesser vestibular glands and ducts (Skene gland)
10. corpus cavernosum

CHAPTER 36

A New Human Life

1. b, p. 1097
2. b, p. 1097
3. d, p. 1098
4. a, p. 1101
5. b, p. 1101
6. a, p. 1097
7. f, p. 1097
8. t, p. 1097
9. t, p. 1101
10. f, p. 1101
11. f, p. 1101
12. f, p. 1103
13. t, p. 1101
14. t, p. 1103

Prenatal Period

15. a, p. 1103
16. b, p. 1103
17. a, p. 1105
18. b, p. 1111
19. c, p. 1113
20. t, p. 1106
21. f, p. 1103
22. f, p. 1111
23. t, p. 1107
24. t, p. 1103

Birth, or Parturition, and the Postnatal Period

25. c, p. 1115
26. c, p. 1115
27. d, p. 1116
28. b, p. 1118

29. b, p. 1117
30. t, p. 1115
31. t, p. 1115
32. f, p. 1115
33. f, p. 1117
34. t, p. 1118

Effects of Aging
35. d, p. 1121
36. d, p. 1122
37. t, p. 1121
38. f, p. 1122

Mechanisms of Disease
39. c, p. 1124
40. a, p. 1124
41. d, p. 1124
42. b, p. 1124
43. h, p. 1125
44. f, p. 1124
45. j, p. 1124
46. g, p. 1124

Applying What You Know
47. Only about 40% of the taste-buds present at age 30 remain at age 75.
48. Identical twins have the same genetic code.

One Last Quick Check
49. g, p. 1101
50. f, p. 1111
51. c, p. 1110
52. b, p. 1107
53. a, p. 1105
54. h, p. 1114
55. e, p. 1115
56. d, p. 1111
57. i, p. 1107
58. j, p. 1110
59. d, p. 1121
60. d, p. 1122
61. d, p. 1122
62. a, p. 1118
63. b, p. 1111
64. d, p. 1122
65. e, p. 1118
66. a, p. 1120

67. c, p. 1119
68. b, p. 1118

Diagram

Fertilization and Implantation
1. ovary
2. developing follicles
3. corpus luteum
4. fimbriae
5. discharged ovum
6. spermatozoa
7. first mitosis
8. uterine (fallopian) tube
9. blastocyst
10. morula
11. blastocyst
12. implantation

CHAPTER 37

The Science of Genetics; Chromosomes and Genes; Gene Expression
1. c, p. 1132
2. c, p. 1132
3. d, p. 1137
4. c, p. 1138
5. a, p. 1133
6. d, p. 1140
7. c, p. 1139
8. d, p. 1132
9. f, p. 1135
10. t, p. 1137
11. f, p. 1137
12. f, p. 1138
13. t, p. 1139
14. t, p. 1138
15. t, p. 1135
16. f, p. 1137

Medical Genetics; Prevention and Treatment of Genetic Diseases
17. b, p. 1141
18. b, p. 1144
19. a, p. 1145
20. c, p. 1137
21. c, p. 1145

22. b, p. 1146
23. d, p. 1148
24. d, p. 1148
25. c, p. 1147
26. b, p. 1147
27. f, p. 1141
28. t, p. 1143
29. f, p. 1142
30. t, p. 1146
31. t, p. 1146
32. f, p. 1142
33. t, p. 1143
34. t, p. 1147
35. t, p. 1141

Applying What You Know
36. In a form of dominance called co-dominance, the effect will be equal, causing "light brown" to occur.
37. One in four or 25%

One Last Quick Check
38. a, p. 1136
39. d, p. 1146
40. c, p. 1136
41. b, p. 1136
42. a, p. 1135
43. c, p. 1132
44. b, p. 1138
45. c, p. 1138
46. a, p. 1147
47. b, p. 1145
48. h, p. 1145
49. k, p. 1147
50. c, p. 1142
51. e, p. 1133
52. a, p. 1142
53. d, p. 1137
54. j, p. 1142
55. l, p. 1143
56. g, p. 1136
57. RNA, p. 1132
58. Transcriptomics, p. 1134
59. p-arm and q-arm, p. 1135
60. Down syndrome, p. 1144
61. viruses, p. 1148
62. ideogram, p. 1140

Solutions to Crossword Puzzles

CHAPTER 1

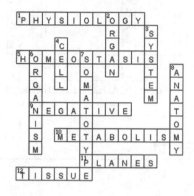

CHAPTER 4

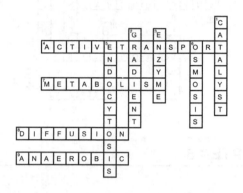

CHAPTER 2

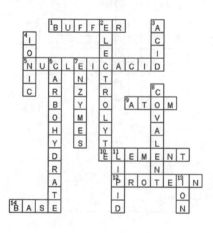

CHAPTER 5

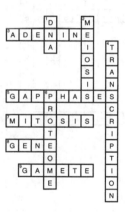

CHAPTER 3

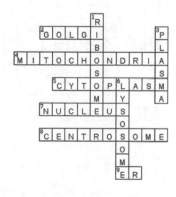

CHAPTER 6

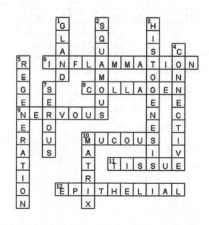

CHAPTER 7

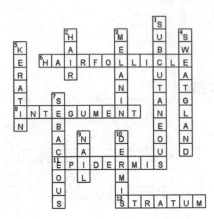

CHAPTER 10

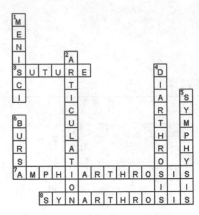

CHAPTER 8

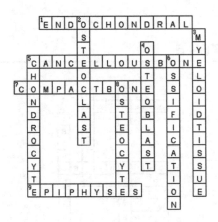

CHAPTER 11

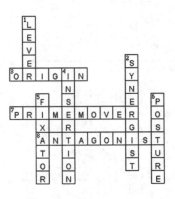

CHAPTER 9

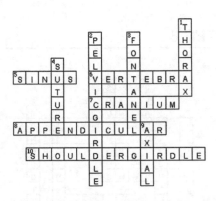

CHAPTER 12

CHAPTER 13

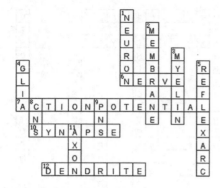

CHAPTER 16

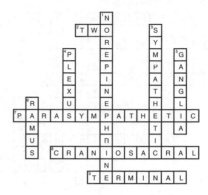

CHAPTER 14

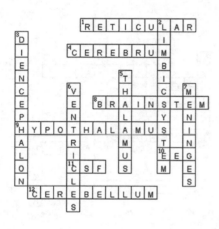

CHAPTER 17

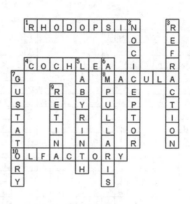

CHAPTER 15

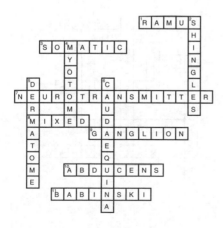

CHAPTER 18

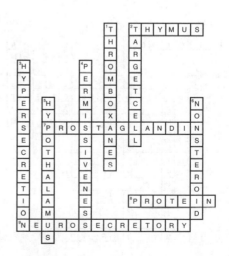

CHAPTER 19

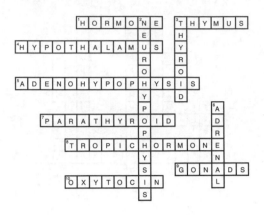

CHAPTER 22

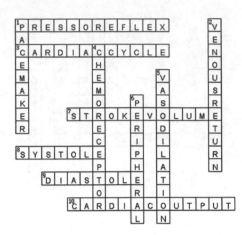

CHAPTER 20

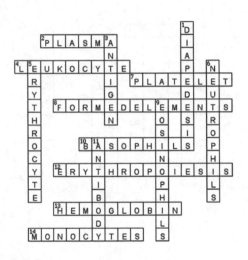

CHAPTER 23

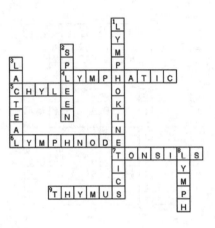

CHAPTER 21

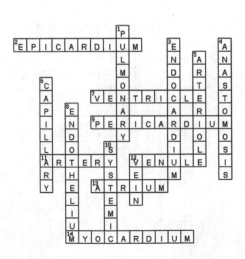

CHAPTER 24

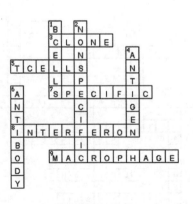

CHAPTER 25

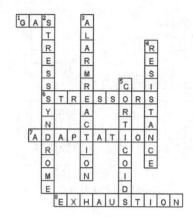

CHAPTER 28

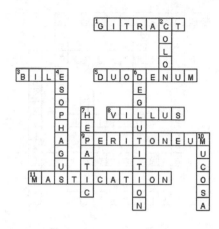

CHAPTER 26

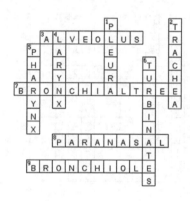

CHAPTER 29

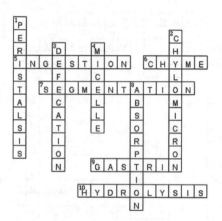

CHAPTER 27

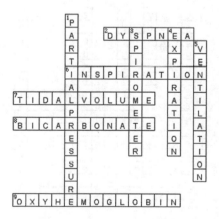

CHAPTER 30

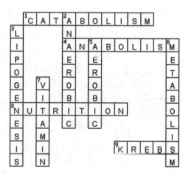

CHAPTER 31

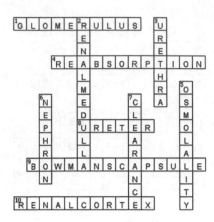

Across

1. GLOMERULUS
4. REABSORPTION
8. URETER
9. BOWMANSCAPSULE
10. RENALCORTEX

CHAPTER 34

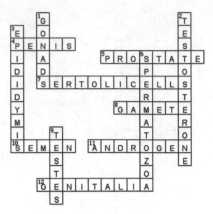

4. PENIS
5. PROSTATE
7. SERTOLICELLS
8. GAMETE
10. SEMEN
11. ANDROGEN
12. GENITALIA

CHAPTER 32

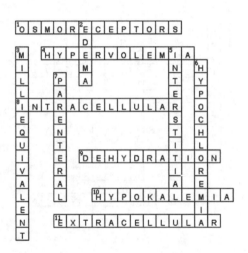

1. OSMORECEPTORS
4. HYPERVOLEMIA
8. INTRACELLULAR
9. DEHYDRATION
10. HYPOKALEMIA
11. EXTRACELLULAR

CHAPTER 35

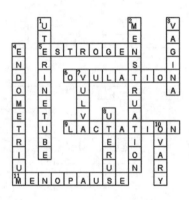

5. ESTROGEN
6. OVULATION
9. LACTATION
11. MENOPAUSE

CHAPTER 33

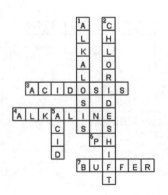

3. ACIDOSIS
4. ALKALINE
7. BUFFER

CHAPTER 36

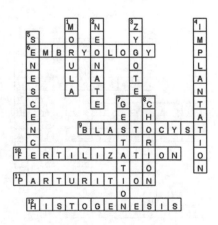

6. EMBRYOLOGY
9. BLASTOCYST
10. FERTILIZATION
11. PARTURITION
12. HISTOGENESIS

CHAPTER 37

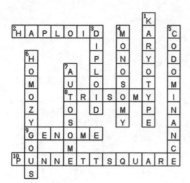